A Bibliography on Herbs, Herbal Medicine,
"Natural" Foods, and Unconventional
Medical Treatment

A Bibliography on Herbs, Herbal Medicine, "Natural" Foods, and Unconventional Medical Treatment

Theodora Andrews
Professor of Library Science
Pharmacy, Nursing, and Health
Sciences Librarian
Purdue University

with the assistance of

William L. Corya
Associate Professor of Library Science
Head, Catalog Department
Purdue University Libraries

Donald A. Stickel, Jr.
Assistant Professor of Library Science
Assistant Life Science Librarian
Purdue University

Libraries Unlimited, Inc.   **1982**
Littleton, Colorado

Copyright © 1982 Libraries Unlimited, Inc.
All Rights Reserved
Printed in the United States of America

No part of this publication may be reproduced, stored in a retrieval system, or transmitted, in any form or by any means, electronic, mechanical, photocopying, recording, or otherwise, without the prior written permission of the publisher.

LIBRARIES UNLIMITED, INC.
P.O. Box 263
Littleton, Colorado 80160

Library of Congress Cataloging in Publication Data

Andrews, Theodora.
　　A bibliography on herbs, herbal medicine, "natural" foods, and unconventional medical treatment.

　　Includes index.
　　1. Herbs--Therapeutic use--Bibliography.
2. Herbs--Bibliography.　3. Herbals--Bibliography.
4. Food, Natural--Bibliography.　5. Folk medicine--Bibliography.　I. Corya, William L.　II. Stickel, Donald A., 1953-　.　III. Title. [DNLM:
1. Plants, Medicinal--Bibliography.　2. Medicine, Herbal--Bibliography.　3. Food--Bibliography.
4. Therapeutic cults--Bibliography.　ZWB 925 A571b]
Z6665.H47A5　[RM666.H33]　016.615'321　82-128
ISBN 0-87287-288-2　　　　　　　　　　　　AACR2

Libraries Unlimited books are bound with Type II nonwoven material that meets and exceeds National Association of State Textbook Administrators' Type II nonwoven material specifications Class A through E.

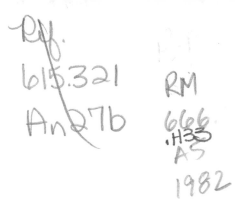

TABLE OF CONTENTS

INTRODUCTION

For the past few years, the use of herbs, "natural" and "health" foods, and various unconventional medical systems has occupied the attention of the news media and the public. A large number of publications concerning them have been made available. This craze and preoccupation with health evidently grew out of the bad publicity given food additives and "junk" food along with the counterculture movement of the 1960s and its distrust of the medical "establishment." The desire has been to return to a simpler life, one which emphasizes a back-to-nature bent. Herbal medicine has gained wide appeal, perhaps because of its simplicity. Early medicines were called "simples" on the theory that there was a simple remedy for every illness; one had only to find it.

It is a paradox that the present irrational approach to better health comes at a time when medical science has developed greatly, the educational level of the people is higher than ever, and more stringent laws are in effect. The health sciences have a great deal to offer, yet misrepresentation and quackery abound.

Despite the negative comments expressed above, a positive side to the current interest in herbs and herbal medicine exists. First, a hobby interest in the plants prevails; they are often grown for enjoyment rather than for any practical purpose. Many are used for flavoring foods rather than for medicine, and serve that purpose nicely. The herbals are handsome; in most cases they contain fine illustrations. Herbals have fascinated people from early times until today. Historians, ethnobotanists, and folklorists have long been interested in them. Scientists have found them to be valuable because they suggest possible uses for constituents that can be extracted from the plants. Modern drugs have their origins in plant substances. In addition to the extracted medicines, plant materials have served as structural prototypes that have inspired chemists to synthesize similar drugs with even more desirable properties. The field is highly developed scientifically as many of the works listed in this bibliography show. It is generally conceded, though, that much work remains to be done. Many plants have not been studied or substances isolated from them, and physiological effects of the constituents must be investigated further.

This bibliography is an attempt to review books that cover a wide range of topics related to herbs, "health" foods, and unconventional medical treatment. Scientific and popular books are included. Many of the latter are of questionable quality and authenticity, although they are widely sold and read. This bibliography includes what are believed to be some of the best works in the field, representative examples of poor ones, and some unusual titles. A number of older works are included because reprinted editions of many of them are available, and the new titles are often similar to the old. There is much repetition in the material published.

Herbs are botanically defined as plants that are not woody but die back to a rootstock in winter, thus excluding some shrubs and other plants commonly thought of as herbs. Most of the books describe herbs as plants of which the leaves, stems, roots, or seeds, and, in some cases, flowers, are used for medicine, scent, or flavor. In a broad sense, they are plants that give service of some kind directly to human beings without undergoing any processing in laboratory or factory.

It is interesting that laypersons speak of "herbs" or "health food" plants and think of them as specific entities with medicinal uses. Scientists seem to prefer instead to use the term "medicinal plants" and view them as sources for desired constituents that can be extracted from unwanted substances and used as drugs. For this reason, books on "herbs" (placed in chapter 5) have been separated from those dealing with "medicinal plants" (placed in chapter 11). The plants involved are much the same, but the emphasis is different.

In one of the books reviewed, Krutch in his *Herbal* (see entry 167) remarks that herbalists have charm and impart a sense of beauty and wonder. He further suggests that although scientists may feel this, they do not communicate it, as it is not their function to do so. Unfortunately, though, herbalists and authors of books on unconventional medicine pass on a great deal of folklore as fact, and feel no need to base judgments on the value of various medicinal herbs on scientific evidence. Furthermore, they encourage self-treatment and treatment by those unqualified to give it. A quotation from Leonardo da Vinci comes to mind: "Those who devote themselves to practice without science are like sailors who put to sea without rudder or compass and who can never be certain of where they are going. Practice must always be founded on sound theory."

It should be pointed out that many of the plants called "herbs" are poisonous if taken in large amounts. Likewise, some of the special diets suggested and the "natural" foods may have harmful effects. "Naturalness" is no guarantee of safety, contrary to popular belief. It is also important to realize that there are no legal controls over herbal products sold as foods, although they may contain toxic materials. It is only when such products are labelled "drugs" (which they seldom are) and sold by a pharmacist that they are subject to control by the Food and Drug Administration.

Many of the books in this bibliography include a disclaimer stating that the suggested remedies are not intended to take the place of treatment by a physician. Text material in them, however, often seems to have just that intent.

Reference works and treatises make up the bulk of the materials reviewed, although a periodicals chapter has been included. Reference works are grouped in Part I; treatises in Part II. A Directory of Organizations, Associations, and Groups concerned with herbs, herbal medicine, "natural" foods, and unconventional medicine is appended. Only English language publications are included in this bibliography.

Each chapter of this bibliography is preceded by a few remarks that attempt to characterize the literature of that chapter. It is hoped that those comments, the comments made in this introduction, and the reviews of the books listed will provide a view of the material under consideration, place it in perspective, and provide insights that will assist librarians and readers in assessing the prevailing viewpoints and literature.

Theodora Andrews

PART I
General Reference Sources

1

BIBLIOGRAPHIES, INDEXES, HANDBOOKS, MANUALS, CATALOGS, DIRECTORIES, FORMULARIES, AND PHARMACOPEIAS

Listed here are a wide variety of reference materials covering the subjects dealt with in this bibliography. A few general works on plants have been included, such as Britton and Brown's *Illustrated Flora of the Northern United States,* Gray's *Manual of Botany* (both classical works), and Plowden's *Manual of Plant Names,* because they are useful in helping to identify herbs and other kinds of plants. In addition, there are works covering only herbal plants, such as *The British Herbal Pharmacopoeia,* the Brooklyn Botanic Garden's *Handbook on Herbs,* and Gabriel's *Herb Identifier and Handbook.* A few titles cover specific plants or classes of plants, such as *Abstracts of Korean Ginseng Studies* and Krieger's *Mushroom Handbook.* (A number of treatises on mushrooms and ginseng may be found listed in other sections of this bibliography.)

There are several scholarly works that deal with plants having medicinal uses, including Burlage's *Index of Plants of Texas,* de Laszlo's *Library of Medicinal Plants,* and Jacobs and Burlage's *Index of Plants of North Carolina.*

Several formulary works are included, for instance Henley's *Formulas for Home and Workshop,* Meyer's *Herbal Recipes,* and Montagna's *PDR, People's Desk Reference.* (Many books listed throughout Part II of this bibliography also include formulas and recipes among text materials.)

A number of titles dealing with unconventional medicine are listed. These include the Berkeley Holistic Health Center's *Holistic Health Handbook,* Kaslof's *Wholistic Dimensions in Healing,* Klein and Meyer's *Chiropractic,* and the titles on acupuncture.

Also included is a title dealing with an unusual aspect of the subject— Conklin's *Folk Classification.*

Listed materials vary in quality and value. Some deal in a scholarly manner with the subject under consideration, and some are classics of their kind. Others have little value except to serve as examples of current popular works.

* * * * *

1.   **Abstracts of Korean Ginseng Studies (1687-1975), World-Wide Collected Bibliography: Citations and Abstracts.** Seoul, Korea: Research Institute, Office of Monopoly, Republic of Korea, 1975. 254p.

Ginseng is a popular herb in the Orient, and it is becoming more so in Western countries. Used as a mysterious, supernatural drug for perhaps 5,000 years, the first written record of it appeared in classical Chinese literature about 2,000 years ago. Ginseng is still playing a part in cultural, commercial, and even diplomatic matters. Many research studies on the plant have appeared.

This book lists the studies which have been reported sporadically in books, journals, magazines, and newspapers. The literature references are grouped under these broad headings: ginseng biology, ginseng chemistry, ginseng pharmacology, ginseng history, ginseng preparation, ginseng markets, and general writing. The subject is further subdivided under each heading. The last chapter, however, divides the material by date. Most works are annotated, and most annotations are in English with a few in German. Titles are given in the original language with translations (and transliterations, if necessary).

This is a valuable compilation which provides an overview of the research carried out so far on ginseng.

2.   Baïracli-Levy, Juliette de. **Herbal Handbook for Farm and Stable.** London: Faber and Faber, 1952; repr. Emmaus, PA, Rodale Press (33 E. Minor St., Emmaus, PA 18049), 1976. 320p. illus. $7.95; $3.95pa. LC 76-2734. ISBN 0-87857-120-5; 0-87857-115-9pa.

This work deals with the use of herbal remedies in the care of farm animals in order to avoid problems stemming from the uncontrolled use of chemicals and vaccines. It is not meant to be an exhaustive volume but is intended as a practical handbook covering the common animal sicknesses that presumably can be treated by common herbal remedies that can be found wild, easily cultivated, or purchased. The author has spent a lifetime learning and using herbal remedies by working among gypsy and peasant herbalists in several European countries, the Near East, Northern Africa, and Mexico.

The book covers the basics of gathering, preserving, and preparing herbs. There is a materia medica botanica section that describes the main medicinal and nutritive herbs, giving medicinal properties, preparation, and dosage of each. Plants are arranged alphabetically by British common names with Latin names following. Identifying descriptions are brief, and full identification would need to come from other sources. There are separate sections for herbal treatment of sheep, goats, cows, horses, poultry, and sheepdogs. Symptoms and treatments are given for specific illnesses suffered by each animal.

Herbal remedies, the author claims, can be used to help bolster food production and keep down farm expenses. "It pays to keep animals healthy," the author says, indicating that herbs can be used to combat disease.

3.   Berkeley Holistic Health Center, comp. **Holistic Health Handbook: A Tool for Attaining Wholeness of Body, Mind, and Spirit.** Edward Bauman, et al. Berkeley, CA: And/Or Press, 1978. 479p. illus. bibliog. index. $9.95. LC 78-54344. ISBN 0-915904-32-2.

"Holistic health" is the name given to the therapeutic system or cult discussed here. The handbook is said to be the definitive statement of the movement, written by those who are bringing about an emerging health revolution. What the cult stands for is difficult to ascertain, except that "wholeness" and "well-being" are involved as is the "continuum from the body to the spirit."

A partial list of topics covered is indicative of the interests and views of the contributors: acupuncture, yoga, homeopathy, naturopathy, polarity, nutrition, iridology, massage, bioenergetics, biofeedback, Reichian therapy, hypnotism, autogenics, meditation, spiritual healing, holistic sexuality, natural birth control, natural childbirth, recreation, dying and death, legal issues, social movements, and establishment of a health center.

4.   **British Herbal Pharmacopoeia, 1972.** London: British Herbal Medicine Association (Walter House, 418/422 Strand, London, W.C. 1), 1971. Produced by the Association's Scientific Committee. 1v. (looseleaf).

The monographs selected for inclusion in this work were chosen because the herbs in question usually have not been described in the *British Pharmacopoeia* or the *British Pharmaceutical Codex.* In addition, little other documentation of them exists, and authentic information on them will be valuable. New monographs and updates are to be added to the looseleaf book from time to time.

The following information about each plant is usually given: synonymous names, definition, description (macroscopical, microscopical, and references to methods of analysis), and therapeutics (including action, indications, uses, preparations, and dosage). The book is not a rewriting of existing material but is based on much original work. The literature references are to recent standard scientific works.

5.   Britton, Nathaniel Lord, and Addison Brown. **Illustrated Flora of the Northern United States, Canada and the British Possessions from Newfoundland to the Parallel of the Southern Boundary of Virginia, and from the Atlantic Ocean Westward to the 102d Meridian.** 2d ed. rev. and enl. New York: Charles Scribner's Sons, 1913; repr. New York: Dover Publications, 1970. 3v. illus. index. $8.00 per v. pa. ISBN 0-486-22642-5; 0-486-22643-3; 0-486-22644-1.

This classical compilation was the first complete work of its kind published in the United States. It attempts to illustrate and describe every species of flora from the ferns upward that are recognized as distinct and that grow wild in the areas indicated in the subtitle. This is an early edition of the work, but it is preferred by many over more recent ones and is the only edition in print at this writing.

The encyclopedic work describes 4,666 species with full botanical information and an illustration (line drawing) for each. Arrangement is by plant family. Common names are indicated, and information about habitat included. Introductory material includes abbreviations of names of authors cited and a general key to orders and families. An index to Latin genera and species, along with an English index including popular plant names, is found in volume 3.

6.   Brooklyn Botanic Garden. **Handbook on Herbs.** Brooklyn, NY: The Garden, 1971. (Repr. of **Plants and Gardens,** Vol.14, No.2, 1958). 96p. illus. index. (World's Best Illustrated Garden and Horticultural Handbooks, No. 27).

The main body of this work is an illustrated dictionary of herbs, covering about 70 plants. Material is arranged by scientific names and includes for each: common names, brief description, uses in general terms (e.g., use in medicine indicated but not specifically how used), horticultural uses (e.g., as a border plant, background plant, etc.), brief culture, and a black and white photograph.

The rest of the work is a compilation of articles contributed by various authors. Special attention is given to propagating herbs, herbs for shaded gardens, spices grown in a window box, mints, geraniums, thymes, herb gardens and their design, ornamental herbs, herbs used by the Indians and early settlers, a short description of herb families (mint, composite, parsley, mustard, and borage families), and a short discussion on whether herb is pronounced with the *h* or not. The emphasis of this work seems to be on plants of the New England states.

7.   Brooklyn Botanic Garden. **Handbook on Japanese Herbs and Their Uses.** Brooklyn, NY: The Garden, 1968. (Special Printing of **Plants and Gardens,** Vol.24, No.2, 1968). 72p. illus.

Herbs have played an important part in Japanese medicine, cooking, and art. This work is a compilation of articles on Japanese herbs, contributed by several authors. Before the introduction of Western medicine, Chinese and native medicinal herbs were relied upon for treatment purposes.

The book covers both medicinal and culinary herbs, including spices. One article is devoted entirely to the cooking of chrysanthemums. There is a section of recipes for Japanese dishes accented with herbs. The history of Japanese herbs and herb gardens is given. Flower arrangement is covered. The work concludes with a summary listing of herbs covered, identifying them by scientific, common English, and Japanese names. Reference is made to author and page number where mentioned in the work. Part of the plant to be used and culinary and medicinal uses are provided for each.

8. Burlage, Henry M. **Index of Plants of Texas with Reputed Medicinal and Poisonous Properties.** Austin, TX: The author, 1968. 272p. bibliog. index.

The late author of this work, a professor at a school of pharmacy, was aware that improved technical methods and equipment were making it possible to reevaluate many old-time botanicals. He thought this work would contribute to plant reevaluation and to the isolation of new compounds of possible medicinal value.

Texas has diversified flora; it has plants that are semi-tropical, those that grow in arid regions, those that are common to mountainous regions, and those found in wooded areas and on the plains. The book is a bibliographic survey. Over 1,200 plants of Texas are grouped by family with scientific names, common names, and, when available, Indian, Aztec, and other Mexican names given. Habitat, use, and constituents are indicated. References to the numbered items of the bibliography are provided with the entries.

The following indexes are included: index to plant families; index to Latin names of genera and species; index to common and generic names of plants; index to American Indian, Spanish and other non-English common names of plants; index of reputed poisonous properties; index of constituents reported; numerical index of references by number; alphabetical author index of references; and alphabetic author index of references consulted but not pertinent.

9. **Combination Tablets.** St. Louis, MO: Luyties Pharmacal Co., 1976. 36p.

This booklet lists diseases alphabetically and indicates the combination tablets the Luyties Pharmacal Company has available for treating the various conditions. Symptoms and dosages are given. The combination tablets are made up of perhaps three or four ingredients, some of which are recognized homeopathic remedies and some of which are standard drugs. The Luyties Pharmacal Company is one of the few remaining companies in the world that still manufactures homeopathic remedies.

10. Conklin, Harold C. **Folk Classification: A Topically Arranged Bibliography of Contemporary and Background References through 1971.** Revised reprinting with author index. New Haven, CT: Yale University Department of Anthropology, 1980. 521p. index. $8.50pa. LC 80-80582. ISBN 0-913516-02-3.

The earlier edition (1972) of this unusual work contained about 1,400 entries; this one includes about 5,000. Arranged alphabetically under ten topical headings are references to: 1) analyses of specific systems of folk classification; 2) discussions and comparisons of such analyses; and 3) theoretical and practical background literature on classification in general and in various subject fields. The purpose of the work is to provide students of folk classification with an introduction to the contemporary and historical literature on the problems, modes of analysis, and types of classificatory relations encountered in various areas.

The bibliographic sections are headed as follows: 1) Principles of Classification; 2) Kinship and Related Topics; 3) Archeological Classification; 4) Anthropological Classification; 5) Ethnobotany; 6) Ethnozoology; 7) Ethnomedicine; 8) Orientation; 9) Color; and 10) Sensation. The sections on ethnobotany and ethnomedicine are of particular interest. The former includes references to various types of ethnobotanical reports and background works on botanical classification as well as analyses of folk systems of plant categorization. Books, journal articles, museum reports, and proceedings of meetings are listed, some in foreign languages. The section on ethnomedicine includes references to ethnomedical and related medical works on disease categorization and treatment, anatomical classification, and similar topics. As in the other section, a variety of materials are listed and several languages represented.

The compilation presents useful scholarly material that is of special value to those interested in folk science or ethnoscience.

11.   de Laszlo, Henry G. **Library of Medicinal Plants.** Cambridge, Great Britain: W. Heffer and Sons, Ltd., 1958. 54p.

The compiler of this bibliography on phytotherapy collected the works listed for his personal library. About 1,500 books, articles, and pamphlets are included. The time span covered is from 1700 until about 1957. The author hoped his collection would help therapeutic chemists discover unknown molecular structures in plants that would be useful to man. References are arranged alphabetically by author in three sections: books; latest additions; and pamphlets, photocopies, and microfilms. The last section lists periodical articles. Foreign language materials are included, particularly those in German and French.

12.   Gabriel, Ingrid. **Herb Identifier and Handbook.** New York: Sterling Publishing Co., 1975. 256p. illus. (part col.). index. $6.95. LC 74-31698. ISBN 0-8069-3069-3. (Adapted from the German book **Die farbige Kräuterfibel**).

This handy guide provides an introduction to some of the most useful medicinal and culinary plants. Many of them grow wild, and some can be cultivated in the home garden. Introductory material in the work includes short general discussions on medicinal uses of plants, drying herbs, the herbarium, and herb teas. The rest of the book is a listing of the plants, arranged alphabetically by common name. Information provided about each plant includes scientific name, other popular names, family, range, description, chemical content (called "elements contained"), medicinal use, and culinary use (if any). Illustrations are provided, about half in color. About 115 plants are included. There are several indexes: general, scientific name, popular name, and geographical.

The book should serve its intended purpose quite well. However, it probably serves best as a field guide for identification of herbs. Medicinal uses suggested should not be taken too seriously.

13.   Gray, Asa. **Manual of Botany: A Handbook of the Flowering Plants of the Central and Northeastern United States and Adjacent Canada.** 8th ed. New York: Van Nostrand Reinhold, 1950. 1,632p. illus. index. $37.95. ISBN 0-442-22250-5.

The first edition of this substantial botanical reference work came out in 1848 as *Manual of the Botany of the Northern United States.* Eight different editions were published within the next 100 years.

This latest eighth edition, rewritten and expanded by Merrit Lyndon Fernald, is still in print and is a much-used authority. In the preface, Fernald claims this eighth edition "has been one of fundamental changes, both in our understanding of our plants and in the requirements of the International Rules of Botanical Nomenclature." The preface covers matters such as the taxonomic system used, the meaning of taxonomic words, and other explanations concerning the text. The text begins with an overview of the orders and families of the vascular plants covered in the work, an analytical key to the families, and explanations of abbreviations used. The "descriptive flora" section is the main body of the book. It is arranged taxonomically and covers more than 8,000 species, varieties, forms, and named hybrids. Common names are included when known. Illustrations are line drawings. Not all genera have drawings, but most large and technical ones do.

14. **Henley's Formulas for Home and Workshop: Containing Ten Thousand Selected Household, Workshop and Scientific Formulas, Trade Secrets, Food and Chemical Recipes, Processes and Money Saving Ideas.** Edited by Gardner D. Hiscox; new Foreword by Anne Hessey. Enl. ed. New York: Avenel Books, 1979. 809p. illus. index. LC 79-21439. ISBN 0-517-29307-2.

This is evidently a facsimilie edition of a work originally published in 1907 and revised in 1927. Although long a classic of its kind and reissued from time to time, at least one intent of this reprint seems to be to bring a touch of nostalgia to the reader. There is a cautionary notice that points out that some of the proposed remedies are now considered by modern medicine to be inadequate and potentially harmful. One is advised to see a physician rather than take advice given in the book.

The range of subjects covered in Henley's is great. There is a formula for virtually everything used in the early 1900s, and some are still of use, although many new materials are now available, synthetics especially. People interested in "natural" products should be delighted with the book. Sections of most interest to readers of this bibliography include those on cosmetics, condiments, balsams, antidotes for poisons, dyes, essences and extracts, food adulterants, hair preparations, and perfumes. Some herbs are listed separately in the index.

This is a fascinating and still somewhat useful book.

15. **Herbalist Almanac, 1980.** Hammond, IN: Indiana Botanic Gardens (Box 5, Hammond, IN 46325), 1980. 62p. illus. $1.95pa.

This little almanac is basically an advertising and promotional pamphlet from an herb supplier. It is included here as an example of the kind of publication issued by several herb suppliers in the United States. This particular almanac has been issued for more than 50 years.

Like many almanacs, this one includes calendars for the year and weather forecasts for specific periods of the month. Descriptions of various herbal preparations available from the company are interspersed throughout, along with some testimonies from satisfied users. Several culinary recipes are included as well as general household hints. How to handle toads and how to make "cookies" for killing rats are examples of the varied information one finds in this pamphlet. There is no index, but a complete list of botanicals and oils is given. These are, of course, available from the company. This is an interesting publication, but not very valuable as a home medical advisor.

16. Jacobs, Marion Lee, and Henry M. Burlage. **Index of Plants of North Carolina with Reputed Medicinal Uses.** Chapel Hill, NC: Henry M. Burlage, 1958. 322p. bibliog. index.

This work is a bibliographic survey undertaken by two professors (both now deceased) to review the evidence for the many plants in North Carolina that have been used in medicine. The task was a formidable one, as about 1,500 plants of the area were found to have had some application in medicine.

The introductory chapter is an essay by George M. Hocking on "The Development of the Crude Drug Industry in North Carolina." The main body of the work contains entries for each plant, arranged alphabetically by Latin name under family name, also arranged alphabetically. Information given about each plant includes common names, habitat, uses, properties, brief description, and reference to works listed in the bibliography of 90 entries. Contents of the main section are indexed by plant family (Latin name), plant family (English name), Latin name of genera and species, common and generic names of plants, reputed therapeutic and other uses, constituents reported, author index of references, and chronological numerical index of references.

17.　　Kaslof, Leslie J., ed. **Wholistic Dimensions in Healing: A Resource Guide.** Garden City, NY: Doubleday, 1978. 295p. illus. bibliog. $7.95pa. LC 76-50874. ISBN 0-385-12628-X.

This useful reference work is a catalog of groups, associations, schools, centers, clinics, journals, publications, products, and services that are concerned with a variety of healing techniques considered under the broad topic of holistic medicine. The concept of (w)holistic medicine emphasizes the responsibility of patients for healing themselves; thus, widely varied self-healing techniques are utilized in holistic medicine. Many of these techniques are discussed in this book.

The book addresses the following topics: childbirth; integrative medical systems; nutrition and herbs; heuristic directions in diagnosis and treatment; biofeedback and self-regulation; psychic and spiritual healing; psychophysical approaches; and humanistic and transpersonal psychotherapies. Each of these sections is followed by introductory essays, specific approaches and techniques involved, and a great number of resources for each technique. All resources include addresses, and many give telephone numbers. Essays are written by experts in the specific topic or technique, and a separate section of the book includes brief biographies of the contributors. A comprehensive bibliography of additional readings is also included.

Although many techniques discussed in the book seem a little "far out," it is a comprehensive guide to what is currently called holistic medicine. Only a brief section of the book is given specifically to herbal medicine, but an impressive list of herb sources is included.

18.　　Klein, Lawrence, and Sharon Meyer. **Chiropractic: An International Bibliography.** Des Moines, IA: Foundation for Chiropractic Education and Research, 1976. 90p. index. $6.00. LC 76-40865. ISBN 0-9601082-1-1.

Included in this bibliography are 1,600 items dealing with the world's literature on chiropractic and manipulative therapy. It is arranged by type of material, for example, directories, popular works, journal articles, to name a few. The largest sections are the book and the journal lists. Foreign titles are translated. Introductory material provides a historical overview, a list of sources searched, and a list of abbreviations used in the bibliography. Appended are a list of chiropractic associations, names and addresses of accredited chiropractic colleges, and chiropractic periodicals. Author and subject indexes are included.

19.   Krieger, Louis C. C. **The Mushroom Handbook.** Illustrated by photographs and drawings by the author with a new Preface and Appendix on nomenclatural changes by Robert L. Shaffer. New York: Dover Publications, 1967. (Repr. of the 2nd, 1936 ed. published by the Macmillan Co. Originally published by the University of the State of New York in 1935 under the title **A Popular Guide to the Higher Fungi [Mushrooms] of New York State**). 560p. illus. (part col.). bibliog. index. $5.00pa. LC 67-28792. ISBN 0-486-21861-9.

This is a reissue of a popular mushroom manual. New nomenclatural changes are listed in an appendix. The book serves as an identification and field guide to edible and poisonous mushrooms, and also as a mycological textbook for amateurs. The work features a bibliography of 38 pages and reproductions of 32 of Krieger's mushroom paintings.

Section headings are: 1) Field study of mushrooms and other fungi; 2) Conditions under which mushrooms grow and thrive; 3) Forest types, with reference to distribution of the higher fungi; 4) How to collect, study, and prepare mushrooms for the herbarium; 5) Life history and general characteristics of mushrooms; 6) Economic importance of fungi; 7) Common edible mushrooms; 8) Growing mushrooms; 9) Poisonous mushrooms; 10) The wood-destroying fungi; 11) The literature on mushrooms and their allies; 12) Systematic account of selected larger fungi; and 13) Names of the principal authors of fungus species. There is a glossary of technical terms. The book contains much miscellaneous information, including some good recipes for cooking mushrooms.

20.   Liao, Allen Y. **Acupuncture: A Research Bibliography.** New York: New York University Medical Center Library, 1975. 66p. index. $3.95pa.

This bibliography is noteworthy because of the recent upsurge of interest in America in acupuncture, although the procedure has been used for hundreds of years in China as a therapeutic tool. Until recently few scientific and objective studies have been attempted to clarify the role of acupuncture in medicine. Although its value is open to question, there is general agreement that acupuncture is useful in certain areas, but not in others, and that it produces physiological changes that warrant serious further study.

This publication covers materials published from 1960 to early 1975. Books, journal articles (in English and foreign languages), and audiovisual materials are included. A list of periodicals, journal abbreviations, and an author index have been supplied. The purpose of the bibliography is to assist health professionals and others interested in acupuncture research. Non-medical materials, such as newspaper and non-scientific articles, are not included in the listing; only information from medical and scientific sources was used.

21.   Lincoff, Gary, and D. H. Mitchel. **Toxic and Hallucinogenic Mushroom Poisoning: A Handbook for Physicians and Mushroom Hunters.** Edited by Wilbur K. Williams, illustrations by Irene E. Liberman, with a foreword by Alexander H. Smith. New York: Van Nostrand Reinhold Co., 1977. 267p. illus. bibliog. index. $16.95 LC 77-24639. ISBN 0-442-24580-7.

The authors of this outstanding work, a mycologist and a physician who is also a mushroom specialist, have prepared an excellent compendium of useful materials as well as a readable book. They summarize the existing knowledge about identity, biological characteristics, chemical composition, toxicology, and therapeutic management where toxic mushrooms are concerned. The book meets a need, as there has been an increase in recent years in the use of wild mushrooms as food; also, some people have begun consuming poisonous and hallucinogenic species for the "trip" that a light dose of the poison produces. Consequently, there has been an increase in cases of mushroom poisoning.

The book is intended for mushroom hunters who may not be familiar with the specific symptoms related to mushroom poisoning, and also for physicians and hospital emergency room personnel who are called upon to diagnose and treat poison cases. The introductory chapter places the topic in perspective; the next six chapters take up types of poisoning most frequently encountered based on types of toxins involved; the next chapter covers a heterogeneous group of mushrooms containing many different poisons, only a few of which have been identified; and the final chapter provides a discussion of the best approaches to diagnosis and treatment of mushroom poisoning. There are also several rather technical appendices of chemical and mycological detail. The work is well illustrated with line drawings and color plates.

Until recently, toxic mushrooms and mushroom toxins remained largely a mystery. Considerable light has been thrown on the subject in the past 20 years, and this book does much in communicating the information.

22.   Linde, Shirley. **The Whole Health Catalog: How to Stay Well—Cheaper.** 1st ed. New York: Rawson Associates Publishers, 1977. 225p. illus. index. $12.95; $6.95pa. LC 77-77890. ISBN 0-89256-012-6; 0-89256-035-5pa.

Written by a well-known medical and science writer, this work is designed to assist the individual in taking charge of his or her own health, a kind of do-it-yourself manual with emphasis on saving money. A variety of topics are covered, such as: diet, exercise, diseases, bad habits, pregnancy, sex therapy, child rearing, aging, medicines, hospitalization, health insurance, first aid, mental illness, and medical tests that can be done at home. Also included is a list of inexpensive or free health information services with addresses.

For the most part, material presented is sensible, practical, and authentic. It is a popular work intended for home libraries, but it is a valuable reference book for institutional libraries as well.

23.   Lloyd, John Uri. **Origin and History of the Pharmacopeial Vegetable Drugs, Chemicals, and Preparations with Bibliography.** v.1, **Vegetable Drugs,** 8th and 9th Decennial Revisions (Botanical Descriptions Omitted). Washington, DC: American Drug Manufacturers' Association, 1921. 449p. illus. bibliog. index.

At a meeting of the Committee on Standards and Deteriorations of the American Drug Manufacturers' Association in 1917, it was decided that a historical investigation of drugs listed in the *Pharmacopeia of the United States* should be published and that such a publication should contain bibliographical data sufficient to allow the reader to obtain access to primary literature on the subject. This work was undertaken to fulfill that resolve.

The author has provided reference data on the earliest uses of each pharmacopeial drug and has related important historical incidents as well. Drugs are listed alphabetically by official name. The following information is usually given about each drug: common names; the edition of the Pharmacopeia in which it had been official; historical background; uses; references to the literature listed in the bibliography; and some appropriate quotations. Use in folk medicine is often mentioned. In one monograph, an attempt is made to identify the Biblical manna that sustained the Israelites in the wilderness. The bibliography contains 707 references. An index of personal names has been provided as well as a plant name index.

The volume is of considerable historical interest. It presents a view of conventional medicines in use at the time it was written and provides a link with past times. The author was a pharmaceutical manufacturer and a novelist. He founded the Lloyd Library of Cincinnati that houses a valuable collection on medicinal plants and products, along with old rare publications about botany and pharmacy.

24.   **Medicinal and Aromatic Plants Abstracts.** New Delhi, India (Publications and Information Directorate, CSIR, Hillside Road, New Delhi 110012, India): 1979- . Bimonthly.

This rather new abstracting journal reports on world literature in the field of medicinal and aromatic plants. Its aim is to cull from important journals the highlights of current research in the field. The advisory committee is made up of scientists from various countries, although most are from India. More than 250 journals were reportedly scanned for pertinent material. Each issue contains a list of journals abstracted; many are Indian in origin.

The abstracts included are short, usually about a paragraph. The entries are grouped by specific subject. Each issue contains a keyword subject index, and annual indexes include authors' names also.

A special bibliography on a subject of current interest is included in each issue. The special bibliographies have references without abstracts. The journal is valuable because there is no other publication that currently serves the same purpose.

25.   Meyer, David C. **Herbal Recipes: For Hair, Salves & Liniments, Medicinal Wines and Vinegars, Plant Ash Uses.** Glenwood, IL: Meyerbooks (P. O. Box 427, 235 West Main St., Glenwood, IL 60425), 1978. 53p. $2.95pa. ISBN 0-916638-04-9.

This small book contains six sections on the topics indicated in the subtitle. Probably the most unique section is the one about uses of ashes from various plants. The hair section gives recipes for stimulating hair growth as well as for coloring and setting hair. Each recipe lists specific ingredients and provides instructions on how to use the product. Most of the recipes have apparently been taken from earlier books and herbals because many have a short but incomplete reference. This is an informally produced, but interesting, book. The publisher apparently offers similar books that are compilations of information from earlier sources.

26.   Montagna, F. Joseph. **PDR, People's Desk Reference: Traditional Herbal Formulas.** Lake Oswego, OR: Quest for Truth Publications, Inc. (16224 S. W. Bonaire, Lake Oswego, OR 97034), 1979. 2v. illus. bibliog. $74.00/set. LC 80-52954.

Although there are few similarities, the title "PDR" for this work is evidently taken in imitation of the *Physicians' Desk Reference*, well known in the conventional medical world as the "PDR."

The author, a Doctor of Herbal Medicine, compiled these large volumes to bring together traditional herbal knowledge developed throughout history. The title page says the work is "a concise treatise on medicinal herbs, their usefullness and combination for the prevention of disease; ailments, their causes and symptoms with herbal formulas for their prevention; vitamins and minerals, their biological functions, deficiency symptoms and sources; book of doses (materia medica) and complete botanical reference especially designed for herbalists and doctors."

Arrangement of the work is complicated, and no index is provided. The intention is that the table of contents will be used to find needed material. The book is divided into seven parts: 1) Traditional herbal formulas (an alphabetical listing of 60 herbal formulas with medicinal properties and dosage); 2) Ailments, their causes and symptoms (ailments listed alphabetically with definitions, causes, symptoms and treatment and with references to herbal formulas); 3) Ailment cross-reference (ailments listed with botanical used for treatment and prevention); 4) Botanical cross-reference (herbs listed with uses; for each herb a number is given which refers to the alphabetical listing of botanicals in part 7, allowing one to find additional information); 5) Book of doses (contains dosages of over 750 botanicals according to infusion, decoction, powder, tincture, fluid extract, aqueous extract, syrup, and oil); 6) Vitamins and minerals (a listing emphasizing their biological functions, deficiency symptoms, and sources); 7) Complete botanical reference (a list compiled in the late 1800s of botanicals known at that time; it lists German, pharmaceutical, and Latin botanical names and includes oils and essences).

Also provided is an appendix in seven parts: 1) Symptoms and underlying causes; 2) A list of medical properties with botanicals used for treatment; 3) Dosages adjusted by age of the patient; 4) Brief explanation of how to formulate preparations such as tinctures, infusions, syrups, ointments; 5) A summary of how to collect and preserve botanicals; 6) Weights and measures; and 7) Medical axioms relating to the action of medicines.

The publication contains a great deal of information, but the arrangement, the many parts, and the lack of an index limits its use for ready reference. The publisher disclaims responsibility for the effectiveness of any remedy mentioned in the book; indeed, many of the herbal formulas given are of doubtful value. The emphasis of the work, though, is said to be on prevention of disease rather than treatment.

27. **The Organic Directory.** Compiled by the editors of **Organic Gardening and Farming** and **Prevention.** Emmaus, PA: Rodale Press, 1971. 165p. $1.95pa.

The first half of the work consists of 16 signed articles on the value of the "organic" approach to food cultivation and preparation, and the dangers of continuing to live with man-made "poisons" in food.

The book includes a 50-page listing of "organic" food sources in the United States by state. Most entries include address, telephone number, type of food product available, and shipping policy. Some are "validated" as to their strict adherence to "organic" principles. Herb sources are included. Another section provides a directory by state of ecology action groups. Entries include individuals connected with universities and state conservation agencies. Addresses are given. The final section is a directory by state of suppliers and manufacturers of natural fertilizers, soil conditioners, and mulches. Most of these entries include address, telephone number, type of product, and shipping policy.

This directory is evidently updated periodically by the Rodale Press staff. It is a good source of information on the availability of "organic" food and plant products.

28. **Pharmacognosy Titles.** Chicago, IL: Department of Pharmacognosy and Pharmacology, College of Pharmacy, University of Illinois at the Medical Center, 1966-1974. Monthly.

Natural products are dealt with in this indexing journal, which, although no longer published, covers the world literature on the subject. About 100 leading journals were used directly to compile the work, with some other references being taken from *Chemical Abstracts* or *Biological Abstracts.* The publication was free to interested investigators or institutions.

Since pharmacognosy includes the study of all natural products of medicinal value, the journal included information about all living organisms, plants and animals. Articles discussed the following: detection; occurrence; distribution; isolation; and structure elucidation of substances from any living organism, including biological activities of extracts and pure compounds. Indexing was done according to the genus and species of each organism mentioned in the articles. Arrangement was by chemical or biological activity group. Abstracts were not included with the references.

29.   Plowden, C. Chicheley. **A Manual of Plant Names.** 2d rev. ed. Winchester, MA: Allen & Unwin (14 Thompson St., Winchester, MA 01890), 1970. 260p. illus. index. $10.00. SBN 8022-1990-x.

The gardener who wishes to have a better understanding of scientific names, descriptions, and relationships between plants will enjoy this work. The author has tried to condense into one manual a lot of information that would normally be found only in a large library with many reference works.

The sections of the book are: 1) A chapter introducing the history and rules of naming plants; 2) An index of generic plant names in which each entry contains the common name, family, translation, derivation, and application (species of importance or interest are included); 3) A vocabulary of specific epithets; an index of common names with botanical equivalents; 4) An explanatory vocabulary of English botanical terms describing plants, plant parts, or plant functions; 5) A descriptive chapter on the flower and inflorescence; 6) A descriptive chapter on the leaf; 7) A chapter on the relationship between plants; and 8) Notes on important and interesting families and genera. The author doesn't claim to have exhausted the subject, but has tried to produce a work of 'hand-book' size that will be of use and interest to gardeners.

30.   Spinelli, William B. **The Primitive Therapeutic Use of Medicinal Products–A Bibliography.** Pittsburgh, PA: School of Pharmacy, Duquesne University, 1971. 106p. index.

This bibliography presents an alphabetical list by author of 1,491 references to literature dealing with the use of natural products (mostly plant) for the treatment of disease and pain. Monographs and periodical articles have been included. Early and modern times are covered, as are all countries, but the author notes that the list is not comprehensive. The references were collected by searching through the literature on pharmacy, botany, anthropology, medicine, chemistry, and folklore. The word "primitive" in the title means popular (not savage or untutored) as opposed to scientific uses. The subject index includes the names of geographical regions and ethnic groups.

31.   Tam, Billy K. S., and Miriam S. L. Tam. **Acupuncture: An International Bibliography.** Metuchen, NJ: Scarecrow, 1973. 137p. index. $5.00. LC 73-5772. ISBN 0-8109-0625-8.

About 900 entries are included in this bibliography, covering the years A.D. 282 to late 1972. The work is intended for laymen as well as for physicians. The citations refer to a variety of materials, including books, journal articles, atlases, dictionaries, handbooks, and publications of societies and institutions. The journal articles are arranged under broad subject headings by type of disease. Also included is a listing of societies and institutions engaged in acupuncture research.

32.   U.S. National Agricultural Library. **Herb Gardening 1970-1979; 112 Citations.** Searched by Jayne MacLean and Ann Juneau. Beltsville, MD: The Library, 1979. 17p. (Quick Bibliography Series, NAL-BIBL.–79-10). (Photocopy available from Technical Information Systems, Science and Education Administration, U.S. Department of Agriculture, National Agricultural Library Building, Beltsville, MD 20705).

This is a bibliography of 112 citations on herb gardening. It is a photocopy of a printout produced by a computerized literature search of the *AGRICOLA* data base via DIALOG Information Retrieval Service, which was performed at the U.S. National Agricultural Library, Reference Division. Citations are arranged by publication date, the latest first. Articles and monographs are included. Most items are in English, and most are of a popular nature suitable for the home gardener.

33.   Weiss, Mark. **The Handbook for Free Materials on Organic Foods.** Chatsworth, CA: Books for Better Living; distr. New York: Resourceful Research, 1972. 222p. $1.95pa. ISBN 0-87056-227-4.

Although information such as that provided here becomes obsolete rapidly, this work may be useful as a guide to sources where one can obtain free samples of organic food, issues of magazines, motion pictures (for rent), recipes, and lists of farms that grow and organizations that sell organic foods. Each source is annotated briefly. Many items are from the U.S. Superintendent of Documents. (These materials may involve some expense.) Most references are to small pamphlets, and recipes seem to make up the bulk of available literature.

2

DICTIONARIES,
ENCYCLOPEDIAS, AND GLOSSARIES

Of the works listed here, one title is a classic general work on plants, Bailey and Bailey's *Hortus Third.* There are also three titles of high quality that deal with medicinal and other economic plants, those by Hocking, Uphof, and Usher. Moerman's dictionary on *American Medical Ethnobotany* examines the uses of medicinal plants by Native Americans. (Other works on the ethnobotany of various cultural groups can be found in following sections of this bibliography.) Rinzler's *Dictionary of Medical Folklore* describes and evaluates folk remedies.

Most titles in this section are on natural and herbal medicine, and include works by Bricklin, Day, Kadans, Law, Stuart, Robert Thomson, William Thomson, and Wren. Titles by Hill and by Walker deal with other forms of alternative or unconventional medicine. The *Encyclopedia of Mushrooms* by Dickinson and Lucas covers most aspects of these fungi. (Other mushroom books are listed in chapter 17.)

Three works are foreign language glossaries, those by Sliosberg, Steinmetz, and Stracke.

A few unusual works have been included in this section. The first, Leung's *Encyclopedia of Common Natural Ingredients Used in Food,* is a scientific work that will help put natural products in perspective. Wedeck's *Dictionary of Aphrodisiacs* is not a scientific work, but covers a subject of interest. Lastly, the two small books on *Legal Highs,* one by Gottlieb and the other with no author given, offer a unique but perhaps unscrupulous approach to the use of natural psychoactive substances.

* * * * *

34.   Bailey, Liberty Hyde, and Ethel Zoe Bailey. **Hortus Third: A Concise Dictionary of Plants Cultivated in the United States and Canada.** Revised and expanded by the staff of the Liberty Hyde Bailey Hortorium. New York: Macmillan Publishing Co., 1976. 1290p. illus. index. $99.50. ISBN 0-02-505470-8.

This monumental work continues a longstanding effort, initiated by Bailey before the turn of the century, to classify cultivated plants. It is a revision of *Hortus* (1930) and *Hortus Second* (1941) and a recent assessment of the kinds and names of plants cultivated in the continental United States, Canada, Puerto Rico, and Hawaii. Included are the descriptions and correct botanical names with their authors for 281 families, 3,301 genera, and 20,297 species. In addition, a large number of subspecies, varieties, forms, notes on uses, methods of propagation, and culture are included with the entries.

The book is arranged alphabetically in dictionary format. Entries are listed under plant family name, generic names, and general subjects. There are line-drawings of various species representing most families. Appendices include a list of authors cited, a glossary of botanical terms, and an index to common names.

This fine work is a standard reference book on the plants of North American horticulture.

35.   Bricklin, Mark. **The Practical Encyclopedia of Natural Healing**. Emmaus, PA: Rodale Press, 1976. 582p. illus. bibliog. index. $12.95. LC 76-25864. ISBN 0-87857-136-1.

The author of this work approaches natural healing in two ways. He describes different schools of healing such as naturopathy and music therapy; he discusses ailments individually and includes "natural" remedies and therapies. Mention is made of herbal medicine and folk remedies and anecdotes of interest are included.

Material is arranged alphabetically by subject. Most entries run several pages and include subheadings. Herbs as remedies are mentioned in many entries in the book, and there is, in addition, a rather long section on herbal medicine. The ten most practical herbs are listed with information on how to grow and use them. Quotations from a number of publications on herbs are included, and recipes for a few concoctions are given. A critical review of correspondence courses in herbalism is included as is a short annotated bibliography of books on the subject.

A rather comprehensive, low-key treatment of the subject is provided. The author is the executive editor of *Prevention* magazine (see entry 118).

36. Carroll, Anstice, and Embree De Persiis Vona. **The Health Food Dictionary with Recipes**. Illustrated by Vincenzo De Persiis Vona. Englewood Cliffs, NJ: Prentice-Hall, 1973. 200p. illus, index. $6.95. LC 72-8935. ISBN 0-13-384495-1.

The authors claim that this work, although pro health foods, is not for the "health food fanatic." It is for those who are overwhelmed and confused by the proliferation of health food literature. The aim is to answer questions so that people won't get "gypped in a health food store." The work, as a dictionary, has entries listed in alphabetical order by common health food name. Each entry gives a short description of the product, where it comes from, health properties, how to use, other foods it goes with, and simple recipes. There are a few drawings scattered throughout, but not one for each entry. Scientific names of plants are not usually included. There is both a subject and a recipe index.

37. Chopra, R. N., S. L. Nayar, and I. C. Chopra. **Glossary of Indian Medicinal Plants**. New Delhi, India: Council of Scientific and Industrial Research, 1956. 330p. bibliog. index. (A **Supplement to Glossary of Indian Medicinal Plants** by R. N. Chopra, I. C. Chopra, and B. S. Varma was published by the Publications and Information Directorate, Hillside Road, New Delhi 12, India, in 1969. 119p.).

Research workers dealing with Indian indigenous drugs and medicinal plants, particularly botanists, chemists, and pharmacologists, will find this work valuable. Plants are arranged alphabetically by botanical names. Vernacular names, synonymous names, distribution, habitat, use, part of plant used, chemical composition (if known), and scientific references are usually given. There are two indexes, common vernacular name and chemical constituent. The supplementary volume is similar to the main work in arrangement and content. It covers the literature from 1955 to 1964. A large number of scientific books and journal articles are cited in the text of this work. Lists of them are provided.

38.   Day, Harvey. **Encyclopedia of Natural Health and Healing.** Santa Barbara, CA: Woodbridge Press Publishing Co., 1979. 206p. illus. $7.95. LC 78-24666. ISBN 0-912800-62-3.

The author says he has written this encyclopedia (really an elaborate dictionary) to give readers access to information about natural approaches to health and well-being and, at the same time, to provide information about foods, diets, and products associated with sound nutrition. He believes in "a balanced diet, fresh air and sunshine, hydrotherapy, acupuncture, homeopathy, osteopathy, chiropractic, herbs, and exercise" to assist the healing process.

The book provides monographs of about a half page on foods, herbs, minerals, vitamins, health cults, and diseases. In addition, many biographical sketches of pioneers in the "natural" health field are included, together with some famous scientists. For instance, the biography of Wilhelm Conrad Röntgen (discoverer of X-rays) follows closely that of J. I. Rodale, an apostle of health foods and organic gardening (see entry 306). Literature references are scattered throughout the text.

The author of the book is evidently British, although references are made frequently to America and continental Europe. It was surprising to find tomatoes referred to as "tropical American plants."

The book provides reasonably complete coverage of matters relating to the "natural" health field.

39.   Dickinson, Colin, and John Lucas, eds. **The Encyclopedia of Mushrooms.** New York: G. P. Putnam's Sons, 1979. 280p. illus. (col.). bibliog. index. $25.00. LC 77-014635. SBN 399-12104-8.

Knowledge about mushrooms is important and needed, the authors of this book claim, and so they prepared this encyclopedia about them for the general reader. They point out that terminology regarding these plants is ambiguous. The book covers the many different kinds of fungi apt to be seen in the field. It is a combination field guide and encyclopedia and includes more than 600 fine color illustrations.

Almost half the book examines the following aspects of the subject: 1) the mushroom in history; 2) the biology of fungi; 3) the lifestyles of fungi; 4) the mushroom habitat; 5) mushrooms and man, 6) mushrooms as food; and 7) the naming of fungi. The largest part of the book, the "Reference Section," lists mushrooms alphabetically by family name. Information about each species includes: common name, description, fruiting body, habitat and distribution, occurrence, culinary properties, and a color photograph. The section on mushrooms and man includes material on mushroom poisoning and hallucinogenic mushrooms. The section on mushrooms as food contains a number of recipes and instructions on preparation of mushrooms for food. The book includes a glossary of specialized terms and three indexes (botanical names, common English names, and general).

40.   Gottlieb, Adam. **Legal Highs: A Concise Encyclopedia of Legal Herbs and Chemicals with Psychoactive Properties.** Manhattan Beach, CA: 20th Century Alchemist; distr. Berkeley, CA, And/Or Press (P.O. Box 2246, Berkeley, CA 94702), 1973. 64p. illus. $2.95pa. (Previously published by High Times/Level Press).

This small book lists substances and plants that are legal although they possess psychoactive properties. Some of the plants are relatively obscure and have attracted little notice; others contain chemicals that are controlled substances, but their plant sources are not controlled. In addition, some are legal for use in religious sacraments, for instance, peyote, because it was used by American Indians in their religious rituals long before white settlers came to the United States.

About 70 herbs and chemicals are listed alphabetically by common name. Information provided about each includes chemical name if a chemical, scientific name if a plant, material (such as part of plant used), usage, active constituents, effects, contraindication, and supplier (in many cases a commercial herb grower). Although the author declares he is not encouraging experimentation with psychoactive substances, the book provides considerable information about how to obtain and use them. Some caution is advised, however.

The title *Legal Highs* (see entry 46) is nearly identical to this one.

41.   Hill, Ann, ed. **A Visual Encyclopedia of Unconventional Medicine.** New York: Crown Publishers, 1979. 240p. illus. (part col.). bibliog. index. $12.95; $6.95pa. LC 78-14009. ISBN 0-517-52613-7; 0-517-53614-5pa.

The editor of this work does not contend that all conventional medicine is wrong or that all unconventional therapies can provide all that is needed to remain well. The two systems should be complementary, she says. She has gathered information on all the unconventional systems that seem useful and has presented them with little bias or evaluation. The material has been written by practitioners of the various systems.

General headings under which the material appears are as follows: 1) Comprehensive systems; 2) Diagnostic methods; 3) Physical therapies; 4) Hydrotherapy; 5) Plant-based therapies; 6) Nutrition; 7) Wave, radiation and vibration; 8) Mind and spirit therapies; and 9) Self-exercise therapies.

Considering the nature of the material, the presentation is good, However, most of the systems and therapies discussed are not only unconventional but unproven, and some are little more than quackery. The work should be useful, however, as it is an excellent source of information about unconventional medicine and will answer many reference questions. Unconventional, unproven remedies are currently receiving a great deal of attention.

42.   Hocking, George MacDonald. **A Dictionary of Terms in Pharmacognosy and Other Divisions of Economic Botany.** Springfield, IL: Charles C. Thomas, 1955. 284p. illus. bibliog. LC 55-7453.

The title page says this is "a compilation of words and expressions relating principally to natural medicinal and pharmaceutical materials and the plants and animals from which they are derived, their chemical composition, applications, and uses, together with some other materials derived from the plant, animal, and mineral kingdoms of current economic interest." The author defines "pharmacognosy" as "the science which treats in detail those medicinal and related products of crude or primary type obtained from the vegetable, animal, and mineral kingdoms as they appear on the market as raw materials, as they occur in folk medical practice, and as they function in chemical manufacturing processes." Professor Hocking hopes his work will be appreciated as a guide through the maze of innumerable Latin terms, biological names, vernacular terms, and other specialized jargons.

At the time the dictionary was compiled, herbal medicine had suffered a decline in usage, at least in the form usually identified as "herbal", although a large number of drugs, then as now, were derived from plant substances. The dictionary was designed primarily for students and practitioners in the health professions, people in trade and industry, and others interested in the useful plants of the world. Many will find it valuable because of the current resurgence of interest in the field.

An explanatory foreword covers definitions, nomenclature, pronunciation, geographical distribution, constituents, and applications and uses of the materials. Other supplementary sections include lists of abbreviations, symbols, references, serials and periodicals, terms describing properties and therapeutic uses of drugs, and material on classification of plants and animals.

43.   Hulke, Malcolm, ed. **The Encyclopedia of Alternative Medicine and Self-Help.** New York: Schocken Books, 1979. 243p. bibliog. index. $12.95; $6.95pa. LC 78-21115. ISBN 0-8052-3713-5; 0-8052-0623-Xpa.

If one is looking for information on a particular alternative system to conventional, traditional, orthodox Western medicine, this encyclopedia can probably provide it. There are articles, some several pages in length, about various therapeutic systems, each written by a person familiar with the movement under discussion. For example, the following are treated: acupuncture, chiropractic, color therapy, flower healing, health foods, herbalism, naturism, osteopathy, reflexology, and yoga. Also included in the alphabetical arrangement are articles on common ailments with suggested treatment.

Most of the alternative forms of medicine emphasize self-help and have a tendency to treat the "whole" person, that is, body, mind, and spirit. Conventional medicine is criticized because it ordinarily concentrates only on the specific malady or condition.

The book contains a directory that lists associations, products, training and treatment centers, health spas and resorts, and health magazines.

44.   Kadans, Joseph M. **Encyclopedia of Medicinal Herbs.** With the Herb-O-Matic Locator Index. New York: Arco Publishing Co., 1978. 256p. index. $1.75pa. LC 79-158469. ISBN 0-668-02487-9.

This work was published previously under the title *Modern Encyclopedia of Herbs.* It lists herbs alphabetically under popular names. In cases where the plants are known by several popular names, cross-references have been provided. Each monograph usually includes botanical name, synonymous common names, effects, reported uses, habitat, growth needs, description, preparation, and any necessary warnings. Over 600 herbs are described. There is a special section on spice and herb cookery. The index provided, called an "Herb-O-Matic Locator Index," is designed to direct the reader to the herb that fits his needs. For example, one can look up an ailment and be directed to pages that give complete information about herbs said to be useful for treating the condition.

45.   Law, Donald. **The Concise Herbal Encyclopedia.** New York: Saint Martin's Press, 1973. 266p. illus. (part col.). bibliog. $7.95. LC 73-87589.

The author says he wrote this book to present "some of the mysteries, magic, myths, and medicinal values of herbs so that the man in the street can benefit." Although called an "encyclopedia," the work does not follow the typical format of other such reference works. These chapters are presented: 1) History of Herbal Medicine; 2) Some Commonly Used Herbs; 3) Health from Herbal Wines; 4) How to Make Cosmetics from Herbs; 5) Herbs for Diets; 6) Herbs of Cooking; 7) Herbs for Veterinary Purposes; 8) Dyes from Vegetable Substances; 9) Herbs in Magic and Witchcraft; 10) Herbal Tobacco; 11) Tropical and Overseas Herbs; and 12) Herbs and Health.

Most chapters present introductory material, then an alphabetical listing of the suitable herbs with short to medium length monographs or definitions. In addition to the history and myths, there are many recipes given for remedies, cosmetics, food, and the like. Also included are many literary passages and poetry. Material presented is of interest mainly for the history and lore. Suggested remedies are of questionable value, but the author does not necessarily present them as lore. Since there is no general index and several separate alphabetical listings, it is difficult to find specific information about any one herb.

46. **Legal Highs: A Concise Encyclopedia of Legal Herbs and Chemicals with Psychoactive Properties.** New York/Hermosa Beach, CA: High Times/Golden State Puslishing, 1973. 32p. illus. $2.00pa.

This booklet provides brief information on various substances that are psychotropic but legal. These include plant materials in crude form and chemicals, either synthesized or extracted from natural materials. Entries are arranged alphabetically. The following is given for each: description, method of preparation, dosage and use, analysis of active constituents, effects, contraindications, and the name of a supplier in letter code. Code letters are identified at the end of the book, and addresses are given. Over 70 materials are listed, including such familiar materials as nutmeg, catnip, dill, hops, and parsley, as well as some exotic and dangerous substances.

The title by Gottlieb, *Legal Highs* (see entry 40), seems to be nearly identical to this one with minor changes only.

47. Leung, Albert Y. **Encyclopedia of Common Natural Ingredients Used in Food, Drugs, and Cosmetics.** New York: John Wiley and Sons, 1980. 409p. bibliog. index. (A Wiley-Interscience Publication). $50.00. LC 79-25998. ISBN 0-471-04954-9.

This is a unique book of high quality. The author was educated as a pharmacist and pharmacognosist and has had extensive experience in industries that deal with natural products. According to the preface, about 500 natural ingredients are currently used in commercial food, drugs, and cosmetic products (not including such materials as vitamins and antibiotics). The book contains information on about 310 of these ingredients used in processed foods, over-the-counter drugs, and cosmetics. Many substances are covered that were formerly official in the *U.S. Pharmacopeia* and *Natural Formulary,* but have been deleted from recent editions (although still used). It is particularly difficult to find up-to-date information on such preparations; and, of course, many products are included which were never official but have been and still are used.

The natural products are arranged alphabetically by the most common name, with each natural ingredient cross-referenced by its scientific and other synonymous names in the general index. There is also a separate chemical index. Information included on each item includes plant or other sources, habitats, parts used or derived from, method of preparation, brief physical description, chemical composition, pharmacological or biological activities, common commercially available forms and their qualities, uses, and regulatory status, if any. Uses are categorized as: pharmaceutical and/or cosmetic, food, folk medicine, and others. The author has provided a glossary of terminology commonly used in the botanical industry. References to scientific literature are provided with each monograph.

The encyclopedia is intended primarily for technical and non-technical members of the food, drug, and cosmetic industries, teachers and students of related sciences, and members of the general public who are interested. The author says he has reported only those folk medicinal uses which are known to him from reliable sources; they are by no means complete or an endorsement of such use, he notes. He has included them because of their popular interest.

48.   Lloyd Brothers. **Drug Treatises,** numbers 1-26. Cincinnati, OH: Lloyd Brothers, 1903-1910. illus.

The Lloyd Brothers, early drug manufacturers of Cincinnati, Ohio, issued short treatises on drugs from 1903 to 1910 for physicians' use. The publications, from 16 to 48 pages each, contain historical and therapeutic information such as descriptions, constituents, uses, and doses. Various authorities, sometimes John Uri Lloyd himself, prepared the booklets.

Following are the materials and/or topics covered: *Thuja (arbor vitae),* *Crataegus* (hawthorn), cactus grandiflors, *Pilocarpus* (jaborandi), *Veratrum Viride* (American hellebore), *Chionanthus Virginica* (fringe tree), asepsin (sodium salt of methyl salicylic acid), *Collinsonia Canadensis* (stone root), nux vomica, *Gelsemium* (jessamine), belladonna (deadly nightshade), *Oenanthe Crocata* (hemlock water parsnip), vegetable caustic, ergot, *Macrotys* (black snakeroot), *Dioscorea* (china root), sulphurous acid, the development of the pharmaceutical still, *Scutellaria* (skullcap), acute poisoning, *Mangifera* (mango), physicians and the National Food and Drugs Act, Libradol (a trade name product), acids and miscellaneous preparations, Cupri Acetas (solution of acetate of copper), charcoal, resin of podophyllum root, insect medicines, opium, golden seal, alkaloids, resins, rhubarb, peppermint, and echinacea.

49.   Maimonides, Moses. **Moses Maimonides' Glossary of Drug Names.** Ed. by Fred Rosner. Translated from Max Meyerhof's French ed. Philadelphia, PA: American Philosophical Society, 1979. 364p. index. (Memoirs of the American Philosophical Society, Vol.135). $20.75pa. LC 79-13875. ISBN 0-87169-135-3; ISSN 0065-9738.

This work is one of a group of medical writings by Moses Maimonides, a noted Jewish physician born in Spain in the twelfth century who later settled in North Africa and attended royal families. His works were originally written in Arabic. The *Glossary of Drug Names* was only relatively recently discovered in a library in Istanbul, Turkey, and was subsequently translated into French (1940). A Hebrew edition has also appeared (1969). The work under review has been translated from the French edition.

The work is essentially a pharmacopeia. Its 405 short monographs are arranged alphabetically by what was considered the best known name of the drug (most of plant origin). The name is usually Arabic (although it may be of Greek, Syriac, or Persian origin); other Arabic and Syriac names follow, as do names in Greek, Persian, Berber, Spanish, and English. Explanatory material, averaging about one-half page, is given on each drug. Many references to early writings about the substances are included. Indexes of Latin, Iberic, Accadian and Syrian, Arabic, Berber, Sanscrit and Indian dialects, and Persian names have been provided.

The translation is a scholarly undertaking and is an important source of information for medical historians and scholars as well as those interested in medicines.

50.   Moerman, Daniel E. **American Medical Ethnobotany: A Reference Dictionary.** New York: Garland Publishing, Inc., 1977. 527p. bibliog. (Garland Reference Library of Social Science, v.34). $51.00. LC 76-24771. ISBN 0-8240-9907-9.

Native American medicinal uses of plants are covered in this reference work, which is also a guide to the literature on the subject. Included are "1,288 different plant species from 531 different genera from 118 different families used in 48 different cultures in 4,869 different ways."

Material is presented in four tables. The first, *Genera,* lists all items in the databank alphabetically by genus and species. The table also lists the botanical family, the tribe, the indication, a common name, and a short note on preparation, use, and a code number which refers to a reference in the bibliography. Table 2, *Indications,* lists all items in the databank according to primary use. Genus, species, common name, tribe, and bibliographic references are given. Table 3, *Families,* lists all items by botanical family, taking into account genus, species, tribe, indication and bibliographic references. Table 4, *Cultures,* lists all the items in the databank for each of the 48 cultures represented. Under each culture is found genus, species, indications, and literature references. The bibliography of coded sources is found following the tables, then a list of common names, and a supplementary bibliography of books and articles on medicinal uses of plants. About half are briefly annotated.

The book reviews uses of specific plants by many cultures, the range of plants and their uses by these cultures, and the taxonomic affinities of the medicinal plants.

51.   Rinzler, Carol Ann. **The Dictionary of Medical Folklore.** New York: Thomas Y. Crowell, 1979. 243p. index. $10.00. LC 78-69518. ISBN 0-690-01704-9.

The author of this work, a science writer, has pulled together more than 500 common medical "old wives' tales," arranged them alphabetically, and then discussed whether there is any truth in the superstitions. Her conclusion? Perhaps 50% to 60% of the old preventives are effective, according to the book.

The author tackles such beliefs as: 1) Chocolate is addictive; 2) Redheads have terrible tempers; 3) Cranberry juice cures or prevents cystitis, 4) Copper bracelets cure arthritis; 5) Cigarettes stunt your growth; and 6) Eating fruit seeds can cause appendicitis. In the book's introduction, the author says she collected material for the book from newspapers, periodicals, and books. She refers to a number of reference books, which she lists, for verification and explanations. For the most part, works cited are authoritative. The book is interesting, and the information is usually correct, although a few errors have been noted, particularly in identifying active constituents of plant materials. It would be impossible for an author to be an expert in all the areas of science that are explored in a book such as this, and errors are probably inevitable.

52.   Singh, Thakur Balwant, and K. C. Chunekar. **Glossary of Vegetable Drugs in Brhattrayi.** Varanasi-1, India: Chowkhamba Sanskrit Series Office (K. 37/99, Gopal Mandir Lane, P. O. Chowkhamba, P. Box 8, Varanasi-1, India), 1972. 544p. bibliog. index. (The Chowkhamba Sanskrit Studies, v.87).

Identification of all medicinal plants mentioned by the authors of three great Samhitas, collectively called Brhattrayi, has not been solved satisfactorily in all cases. The authors of this work have attempted the task and present here an alphabetical list of all the Sanskrit names of the food and drug plants, including references. Latin names have been given when positive identification of the plant was possible. Botanical identities of others are discussed. Descriptions, properties, and uses of the plants are included. There is an index of Latin and English names, a general index of Sanskrit and other Indian names, and a list of books and journals referred to.

The book is of special value for those seeking information on Ayurvedic plants.

53.   Sliosberg, A., comp. **Elsevier's Dictionary of Pharmaceutical Science and Techniques in Six Languages: English, French, Italian, Spanish, German, Latin: Volume 2, Materia Medica.** Amsterdam: Elsevier Scientific Publishing; distr., New York, Elsevier/ North-Holland, 1980. 552p. $116.25. ISBN 0-444-41664-1.

The first volume of this set, which was published in 1968, covered pharmaceutical technology. This one is limited to terms in the area of materia medica, especially substances of vegetable and animal origin used in the preparation of drugs. It is a polyglot dictionary providing synonymous terms in the six languages indicated above.

The main section of the work, the "Basic Table," lists alphabetically by English term 4,688 numbered entries and provides corresponding terms in the other five languages. There are six thumb-indexed sections, one for each language, where terms are listed alphabetically with the number given for the entry in the basic table. Each section seems to contain more entries than are in the basic table because synonymous terms have been added that refer to a basic term.

This should prove to be a valuable work, as few foreign language lists of such terms exist; and there is a growing interest in herbal medicine and medicinal plants by scientists and laypersons alike.

54.   Steinmetz. E. F. **Codex Vegetabilis.** 2d ed. Amsterdam: E. F. Steinmetz, 1957. 1v. (various paging). index.

The late author of this work, an herbalist, compiled the book over a course of many years. It is a list of 1,216 plants with equivalent names in Latin, English, French, German, Dutch, and other European and some Oriental languages. Also included is brief information about the natural habitat, the constituents, and actions of the botanicals. A numbered list comprises half the book; the other half is an index of all the names mentioned.

The work is intended for physicians, botanists, herbalists, chemists, druggists, students, and all others interested in botanical drugs. It serves as a special polylingual dictionary, although perhaps not a very authentic one. There are no literature references.

55.   Stracke, J. Richard, ed. **The Laud Herbal Glossary.** Amsterdam: Rodopi N.V., 1974. 208p. bibliog. index. $24.00. LC 72-93569. ISBN 90-6203-497-7.

Although there is little easy-to-understand material in the introduction of this book, it does say that the Laud Glossary is found on ff. 67-73 of MS Laud Misc. 567, "a manuscript of s.xii containing the Viaticus of Constantinus Africanus and other medical texts." It was given to the Bodleian Library in 1635 by Archbishop Laud and has been used in various compilations of names of plants. The text's dialect is difficult, partly because English was in transition at the time the glossary was prepared (mid-twelfth century). The scribe apparently was Norman.

The text of the glossary is a listing of 1,553 terms, followed by about 40 pages of explanatory notes. Indexes make up about half of the book and include an index of Latin and Latinized words, an index of Old English words, and an index of Old French words.

The book should be useful to those making a serious study of early sources of herbal information.

56.   Stuart, Malcolm, ed. **The Encyclopedia of Herbs and Herbalism.** New York: Grosset & Dunlap, 1979. 304p. illus. (part col.). bibliog. index. $35.00. LC 78-58101. ISBN 0-448-15472-2.

Six substantial articles with up-to-date information about many aspects of herbs and herbalism comprise this book. Titles of the articles (by British experts and scholars) are: The Biology and Chemistry of Plants; The Medicinal Uses of Plants; Herbs in the Kitchen; The Domestic and Cosmetic Uses of Herbs; and The Cultivation, Collection and Preservation of Herbs.

All of these discussions are illustrated with excellent color photographs, drawings, and diagrams. Several charts of herbs and their specific uses for various applications (e.g., food, medicine, and cosmetics) are found throughout the articles, as are recipes for products with various uses. The articles make up about one-half the book. The remainder of the work includes an alphabetical listing of 420 herbs by Latin name. Each entry provides the common name of the plant, a brief historical note, a description, distribution and cultivation, chemical constituents, uses, and, when appropriate, contraindications. Most entries are illustrated by a color photograph of the plant in bloom. A glossary, an extensive bibliography, and good general and plant indexes complete this work.

This work is a good, general purpose and comprehensive reference source about the world of herbs, but the cost is somewhat high. It is not, however, a good choice for a practical field identification guide because of its size.

It is noteworthy that this book does not encourage self-treatment with herbs, as can be seen by the following quotation: "Simply because herbs are natural products it does not follow that their use in medicine is any easier than the use of synthetic substances--in many ways, indeed, it is more complicated. It is for these reasons therefore, that self-medication cannot be recommended and why so many popular modern 'herbals' may be considered with interest, but not as medical manuals."

57. Thomson, Robert. **The Grosset Encyclopedia of Natural Medicine.** New York: Grosset and Dunlap, 1980. 291p. illus. bibliog. index. $9.95pa. LC 79-56186. ISBN 0-448-14897-8.

Thomson, compiler of this work, evidently holds doctoral degrees in naturopathy and naprapathy, two branches of natural medicine. The encyclopedia contains about 600 entries covering many natural healing practices and remedies. A comprehensive range of subjects is presented, including some material from other countries and cultures.

In the alphabetical arrangement will be found short monographs on acupuncture, iridology, herbalism, hydrotherapy, biographies of proponents of various systems of natural medicine, and descriptions of herbal plants. Some physiology and anatomy is also included. There are appended tables of composition of foods, a summary of vitamins, and digestion times of foods. The bibliography is long and is divided by these topics: childbirth, food and nutrition, herbology, history and philosophy of natural medicine, homeopathy, iridology, Islamic healing, magnetics, natural healing systems, reference works, spiritual healing, traditional internal medicine, traditional Eastern medicine, unorthodox cancer therapies, and Western medicine.

58. Thomson, William A. R., ed. **Medicines from the Earth: A Guide to Healing Plants.** New York: McGraw-Hill, 1978. 208p. illus. (part col.). bibliog. index. $29.95. LC 78-8307. ISBN 0-07-056087-0.

This book is an attractive encyclopedia of what are claimed to be the 247 most beneficial plants known. The subject is approached from both the botanical and the medical point of view; that is, the user can find information about a plant, or he can find information about an illness for which there is an herbal remedy.

The book is in eight parts, each prepared by an expert, as follows: 1) The kingdom of plants; 2) The 247 most beneficial plants; 3) Lexicon of the healing plants; 4) Complaints and illnesses; 5) the heritage of folk medicine; 6) The basic techniques of herbal preparations; 7) Healing substances and their effectiveness; and 8) Epilogue: the future.

The plant lexicon is the longest part of the book, and it contains fine color illustrations and descriptions of the 247 plants. They are arranged alphabetically by Latin name. The following information is usually given for each: Latin name, common name, geographic distribution, morphological description, medicinal and other economic uses, and chemical constituents. Three cross-referenced sections are included, giving information in tabular form. One section lists the plants alphabetically by common name and gives the most important medicinal uses. The reader is referred to the plant lexicon section for full information. Another section lists major illnesses alphabetically and the plant alleged to be useful for the condition named. The third reference section lists each plant as in the previous sections, but gives more detail on chemical constituents, harvesting, and pharmacological properties.

While the book is attractive and has other good features, some criticisms can be made. Like most recent works on herbs and folk medicines, the book bears a disclaimer stating that it is not intended as a guide for prescribing medicines and is not a substitute for a physician's services. However, like other such books, it has little other real value except perhaps for the history and folklore it contains. It includes some information on toxicity and medicinal chemistry that health professionals might use, but there are far more reliable scientific sources available.

59.   Uphof, J.C. Th. **Dictionary of Economic Plants.** 2d ed. rev. and enl. Monticello, NY: Lubrecht and Cramer (RFD 1, Box 227, Monticello, NY 12701), 1968. 591p. bibliog. $28.00.

A major authoritative and comprehensive work in dictionary form, this book gives short descriptions of economic plants, covering their distribution, products, and main uses.

Included are plants important to agriculture, forestry, fruit and vegetable growing, pharmacognosy, and those important in world trade, as well as some that are of local value only. In addition, a number of plants of ethnological interest are included because they furnish food, medicine, and other materials of value to primitive people. About 9,500 species of both lower and higher plant forms are included, arranged alphabetically by Latin name. Each entry includes the name, synonymous Latin names if any, and descriptions as mentioned above. Plants were not included if sufficient information was not known about them.

The 27-page bibliography is divided by broad subject and geographical headings. Subjects of particular interest are spices and herbs; medicinal plants; essential oils; and narcotic, hallucinogenic and ordeal plants.

60.   Usher, George. **A Dictionary of Plants Used by Man.** New York: Hafner Press, A Division of Macmillan Publishing Co., 1974. 619p. $15.95. LC 74-2707. ISBN 02-853800-5.

This dictionary provides such information as what a given plant is used for, its habitat, botanical family, and correct scientific name. Plants from all over the world are listed, including trees, shrubs, weeds, herbs, and agricultural plants. A great many tropical and subtropical species are included. A full system of cross-references, covering Latin and common names, has been provided.

61.   Walker, Benjamin. **Encyclopedia of Metaphysical Medicine.** Boston, MA: Routledge & Kegan Paul, 1978. 323p. bibliog. index. $17.50. ISBN 0-7100-8781-0.

Although reviewers have criticized this book as being poorly done, it is included here because of the current interest in alternative medical systems. While the volume contains sections on some non-metaphysical subjects, such as microbes and molecular biology, and omits some which might well have been included, such as alchemy, astrology, and witchcraft, it provides a view of a number of unusual medical philosophies and their history. Bibliographies are provided after each section.

62.   Wedeck, Harry E., ed. **Dictionary of Aphrodisiacs.** New York: Philosophical Library, 1961. 256p. illus. bibliog. $10.00. LC 61-12626. ISBN 0-8022-1828-8.

It has been considered important throughout time that man maintain his amorous abilities. Virility has been presumed to be sustained, preserved, and recaptured by various means, including the use of exotic foods and drink, rare herbal concoctions, and the like. This book surveys and classifies the means to this end, including the herbal, scientific, legendary, medicinal, and culinary methods. (NOTE: Since scientists generally agree that there is no such thing as a true aphrodisiac, the materials listed are of reported or supposed value only.)

Entries are arranged alphabetically with definitions ranging from a few lines to a few paragraphs. Most entries are substances (usually herbs or foods), but some are names of individuals, places, books, and other terms associated with the subject.

63.   Wren, R. C. **Potter's New Cyclopaedia of Botanical Drugs and Preparations.** New ed., re-edited and enlarged by R. W. Wren. Foreword by T. E. Wallis. Holsworthy, England: Health Science Press, 1975. 400p. illus. index. £5.95. ISBN 0-85032-009-7.

The first edition of Potter's work appeared in 1907, the second in 1915, another in 1923, the fourth in 1932; then a fifth, sixth, and seventh edition appeared before this one was published. Various compilers worked on the different editions, and each one was an outstanding success.

The foreword points out that many plants are still used in Great Britain as household remedies or as ingredients of conventional medicines. It was felt that a reliable source of information should be available for dealers in remedies, physicians, pharmacists, and analysts. The encyclopedia serves this purpose, it is hoped, by supplementing the official *British Pharmacopoeia* and the *British Pharmaceutical Codex*.

The work provides a rather comprehensive list of drug plants and plant materials. Arrangement is alphabetical by common name. Each monograph usually includes the following: scientific name, family, synonyms, habitat, flowering time, description, part used, medicinal use, commercial use, preparations, and perhaps a literature reference (often from an old source such as the Bible or an ancient herbal). There are several appendices as follows: guide to therapeutic action, forms of medicinal preparations, weights and measures, domestic doses and their equivalents, herbal compounds (continental), glossary of medical terms, and abbreviations of names of authors of botanical works. Indexes of botanical names, common names, and synonyms are included.

Illustrations in this edition are not as attractive as those in some earlier editions. It's a good work in most respects, although not very critical of the supposed value of the herbs discussed.

3
HISTORIES

History is important in the study of herbs because use of these plants goes back to earliest times, and they still play a role in modern medicine. This section lists a number of historical works on medicine, particularly plant medicine. Also included are histories of botany and early herbals, accounts of plant hunters and their expeditions, and biographies of botanists and herbalists. An unusual title is the Pharmaceutical Society of Great Britain's *Historical Collection of Sixteen Picture Postcards.* An outstanding feature of most of the historical books is the illustrated material. Pictures reproduced from ancient herbals reveal a great deal about the culture and society of early times as well as about medicines.

Most of the books in this section are of high quality.

* * * * *

64.   Ackerknecht, Erwin H. **Therapeutics from the Primitives to the 20th Century. With an Appendix: History of Dietetics.** New York: Hafner Press, 1973. 194p. bibliog. index. $12.50. LC 72-88252. ISBN 02-840060-7.

This is a translation of a German work first published in 1970. The author is a noted medical historian. The "therapeutics" mentioned in the title refers primarily to therapeutics in internal diseases, especially pharmacotherapy. Quackery and secret remedies are included in the discussion. Also a special appendix on the history of diet in health and disease has been included.

Chapter headings are as follows: 1) Primitive Therapeutics; 2) Egyptian Therapeutics; 3) Hippocratic Therapeutics; 4) From the Alexandrians to Dioskorides; 5) Galen and Theriac; 6) Middle Ages; 7) Renaissance; 8) Therapeutics in the Seventeenth Century; 9) Therapeutics in the Eighteenth Century; 10) Therapeutics at the Beginning of the Nineteenth Century: Traditionalism, Skepticism, Physiologism; 11) Middle of the Nineteenth Century: The Acme of the Chaos, Sects, Errors of Pharmacology, Synthetic Drugs; 12) End of the Nineteenth Century: The Breakthrough to Modern Therapeutics by Way of Serum Therapy: Psychotherapeutic and Psychosomatic Endeavors; 13) Twentieth Century: Chemotherapy, Antibiotics, Hormones, Vitamins, Psychopharmacology, Iatrogenic Diseases; 14) Final Discussion.

In the final discussion, the author remarks that certain fashions in treatment are to a large extent developed under the pressure of the patients. Patients have a strange inclination toward "magic procedures," or they interpret scientific procedures as magic. The irrational is often psychologically more satisfying than the rational. History also shows the patient and the physician as willing victims of propaganda.

The book is of high quality.

65.　　Anderson, Frank J. **An Illustrated History of the Herbals.** New York: Columbia University Press, 1977. 270p. illus. bibliog. index. $21.20. LC 77-8821. ISBN 0-231-04002-4.

The author of this work writes that herbals are the most fascinating of books, but also among the least familiar to the layperson. He believes this is because they are rare and, in the past, were usually written in Latin or medieval German, French, or English. He has prepared this book as a partial remedy to that situation. The book presents chapters on 30 major classical works, most of which can be found in the Library of the New York Botanical Garden, where Anderson is Honorary Curator of Rare Books and Manuscripts. The herbals date from the first to the sixteenth century. The special character of each is emphasized, and biographical notes about the authors, along with bibliographic material about publishers, illustrators, printers, and editions, are included. Botany, medicinal uses, and early printing are all considered. In addition, the book includes a number of stories of old legends. Over 100 woodcuts are included to show how the herbals are illustrated.

The author notes that herbals are not only useful in the study of medicine and botany, but also in the history of printing, philology, social history, and folklore. "They present a close-up view of the manners and beliefs of the classical and medieval worlds" and show the change from the "era of empiricism and superstition to the era of science."

66.　　Arber, Agnes. **Herbals: their Origin and Evolution; a Chapter in the History of Botany 1470-1670.** 2d ed. rewritten and enlarged. London: Cambridge University Press, 1938; repr. New York, Hafner, 1970. 326p. illus. bibliog. index. $12.95.

The purpose of this work is to "trace in outline the evolution of the 'printed herbal' in Europe between the years 1470 and 1670." The botanical and artistic areas are the main areas covered; the medical and gardening literature has been generally excluded. Information used in the work was taken mainly from the herbals themselves, although some was obtained from the historical and critical literature of the time. Most illustrations are photographic reproductions of the originals; most sources were found in the Printed Books Department of the British Museum.

The book starts with a short chapter covering the pre-1470 history of botany, followed by a chapter on the earliest printed herbals in the fifteenth century as a result of the invention of printing. The next two chapters deal with the early history of herbals in various geographical locations, the origin of herberia, and the revival of Aristotelian Botany. Also included are chapters on the evolution of the art of plant description, classification, and illustration, and on the doctrine of signatures and astrological botany. Appendix I is a bibliography of the principal herbals and botanical works published between 1470 and 1670; Appendix II is a list of the historical and critical references used by the author; Appendix III is a subject index to the works in Appendix II. The "Index" covers text, plates, figures, and the entries in Appendix I.

67.　　Blanton, Wyndham B. **Medicine in Virginia in the Eighteenth Century.** Richmond, VA: Garrett and Massie, Inc., 1931; repr. New York, AMS Press, 1976. 449p. illus. bibliog. index. $64.50. LC 80-12669. ISBN 0-404-13238-3.

The first chapter of this scholarly work says that medicine in America in the eighteenth century was not greatly different from that of the preceding century. Doctors born and educated in England dominated the profession and, at the same time, quacks were more numerous. The latter years of the century witnessed the rise of American medicine.

The book provides rather complete coverage of the field, and several chapters cover topics of concern in this bibliography. Contents is as follows: 1) The eighteenth century; 2) The three arts; 3) The handmaids of medicine (pharmacy, dentistry, nursing); 4) Epidemic diseases; 5) Medical education; 6) Reading and writing; 7) Botany and medicine; 8) Plantation medicine; 9) Lay contributors to medicine; 10) Advertising and quackery; 11) Men of mark; 12) Doctors of the colonial wars; 13) Revolutionary medicine; 14) Hospitals; 15) Washington's physicians, diseases and death; 16) Town and town doctors; 17) Country doctors; and 18) Medical legislation.

Nostrums and cure-alls caught the popular imagination to an astonishing extent during the eighteenth century. The book contains tales of legislative bodies purchasing recipes for remedies such as Seneca Rattle Snake Root and a concoction for bladder stones which proved to be a mixture containing egg shells, garden snails, soap, burdock seeds, hips, and haws.

68.   Brockbank, William. **Ancient Therapeutic Arts: The Fitzpatrick Lectures Delivered in 1950 & 1951 at the Royal College of Physicians.** Springfield, IL: Charles C. Thomas, 1954. 162p. illus. bibliog. $5.00.

This work discusses several now unconventional medical remedies and treatments that for centuries played a major rule in medicine. The main methods covered are the ancient arts of enema administration, cupping and leeching, counterirritation, and the less ancient art of intravenous injection of drugs. The book is a scholarly presentation on the history of medicine, and the therapeutic arts discussed are not, for the most part, appropriate for use today, at least not on a regular "do-it-yourself" basis.

69.   Budge, E. A. Wallis. **The Divine Origin of the Craft of the Herbalist.** London: Culpeper House by the Society of Herbalists, 1928; repr. Detroit: Gale Research Co., 1971. 96p. illus. index. $12.00. LC 17013. ISBN 0-8103-3794-0.

The author of this work, once keeper of Egyptian and Assyrian antiquities in the British Museum, wrote the book from the point of view of the archeologist and describes briefly the attributes and works of the earliest gods of medicine in Mesopotamia and Egypt. He also shows how the Sumarian, Egyptian, Babylonian and Assyrian herbals formed the foundation of the Greek herbals and how these were in turn translated into Syriac and Arabic and became known throughout Western Asia. Because of the Nestorian missionary doctors, the herbals also became known in Turkestan and China. The book is illustrated with photographs made from manuscripts in the British Museum.

Chapter headings are: 1) The Old Gods as Herbalists and Their Divine Medicines; 2) The Divine Herbalists; 3) Water a Divine Element; 4) Vegetable Substances of Divine Origin; 5) Ancient Egyptian Herbals and Books of Medicine; 6) Holy Oils and Medicated Unguents, 7) Sumerian and Assyrian Herbals, 8) The Greek Herbals; 9) The Latin Herbals; 10) The Herbal in Syriac, 11) The Herbal in Arabic, 12) Coptic Lists of Plants; and 13) The Ethiopian (Abyssinian) Herbal.

70.   Dodge, Bertha S. **It Started in Eden: How the Plant-Hunters and the Plants They Found Changed the Course of History.** New York: McGraw-Hill Book Co., 1979. 288p. bibliog. index. $10.95. LC 79-15049. ISBN 0-07-017290-0.

Plants and their products have pervaded all aspects of our increasingly complex human existence. This book is a popular account of explorers, plant-hunters, and botanists, along with plants, that have played a crucial role in world history.

The first chapter, "The Staff of Life," discusses wheat, rye, corn, potatoes, and breadfruit. Chapter 2, "The Spice of Life," covers the history of the spice trade. The next chapter tells the story of tea, coffee, and chocolate. Chapter 4, "Plant

Enemies," tells of various blights, diseases, and insects that have attacked crops. "Plants on the People's Side" is on medicinal plants such as those yielding quinine, chaulmoogra oil, and curare. The last chapter, "Plants Divine and Otherwise," covers the history and use of coca and opium.

The author concludes that all kinds of people--the adventurous, the greedy, the ambitious, the imaginative, the self-seeking, and the self-sacrificing--have, by exploiting plant virtues, determined their own future and the course of world history. A plea is made for protection of endangered plant species.

71.   Dodge, Bertha S. **Plants that Changed the World.** Illustrated by Henry B. Kane. Boston, MA: Little, Brown and Co., 1959. 183p. illus. bibliog. index. LC 59-5279.

At the time this book was written more attention was being given to synthetic chemicals and drugs than to those from plant sources, although in many cases laboratory workers did little more than copy plant materials. The fact that chemists sometimes managed to improve upon natural products does not lessen the importance of plants or their collectors, the author says. Her book is an attempt to describe a number of plant products that have helped make history. Focus is on adventurous individuals who sought the plants in remote parts of the world as well as on the plants themselves.

Contents of the book is as follows: 1) Lilacs and lilies (about medicinal plants); 2) Joseph Banks and the breadfruit; 3) Food for the gods (cacao or cocoa beans); 4) The fever bark tree (chinchona, the source of quinine); 5) Kalows and kings (about chaulmoogra oil for leprosy); 6) The weeping tree (rubber tree); 7) Enough rope (discusses plants used for rope making, including Cannabis sativa and the abacá plant); 8) The big leaf (wax-bearing plants); 9) Life from the flying death (curare); and 10) A look ahead.

The book is interesting and contains many anecdotes. The approach is somewhat elementary.

72.   Erichsen-Brown, Charlotte. **Use of Plants for the Past 500 Years.** Aurora, Ontario: Breezy Creeks Press (Box 104, Aurora, Ont., Canada, L4G 3H1), 1979. 510p. illus. bibliog. index. ISBN 0-9690007-3-1; 0-9690007-0-7pa.

This impressive, unique work is a record of man's use of plants, trees, and shrubs that grow in eastern North America. These plants supplied the various Indian peoples with food, fuel, fiber, clothing, shelter, utensils, transportation, and medicine. Many were slowly accepted by white settlers as medicinal and food plants.

An introductory essay presents an overall view of the subject and makes a plea for a return to the study of our native plants. The author feels the public is experimenting with dangerous drug plants with little knowledge about their properties. The specific purpose of the work is to list available sources of information about native plants, explore the earliest and the original materials, and to present the chronology of the recorded material in original form. The intended audience includes historians, ethnologists, botanists, archaeologists, pharmacists, and the interested public.

The bulk of the book is a listing of the plants divided into sections on evergreen trees, deciduous trees, shrubs and vines, plants found in wet open places, plants found in woods and thickets, and plants found in dry open places. In each section, plants used for the same purpose are grouped together. The plant monographs include common and Latin names, descriptions, range, and habitat. Then, as a unique feature, many well-chosen quotations from the literature regarding the plant are presented in chronological order. Early as well as recent sources have been used. In addition, line drawings are provided. Appended is a glossary and a long list of all sources quoted in the text. Most references are annotated.

73.   Fairchild, David. **Exploring for Plants.** From Notes of the Allison Vincent Armour Expeditions for the United States Department of Agriculture, 1925, 1926, and 1927. New York: Macmillan, 1930. 591p. illus.

The author of this older work has attempted to interest the layperson "with adventures that are not any of them hairbreadth escapes" and to give information about plants to botanists and horticulturists in a popular manner. He hopes he can at least "convert a single person to the romantic life a deep study of plants can give." Collections of plants gathered on the described expeditions were to be used for improving American agriculture.

The book describes explorations for plants in a great many exotic places in the world. These include: Panama, Sweden, Great Britain, Holland, Belgium, France, Switzerland, Algeria, Morocco, island of Palma, island of Grand Canary, Balearic Islands, Italy, Ceylon, Sumatra, Java, Singapore, West Africa, French Guinea, Liberia, Camaroons, Gold Coast, Spain, and Portugal.

The book is illustrated with photographs of plants and scenes from the various areas. It is quite nicely done.

74.   Goodspeed, T. Harper. **Plant Hunters in the Andes.** New York: Farrar and Rinehart, Inc., 1941. 429p. illus. index.

The work is an account of the author's search for little-known plants in the high ranges of the Andes in Peru and Chile. Of particular interest to Goodspeed were South American relatives of the tobacco plant. Goodspeed's wife and eight other botanists and assistants accompanied him on two expeditions, one in 1935-36 and another in 1938-39.

The book is a detailed, personal account of travel by boat, train, airplane, automobile, horseback, and on foot. Expedition members experienced such difficulties as shipwreck, rockslides, and earthquakes. Landscapes, peoples, and customs are discussed as well as vegetation of areas covered. The book is illustrated with a large number of photographs, including plant species rarely seen and scenes of the locale.

75.   Haughton, Claire Shaver. **Green Immigrants: The Plants that Transformed America.** Drawings by Russell Peterson. New York: Harcourt Brace Jovanovich, 1978. 450p. illus. index. $12.95. LC 78-53870. ISBN 0-15-137034-6.

The preface of this book says that most plants of the United States, cultivated flowers, vegetables, fruits, grains, grasses, and clovers, and nearly 70 percent of weeds, have come from other nations. This book relates the history and romance, the legend and folklore, of about 100 plants, many of them herbs and medicinal plants, that are "immigrants."

Chapters are arranged alphabetically by name of the plant discussed. Each discussion runs several pages. Among the plants included are asparagus, eucalyptus, foxglove, plantain, quince, rhubarb, tansy, watercress, and yarrow. The treatment is light and entertaining.

76.   Hawks, Ellison, and G. S. Boulger. **Pioneers of Plant Study.** New York: Macmillan, 1928; repr. (facs. ed.). New York: Arno, 1975. 288p. illus. index. (Essay Index Reprint Series). $17.00. LC 75-86759. ISBN 0-8369-1139-3.

Although the preface to this work says it makes no attempt to be a complete history of plant study, a good deal is covered, although as is said in an episodic fashion, down to the nineteenth century. The book shows that the earliest studies of plants were economic or medical. The culture of plants for their own sake was a later development and was largely brought about by ordinary people, rather than by scholars, because they loved plants and needed them. Illustrations in the book are portraits of men whose biographies are presented.

Chapter headings are: 1) In Explanation of Technical Terms; 2) Plants of Ancient Egypt; 3) Plants of Assyria and China; 4) Plants of the Old Testament and the Wisdom of Solomon; 5) Phœnician Commerce and Greek Myth; 6) Plants of Homer; 7) The Father of Medicine and the Early Greek Philosophers; 8) Father of Natural History and His Favourite Pupils; 9) Greek scholars at Alexandria; 10) Pliny, the Encyclopaedist of the First Century; 11) A Choice Manuscript of a Little-known Physician; 12) Arab Physicians and Merchants; 13) The School of Salerno; 14) From Charlemagne to Albertus Magnus; 15) Two Great Travellers; 16) The New World; 17) The Renaissance; 18) A Truculent Protestant; 19) First Investigators in India; 20) Conrad Gesner and the Bauhins; 21) The School of Montpellier and Flanders; 22) An Historic Printing House: Plantin and Clusius; 23) The Barber-Surgeon of Holborn and His Editor; 24) The First Systematist; 25) "Paradisi in Sole Paradisus Terrestris"; 26) The First Terminologist; 27) Some Early Days at the Royal Society; 28) John Ray; 29) Sir Hans Sloane and the Chelsea Physic Garden; 30) Sexes of Plants and Some Jacobite Botanists; 31) Some Early Physiological Experiments; 32) Linnaeus; 33) The Natural System in France; 34) Kew; 35) Physic: Farces and Feuds; 36) Robert Brown; and 37) Plant-collecting in the Tropics, Its Suggestions and Its Dangers.

77.   Kelly, Howard A. **Some American Medical Botanists Commemorated in our Botanical Nomenclature.** New York: D. Appleton and Co., 1914; repr. Kennebunkport, ME, Longwood, 1977. 215p. illus. $25.00. LC 77-3485. ISBN 0-89341-145-0.

A doctor who had a lifelong interest in botany has written in this book brief sketches of the lives of some of his forebears who made a contribution to medical botany.

In the introduction, Kelly mentions a large number of background publications, although no formal bibliography is provided. Then he presents biographical sketches on 30 individuals he considers outstanding medical botanists. Each botanist's works are discussed, and plants named for him are mentioned. A portrait is often included as well as pictures of the plants.

The sketches are interesting, although the writing seems a bit quaint and old-fashioned today, with many references to God and the Bible. The selection of biographees may seem curious to some because a number of them are well-known botanists in a general sense, not just medical; for instance, Asa Gray and John Torrey. Gray and Torrey held medical degrees, however, as was common with scientists of their day.

78.   Kreig, Margaret B. **Green Medicine: The Search for Plants that Heal....** Chicago, IL: Rand McNally and Co., 1964. 462p. illus. bibliog. index. LC 64-14403.

This book is perhaps the first to deal with the recent resurgence of interest in medicinal plants and herbs. In the early 1900s, about 80% of all medicines were obtained from roots, barks, and leaves of plants, and today nearly half continue to be derived from natural sources rather than made synthetically. (Not quite all natural products are derived from plants, however.) A great many potential drugs remain to be identified, and there is still a search for new plants that will yield valuable substances.

This book was written mainly for the scientist, but since the general public has become so interested in the subject, it has popular appeal. The author is a journalist who accompanied a scientific expedition to the Amazon and observed field botanists at work in remote areas of Mexico. The book is an account of these expeditions.

Chapters are divided into three sections: 1) Medicine scouts and their methods; 2) Biographies of botanicals; and 3) Frontiers of research. There are chapters on the history of quinine, digitalis, curare, chaulmoogra, sarsaparilla, and the wild Mexican yams. The following are treated in the section on research frontiers: periwinkles, rauwolfia, LSD, ololiuqui, mushrooms, and drugs from the sea.

The author acknowledges a great deal of cooperation and information from scientists and pharmaceutical producers. In addition, members of the American Society of Pharmacognosy reviewed the manuscript for technical accuracy.

Many photographs of noted researchers in the field are included in the book as well as accounts of their work. The book is well-done, and it has been well-received by the lay public and the scientific community.

79.   Kremers, Edward, and George Urdang. **Kremers and Urdang's History of Pharmacy.** 4th ed. revised by Glenn Sonnedecker. Philadelphia, PA: J. B. Lippincott Co., 1976. 571p. illus. bibliog. index. $28.50. LC 75-40104. ISBN 0-397-52074-3.

This classical work has traditionally been used as a textbook by pharmacy students and as a reference work in the history of pharmacy. The growth and development of pharmacy from ancient Egypt to the present in the United States is traced to form an integrated view of the subject. An important antecedent in the development of modern pharmacy was the early use by man of natural resources as "drugs" to fend off disease. In addition, "supernatural" countermeasures were needed. The book considers these matters in the early chapters.

The work is in four parts: 1) Pharmacy's early antecedents; 2) The rise of professional pharmacy in representative countries of Europe; 3) Pharmacy in the United States; and 4) Discoveries and other contributions to society by pharmacists.

A number of sections are of particular interest to users of this bibliography. They include a discussion of Babylonian, Assyrian, Egyptian, Greek, and Roman contributions to medicine. Early literature is covered in these sections. The evolution of plant drugs to chemical drugs is taken up. There is a section on the search of the flora of the New World for aromatics, spices, and medicinal plants. Important ones discovered include curare, tobacco, coca, and cinchona. Homeopathy is discussed as are the Thomsonians and the Eclectics.

There is an excellent appended section on early pharmaceutical literature with references to herbals, pharmacopeias, formularies, and other materials. In addition, there is a glossary and a list of representative drugs of the American Indians. Illustrations are well selected and include photographs of works of art dating back several centuries.

80.   Leake, Chauncey D. **The Old Egyptian Medical Papyri.** Lawrence, KS: University of Kansas Press, 1952. bibliog. index. (Logan Clendening Lectures on the History and Philosophy of Medicine. Second Series.).

Ancient Egyptian medical practice can be satisfactorily reconstructed from an analysis of available sources. These are mainly eight papyri known as the Kahun, the Edwin Smith, the Ebers, the Hearst, the Erman, the London, the Berlin, and the Chester Beatty. These documents have been analyzed by Egyptologists and medical historians.

This small book presents some high points regarding the papyri in the following chapters: 1) The Chief Egyptian Medical Papyri; 2) Old Egyptian Weights and Measures; 3) Drug Measurement in the Old Egyptian Medical Papyri; 4) Ancient

Egyptian Therapeutics; 5) The Hearst Medical Papyrus; 6) Organization of the Hearst Medical Papyrus; 7) Diseases in the Hearst Medical Papyrus; 8) The Ingredients of the Hearst Papyrus Prescriptions; and 9) Summary. There is also an appendix which lists prescriptions in the Hearst medical papyrus.

The chapter on ingredients of papyrus prescriptions is particularly interesting. Most have been identified; of 200 separate materials only eight were without some sort of identification at the time this book was written. About half the ingredients of the prescriptions are of plant origin. About half of these have been satisfactorily identified. The remainder are known to be of plant origin and to refer to some part of a plant, such as seeds, leaves, or fruit. The most widely used of plant ingredients in the papyrus is the gourd, but it is not clear whether reference is made to the ordinary edible gourd or to the bitter gourd (colocynth). Also, references are frequently made to acacia, anise, coreander, cumin, barley, beans, peas, wheat, figs, garlic, leek, juniper berries, castor plant petals, dates, opium poppy, frankincense, gum, and myrrh. Materials from mineral and animal sources comprise some ingredients. "Dragon's blood" has never been satisfactorily classified.

The summary chapter points out that the relatively high character of medical knowledge possessed by the old Egyptian physicians is astonishing, particularly when contrasted with the superstitious attitude about sickness on the part of the people. Leake, who was a noted pharmacologist and physiologist, says this dichotomy between the rational, empirical, and scientific approach to disease by professional physicians, and the anxiously confused, irrational and superstitious attitude about disease on the part of the people generally, persists in civilized countries still. Two factors are chiefly responsible for the popular attitude: 1) the tendency for sick people to improve regardless of treatment; and 2) the fallacy of confusing mere sequence of events with a supposed cause-effect relationship. These factors promote magic, quackery, and cultism in medical matters. Achievements of physicians and attitudes of people should be differentiated clearly.

81.   Le Strange, Richard. **A History of Herbal Plants**. Illustrated by Derek Cork; Foreword by Anthony Huxley. New York: Arco Publishing Co., 1977. 304p. illus. bibliog. index. $15.00. LC 77-3360. ISBN 0-668-04247-8.

After an introductory section on the general history of herbal plants, this book presents under the heading "Botanical Notes" a historical survey of about 750 plants used by man through the ages. Most plants are illustrated with a good line drawing, made from life.

For each plant there is a monograph of about a column in length, arranged alphabetically by common name. The following information is usually provided for each herb: scientific name, other common names, and a well-written paragraph which includes a description, habitat, historical uses, and modern uses (if any). Various species of the same genus are often compared. Emphasis is on history. The book also contains a section of cultivation notes for those who wish to grow herbs, and a glossary of medicinal terms is provided. The index gives botanical and vernacular names.

The book is outstanding in many respects, but notably for "the sorting out of real medicinal values from imagined ones which have accrued over centuries of witchcraft, folk use, and through the 'doctrine of signatures', whereby the resemblance of a plant to a part of the body decreed its medical potential, often with no real basis" (from the foreword). In addition, the author states, "Today it is more for enjoyment than for any practical use that most of us care for the flowers, shrubs and trees growing wild about us."

82.   Mathison, Richard R. **The Eternal Search: The Story of Man and His Drugs.**
New York: G. P. Putnam's Sons, 1958. 381p. illus. bibliog. index. LC 58-8060.

Quackeries, gossip, old wives' tales, myths, superstition, witchcraft, and the
lore of medicine are covered in this book as well as some valid cures. This work is an
anecdotal history and survey of drugs and medicines through the ages. It is arranged
by drug categories or ailments rather than chronologically.

Following is a synopsis of what the chapters cover: 1) Witches, sorcerers, and
magic; 2) The search for everlasting truth; 3) Drug plants; 4) The role of metals in
healing; 5) The alchemists; 6) Drugs of animal origin; 7) The use of human parts as
medicine; 8) Food; 9) Poisoning; 10) Midwifery and early gynecology; 11) Cleanliness
practices; 12) Pain relievers; 13) Plagues and pestilences; 14) Syphilis; 15) Purging;
16) Love potions; 17) Feuds, debates and battles over drugs; 18) Patent medicines;
19) Medicine shows; 20) Cosmetics; 21) Embalming and death rites; 22) Narcotics and
other drugs of abuse; 23) Insanity and hallucinations; and 24) The future of pharmacy.

The book was written by a journalist in entertaining fashion, although some
of the tales are revolting and many remedies are stupid and cruel. The purpose of the
work, according to the preface, is to warn against the dangers of self-satisfaction and
dogmatism. We shall, the author thinks, seem as superstitious and strange to generations to come as earlier generations seem to us.

83.   Maxwell, Nicole. **Witch Doctor's Apprentice.** Rev. ed. New York: Collier
Books (a division of Macmillan Publishing Co.), 1975. 406p. illus. $3.95pa. LC 74-
18120. ISBN 0-02-096020-4.

The author of this work, an anthropologist and ethnologist, is a Research
Associate of the Museum of the American Indian and a Fellow of the Royal Geographic
Society of London. She explored the Amazon River basin for a number of years, made
friends with native tribes, and searched for medicinal plants of value. This book is an
interesting personal account of a trip she made alone in 1958, financed by a pharmaceutical company, to gather more data on the drug plants.

She compiled notes on hundreds of plants used in Amazonia, although she
admits that only a small percentage would ever be worth developing. Some would be
too toxic, and some would accomplish about the same results as other drugs in common
use. The others, she thinks, should be developed. There is one that stops bleeding, one
that dissolves kidney stones, one that cures skin diseases, one for burns, and one contraceptive.

The author is disappointed that those who do medicinal drug research did not
follow up on more of her findings, particularly on the contraceptive plant that seems
so needed because of today's overpopulation problem.

84.   Mességué, Maurice. **Of Men and Plants: The Autobiography of the World's
Most Famous Plant Healer.** New York: Macmillan, 1973. 327p. $6.95. LC 72-81079.
(First published in Paris in 1970 by Éditions Robert Laffont under the title **Des Hom-
mes et des Plantes**).

This autobiographical account of a plant healer begins with the story of how
Mességué, reared in a remote French village, learned plant lore from his father, knowledge which had been handed down for several generations. Mességué later made up a
pharmacopoeia of his remedies, and the book contains an appendix of his basic preparations for the principal chronic diseases.

The story is told how the author met the actress Mistinguett, beloved of actor
Maurice Chevalier. She had been suffering from rheumatism. Mességué's treatment
cured her, the account goes, and she introduced him to other celebrities. He treated

Ali Khan, King Farouk, the cardinal who was to become Pope John XXIII, Utrillo, Cocteau, and others of fame. The book is full of interesting anecdotes, but scattered through it is information about herbal products Mességué used and how he applied them.

The author apparently has been respected in Europe as an herb doctor. The book was a best seller there. It is an interesting tale, although many remedies are not entirely believable.

85. Pachter, Henry M. **Paracelsus: Magic into Science.** New York: Henry Schuman, 1951. 360p. illus. bibliog. index. (A reprinted edition of 1979 with the title **Magic into Science: The Story of Paracelsus** is available from Arden Library, Darby, PA: $30.00. ISBN 0-8495-4335-5).

Paracelsus, a famous Swiss physician and chemist (1493-1541), was one of the controversial characters of the Renaissance. This book is a biography and account of his work. He reportedly delved deeply into alchemy, cured patients ordinary doctors had abandoned for doomed, and knew about wonderful elixirs that could restore youth. More realistically, Paracelsus was highly learned, pious, a professor of theology, and a defender of liberty. He promoted the use of specific remedies and was the author of many medical and occult works.

This book is a well-documented account of Paracelsus' ideas and life. His significance was apparent to contempraries who identified him with the legendary Dr. Faustus, the symbol of man's striving to know the unknowable without the help of a diety. The conclusion of the book remarks that he has been remembered more for his fight against orthodoxy than for his achievements. "Whenever science seemed to have become estranged from nature and medicine disappointed the people, his name as a great healer and friend of the common man re-emerged out of the undercurrents of folk memory," the author states.

86. Pharmaceutical Society of Great Britain. **Historical Collection of the Pharmaceutical Society of Great Britain: Sixteen Picture Postcards.** London: Jarrold and Sons, 1975. 11p.; 16 cards. illus. (col.). bibliog.

The subjects pictured on this set of 16 handsome postcards are from the Pharmaceutical Society of Great Britain's historical collection, which includes many early works on botany, materia medica, and pharmacy. An accompanying pamphet provides notes on the pictures.

Cards 1-4 have illustrations from *Ortus Sanitatas* (1491) that include male and female mandrake, an apothecary compounding theriac, the frontispiece to *Tractatus de Animalibus,* and the frontispiece to *Tabula Super Tractatu de Herbis.* Cards 5-8 depict English Delftware drug jars (1650-1725). Card 9 shows an apothecary's tile, English Delftware (1670). Card 10 shows Italian Maiolica drug jars (sixteenth and seventeenth centuries). Card 11 shows a bell-metal mortar of Charles Angibaud, apothecary to Louis XIV (1678); card 12 pictures lignum vitae mortars and pestles (English, eighteenth century). Cards 13-16 have botanical illustrations from J. J. Plenck's *Icones Plantarum Medicinalium* (Vienna 1788-94). The hand-colored copper engravings are of *Piper Nigrum L.*, *Atropa belladonna L.*, *Rheum palmatum L.*, and *Theobroma cacao L.*

87. Rohde, Eleanour Sinclair. **The Old English Herbals.** London: Longmans, 1922; repr. New York: Dover, 1971. 243p. illus. bibliog. index. $3.00 pa. LC 75-166433. ISBN 0-486-21106-1.

This work, as the title suggests, is a history of old English herbals. They are covered from the eighth through the seventeenth century. Included are: Anglo-Saxon herbals; later manuscript herbals and the early printed herbals; Turner's herbal and the influence of the foreign herbalists; Gerard's herbal; herbals of the New World; John Parkinson, the last of the great English herbalists; and later seventeenth century herbals and sixteenth and seventeenth century still-room books. The comprehensive bibliography includes over 430 descriptive entries. It is divided into three sections: English manuscript herbals, English herbals (printed books), and major foreign herbals which have something to do with the history of herbals in England. In regard to the latter list, copies in American libraries are noted.

There is little mention made in the text of specific uses of plants. The emphasis is on descriptions of herbals mentioned.

88.   Simons, Corinne Miller. **John Uri Lloyd, His Life and His Works, 1849-1936; with a History of the Lloyd Library.** Cincinnati, OH: privately printed by the author, 1972. 337p. illus.

The author of this biographical work was librarian for many years at the Lloyd Library in Cincinnati, an important institution founded by John Uri Lloyd and his brothers. The library houses a large collection of reference works of particular value to research workers interested in medicinal agents in plants and to those interested in rare old publications in the field. An attempt has been made to acquire all materials on the subject of plant medicines for the library.

The biographee was one of the three Lloyd Brothers who founded the pharmaceutical manufacturing firm which bore their name. The book tells in glowing terms of Lloyd's life and accomplishments that included, in addition to his business activities with the company, scientific research and writings in plant medicine and chemistry, inventions, philanthropy, travel, and literary writings. The latter include folklore material, about 60 short stories, and eight novels. The novels all became best sellers, and his fantasy novel, *Etidorpha*, is still in print.

89.   Singer, Charles. **From Magic to Science: Essays on the Scientific Twilight.** London: Ernest Benn Ltd., 1928; repr. New York: Dover, 1959. 253p. illus. (part col.). bibliog. index.

The process by which a rational conception of the world gradually comes to possess the mind is addressed in this work by a noted science historian. The record we have of this rationalization of thought which affects our whole civilization is found in the documents which display the passage of medieval thought into the modern way of thinking. The book is a collection of essays dealing with the early steps in the process and covers until about the twelfth century.

Following are chapter headings: 1) Sciences under the Roman Empire; 2) The Dark Ages and the Dawn of Science; 3) The Lorica of Gildas the Briton; 4) Early English Magic and Medicine; 5) Early Herbals; 6) The Visions of Hildegard of Bingen; and 7) The School of Salerno and Its Legends.

The essay on herbals is of particular interest. Singer studied many surviving manuscripts and his view was that the history of the herbal is continuous from Greek to modern times. He found herbals of great value in his study of folklore because their texts are simple, their ideas comprehensible, their motives obvious, and the tradition of their illustrations can easily be traced. In addition, the entry and recession of the magical element can be closely watched in the herbals, Singer maintains. At the time this book was written, herbal medicine and folklore had been little studied, and the author felt it was an interesting area for exploration.

The very fine illustrations included in the book are from classical books and manuscripts of the past, and most are beautiful.

90.   Spruce, Richard. **Notes of a Botanist on the Amazon and Andes.** Edited and condensed by Alfred Russell Wallace. London: Macmillan, 1908; repr. New York and London: Johnson Reprint Corp., 1970. 2v. illus. bibliog. index. (Landmarks in Anthropology; a series of reprints in cultural anthropology). $61.50. LC 78-117251.

Spruce (1817-1893) was a botanist who spent much of his life exploring plants of the New World tropics. This work was produced after his death from his notes, diaries, and letters. First printed in 1908, the work was almost a collector's item before this reprint was published.

Spruce's notes contained references, descriptions, discussions, and theories concerning the plants and vegetation he studied. Also included is material about the geological, ahthropological, linguistic, historical, sociological, and zoological aspects of the regions he explored. Many plants Spruce investigated played important roles in the lives of the natives. He gave special attention to narcotics and stimulants such as aya-huasca, caapi, coca, guaraná, guayusa, and niopo. He also commented on the use the Indians made of plants in pottery, ropes, bark objects, and blowguns, and in agricultural practices and witchcraft. An important contribution he made was in his study of the rubber-yielding plant *Hevea*. Since much of Spruce's work was done before the field camera was used, the book's illustrations include his pencil sketches, very nicely done, of plants, people, and scenes. A glossary of native names is included as are several maps of the areas he visited.

91.   Whittle, Tyler. **The Plant Hunters: Being an Examination of Collecting with an Account of the Careers and the Methods of a Number of Those Who have Searched the World for Wild Plants.** Philadelphia, PA: Chilton Book Co., 1970. 281p. illus. bibliog. index. $8.95. LC 77-104717. SBN 8019-5472-X.

Lively stories of the exploits of some of the great plant explorers are presented in this accurate and well-written work. Accounts are necessarily brief because a comprehensive history would have to be voluminous. The book covers early explorations to modern times, and the gradual development of the methods modern botanists use are related.

The introductory section on the powers of plants emphasizes important economic plants. The author concludes the section stating that not all plant hunting has been successful and that the pursuit of plants was never an easy or comfortable undertaking. Part 1, "Collecting in the Pre-Wardian Days from 1482 B.C.," covers old civilizations, the Dark and Middle Ages; the Renaissance; English collectors of the Orangery Era; the golden age of botany; Kew and Cathay; and David Douglas of Scone. Part 2, on the techniques of collecting, contains a chapter on fieldwork and one on Nathaniel Ward of Wellclose Square. Ward invented the first portable greenhouse about 1827. Part 3, called a "Scramble for Green Treasure," covers the following topics: from Mexico to Patagonia, in India and Africa, the Eastern tropics, the Land of the Rising Sun, and Post-Wardian China. Part 4, "The Edge of the World," presents these chapters: 1) The Mecca for Botanical Explorers; 2) A Revolution in Western Gardening; 3) Private Travelers, Consular Officials, Honored Commissioners and Military Plant Hunters; 4) Archetype of Missionary-Botanists; 5) Some Changes in the Mode of Plant Hunting; 6) Doyen of Modern Collectors; 7) An Economic Botanist; 8) The Professor of Chinese and Botany; 9) The Prince of Alpine Gardeners; and 10) South of the Cloud. There are appendices on plant distribution, plant names, and plant collecting.

92.   Wootton, A. C. **Chronicles of Pharmacy.** London: Macmillan, 1910; repr. Boston, MA: Milford House, Inc. for USV Pharmaceutical Corp., 1972. 2v. illus. index. LC 72-77662.

This work was difficult to obtain until a special facsimile edition was made available by the USV Pharmaceutical Corporation. The preface identifies pharmacy as the art of selecting, extracting, preparing, and compounding medicines from vegetable, animal, and mineral substances. Pharmacy is said to be almost as ancient as man. The author's view is that the manipulation of drugs has through the ages been "associated with magic, with theology, with alchemy, with crimes and conscious frauds, with the strangest fancies, and dogmas, and delusions, and with the severest science." He further states that "deities, kings, and quacks, philosophers, priests, and poisoners, dreamers, seers, and scientific chemists have all helped to build the fabric of pharmacy." Their work is sketched in the chronicles presented in this fascinating work. In addition, formulas and directions for making old medicines are provided.

Chapter titles are: 1) Myths of Pharmacy; 2) Pharmacy in the Time of the Pharaohs; 3) Pharmacy in the Bible; 4) The Pharmacy of Hippocrates; 5) From Hippocrates to Galen; 6) Arab Pharmacy; 7) From the Arabs to the Europeans; 8) Pharmacy in Great Britain; 9) Magic and Medicine; 10) Dogmas and Delusions; 11) Masters in Pharmacy; 12) Royal and Noble Pharmacists; 13) Chemical Contributions to Pharmacy; 14) Medicines from the Metals; 15) Animals in Pharmacy; 16) Reminiscences of Ancient Pharmacy; 17) Pharmacopoeias; 18) Shakespeare's Pharmacy; 19) Some Noted Drugs; 20) Familiar Medicines and Some Notes of Their Histories; 21) Noted Nostrums; 22) Poisons in History; 23) Pharmacy in the Nineteenth Century; and 24) Names and Symbols.

The last chapter is a useful glossary of technical terms limited to names of pharmaceutical processes, products, and applications. Many of the terms were obsolete even in 1910, but they have been included because they are found in old treatises. Apothecaries' weights and measures signs are defined.

4

PERIODICALS

Because many popular periodicals concerning "health" foods, herbs, and unconventional systems of medicine are produced by small, little-known publishers, it was difficult to obtain review issues of some of them. However, a representative sample of such publications is included in the list below. Some of the magazines look like patent medicine promotional materials of yesteryear, but others are more objective in approach, and some scientific.

Included are publications for the lay public interested in herbs and herb growing and in "health" food and the health food business, vegetarians, and proponents of holistic and other types of unconventional medicine.

There are several good research-level scientific periodicals in existence. Titles in this category include: *Economic Botany, Journal of Ethnopharmacology, Journal of Natural Products, Phytochemistry, Planta Medica,* and *Qualitas Plantarum.* The *FDA Consumer* presents reliable information for the public on such matters as "health" foods and quick "cures."

* * * * *

93.   **American Society of Pharmacognosy News Letter.** Baltimore, MD: American Society of Pharmacognosy, 1963- . Irregular.

Members of the American Society of Pharmacognosy receive this publication. It contains the following sections: editorials, commentary, letters to the editor, meeting reports, articles, Society news, reviews of major review articles, descriptions of new equipment, and news and notes.

94.   **Bulletin of the Oriental Healing Arts Institute of U.S.A.** Los Angeles, CA: Oriental Healing Arts Institute of U.S.A. (8820 South Sepulveda Blvd., Suite 210, Los Angeles, CA 90045), 1976- . Bimonthly. $2.50 per copy.

This bulletin is said to be "dedicated to introducing and furthering research and understanding of the centuries-old Chinese traditional system of medicine." It publishes original articles and their English translations. Since much translated material already exists on acupuncture, the focus of the bulletin is primarily on herbal medicine. Recent issues have presented articles on Chinese herb treatment and hepatitis, cirrhosis, hypertension, obesity, and diabetes. An issue also included a study of drug resources and Chinese herbs in Taiwan.

95.   **Economic Botany.** Bronx, NY: Society for Economic Botany, 1947- . Quarterly.

This journal is "devoted to past, present, and future uses of plants by man." It specializes in scientific articles with emphasis on uses rather than on the growing of plants. Each issue has a section of book reviews and includes reports of annual meetings and other notices of the society. Articles on medicinal uses of plants are frequently published.

96.   **FDA Consumer.** Rockville, MD: U.S. Food and Drug Administration, 1967- . Monthly.

Formerly called *FDA Papers,* this is the official magazine of the U.S. Food and Drug Administration. It provides factual, reliable information for consumers on health, medicine, cosmetics, and foods. It helps put such matters as "natural" and "health" foods, patent medicines, anti-cancer drugs, vitamins, nutrition, and medical devices in perspective.

Each issue contains several articles; notices of legal actions, judgments, and seizures; and news. There is no advertising. The publication is valuable for health professionals as well as for the lay public.

97.   **Good Earth.** Melbourne, Australia: Organic Farming and Gardening Society (Box 2605 W, Melbourne, 3001, Victoria, Australia), 1947- . Quarterly.

Formerly called *Victorian Compost News,* this small publication contains articles of interest to those involved in organic farming and gardening. Included are articles on plants in general and some dealing specifically with organic farming, such as the use of fertilizers, herbicides, and pesticides. (Organic farmers use such materials, but only those that are not synthetic chemicals and which are presumed to have few "side effects.")

The publication contains advertising, book reviews, and official notices of the Society.

98.   **Health Food Trader.** Surrey, United Kingdom (Beaver House, York Close, Byfleet, Surrey KT14 7HN, United Kingdom), 1960- . Monthly.

This tabloid is distributed free to health food retailers in the United Kingdom and is available on subscription to others. It publishes news and views on the European health food market and provides information on new products, legislation, books, and personal views of members of the trade. Many advertisements are included, and a monthly guide to price changes in the health food trade is included.

99.   **Healthways: Magazine Digest.** Des Moines, IA: American Chiropractic Association, Inc., 1946- . Bimonthly.

Although issues contain fewer pages, this publication is similar to *Reader's Digest* in that a number of articles are reprinted or digested from material appearing in other publications. All articles are in some way concerned with health, particularly matters of chiropractic interest and "natural" foods, cosmetics, and healing. Advertising, book reviews, and illustrations are included.

100.   **Herb Grower Magazine.** Falls Village, CT: The Herb Grower (Falls Village, CT 06031), 1947- . Quarterly.

This small periodical, produced by a limited staff, is a delightful publication that does not recommend any medicinal uses for herbs. It is mainly for home growers of culinary herbs. The issues of about 28 pages usually contain several short articles, illustrations, recipes, readers' comments, and book reviews.

101.   **The Herb Quarterly.** Wilmington, VT: The Herb Quarterly (Box 576, Wilmington, VT 05363), 1979- . Quarterly.

New ideas and techniques in growing and using herbs are reported by amateur and professional botanists in this journal. Most aspects of the subject are covered, including history, folklore, recipes, and artistic use of pictures of herbs. There are attractive illustrations and a good deal of advertising. Special features include letters, book reviews, questions and answers, and a column about public herb gardens.

102.   **The Herbalist New Health.** Springfield, UT: Thornwood Communications, Inc. (1680 S. Main St., Springfield, UT 84663), 1976- . Monthly.

This publication has had a variety of subtitles during its existence. It covers a variety of topics related to herbs. History, medicinal uses, cookery, ethnic uses, herb growing, and folklore are all handled in a popular manner.

Each issue contains several articles and a number of features, including editorials, letters to the editor, news, and book reviews. Illustrations (many in color) are well done, and there are many advertisements. There have been several special issues, for example, a Christmas number. Cinema and TV stars have been featured with comments about their uses of herbs. The uses of herbs as food is dealt with more satisfactorily than herbs as medicine. Articles on unconventional treatments are frequently published.

103.   **The Herbarist.** Boston, MA: Herb Society of America, 1935- . Annual.

Each issue of this attractive publication contains some official information about the Herb Society of America, such as a list of officers, directors, and committee chairmen, and notes about the annual meeting. In addition, there are several articles, book reviews, illustrations, poetry, and advertisements. The material included is well chosen. The articles do not contain exaggerated claims regarding the value of herbs; the approach taken is sensible. The articles cover history, techniques of growing herbs, herbal gardens, folklore, recipes, and artistic use of the plants. The 1978 issue contained a list of herb nomenclature changes from *Hortus II*, 1941 edition, to *Hortus III*, 1976 edition (see entry 34).

104.   **Here's Health.** Surrey, United Kingdom (Beaver House, York Close, Byfleet, Surrey KT14 7HN, United Kingdom), 1956- . Monthly.

This publication covers virtually all aspects of living "naturally," including recipes and cookery ideas, natural treatments, beauty, gardening, ecology, exercise, and environmental subjects. Each issue usually contains several articles and features, advertisements, letters to the editor, book reviews, and a directory of health food stores (in the United Kingdom).

105.   **Holistic Health Review.** New York: Human Sciences Press (72 Fifth Ave., New York, NY 10011), 1977- . Quarterly.

The aim of this publication is to "increase awareness of perspectives in health care that address the whole individual, seen as a multidimensional and integrated being existing in relationship to the surrounding social, political, cultural and physical environment." It provides a forum for those who wish to discuss the concepts, methods, and social policy issues that emerge from the practices of the growing holistic health movement. Each issue usually contains an editorial, several articles, book reviews, and letters to the editors.

106.   **The Jewish Vegetarian.** London: Jewish Vegetarian Society (855 Finchley Rd., London NW11 8LX, England), 1965- . Quarterly.

This small publication contains short articles on vegetarianism, health, and "natural" remedies, news of the Society, travel topics, vegetarian recipes, book reviews, and advertisements (including the classified). Frequent references are made to Jewish teachings concerning vegetarianism and the vegetarian movement in Israel.

107.   **Journal of Ethnopharmacology: An Interdisciplinary Journal Devoted to Bioscientific Research on Indigenous Drugs.** Lausanne, Switzerland, Elsevier Sequoia S.A., 1979- . Quarterly.

This publication is primarily concerned with the investigation and description of the biological activities and the active substances of plants used in traditional medicines of past and present cultures. Many of these substances are drugs of abuse. Full-length papers describing original research, review articles, short communications describing limited investigations, and letters to the editor are published.

108.   **Journal of Natural Products (Lloydia).** Cincinnati, OH: American Society of Pharmacognosy and the Lloyd Library and Museum (917 Plum St., Cincinnati, OH 45202), 1938- . Bimonthly.

From 1938 to 1960, this journal was published by the Lloyd Library and Museum (a privately endowed library) and called *Lloydia*. In 1961 the American Society of Pharmacognosy joined with the library to produce a somewhat different publication. The title was changed to the present one in 1979, although the subtitle "Journal of Natural Products" was used for some years previously.

Early issues were devoted to the biological sciences, drug plants in particular. Frequently, bibliographies of old, rare works on drug plants, herbal medicine, and pharmacopoeias appeared. More recent issues include papers on all aspects of natural products research. The highly scientific contributions relate to the chemistry and biochemistry of naturally occurring compounds or the biology of living systems from which they are obtained. Some specific areas covered are: secondary metabolites of microorganisms (such as antibiotics and mycotoxins); physiologically active compounds from higher plants and animals; biochemical studies (such as biosyntheses); fermentation and plant tissue culture; the isolation, structure elucidation and chemical syntheses of new compounds from nature; and the pharmacology of compounds of natural origin. Each issue contains from 10 to 12 scientific papers, several "notes" (brief communications), and book reviews. Abstracts of the papers of the Society's meetings are included from time to time.

109.   **Journal of Research in Indian Medicine, Yoga and Homoeopathy.** New Delhi, India: Central Council for Research in Indian Medicine and Homoeopathy (Banaras Hindu University, Varanasi-5, India), 1966- . Quarterly.

The text of this periodical is printed in English, Hindi, and Sanskrit with summaries in English and Hindi. Each issue contains several scientific articles, most dealing with medicinal plants. Also included are short research communications and book reviews. The publication is indexed in *Biological Abstracts* and *Chemical Abstracts*.

110.   **Journal of the American Institute of Homeopathy.** Falls Church, VA: American Institute of Homeopathy (7297-H Lee Highway, Falls Church, VA 22042), 1907- . Quarterly.

Much material is this official publication of the American Institute of Homeopathy deals with organizational matters, such as meeting notices and reports, remarks of the president, and obituaries of members. However, the journal also publishes articles, book reviews, letters to the editor, and commentaries that are directed to the interests of those engaged in the practice of homeopathic medicine. Many of the articles report on herbal and folk remedies said to be valuable for various conditions.

111.   **Journal of the John Bastyr College of Naturopathic Medicine.** Seattle, WA: John Bastyr College of Naturopathic Medicine (518 1st Ave. North, Suite 28, Seattle, WA 98109), 1980- . 2 issues per year.

This journal publishes articles on "natural" health and the practice of "natural" medicine. Recent issues have included articles on yeast and health, clinical uses of ginseng, the nutritional value of sprouts, garlic as a therapeutic agent, yoga and the cardiovascular system, and the self-selection of diet by children.

112.   **Let's LIVE: America's Foremost Health and Preventive Medicine Magazine.** Los Angeles, CA (444 N. Larchmont Ave., Los Angeles, CA 90004), 1933- . Monthly.

Distributed through health and dietary food stores, this publication contains articles, book reviews, advertisements, letters to the editor, recipes, and columns regarding nutrition, diet, vitamins, minerals, exercise, disease, and miscellaneous matters of health. Materials published emphasize "health" foods. Lists of health food stores are included.

113.   **Mother Earth News.** Hendersonville, NC: Mother Earth News, Inc. (Box 70, 105 Stoney Mountain Drive, Hendersonville, NC 28739), 1970- . Bimonthly.

The emphasis of this periodical is on alternative lifestyles, ecology, and working with nature. Each issue contains 150 pages or more. Most issues feature a special subject, and include material of practical value. In addition to regular articles, the publication has a number of short ones, many advertisements, and letters to the editor.

Recent issues have covered such topics as hybrid electric cars; wild foods; "natural" home-produced first aid kits, perfumes, and herbal remedies; cheap energy; cultivating plants; and subsistence homesteading.

The publication has been popular. It is indexed in _Readers' Guide to Periodical Literature._

114.   **Natural Health Bulletin.** West Nyack, NY: Parker Publishing Co. (P. O. Box 14, West Nyack, NY 10994), 1970- . Biweekly.

This four-page newsletter reports recent research on health and presents brief paragraphs of advice, news, tips, and medical information. Recent issues have included reports on environmental lead; jogging; the importance of calcium; vitamin E; weight loss programs; pain relief without drugs; home beauty products; natural treatments and preventive measures; how to settle an upset stomach; and farmers and cancer.

The material seems authentic and reliable; exaggerated claims are not made.

115.   **Natural Life News.** Jarvis, Ontario, Canada: Natural Dynamics, Inc., 1976- . Quarterly.

This publication was formed by a combination of three publications, _Natural Life, Energy Efficient Homes,_ and _Natural Foods._ It is a 16-page tabloid said to be dedicated to presenting useful information "to enable readers to live a simple, healthier, more energy efficient and environmentally conscious wholistic life."

A recent issue presents material on "natural" foods such as soya products and yogurt. Recipes are included. Also included are appropriate news items; letters to the editor; material on solar and wood stove heating; greenhouses; health food retailer advice; book reviews; and many advertisements.

116.   **Phytochemistry: An International Journal of Plant Biochemistry.** Oxford: Pergamon Press, 1961- . Monthly.

The intention of this highly scientific journal is to cover all aspects of pure and applied plant biochemistry, especially those which elucidate factors underlying the growth, development, and differentiation of plants, and the chemistry of plant products.

The contents is grouped in sections as follows: biochemistry, biosynthesis, chemotaxonomy, phytochemistry, and short reports. An attempt is made to group together papers of like subjects. A substantial number of papers appear in each issue; issues often contain nearly 200 pages. Book reviews are included.

117.   **Planta Medica: Journal of Medicinal Plant Research.** Stuttgart, Hippokrates Verlag (Neckarstrasse 121, 7000 Stuttgart 1, Germany), 1953- . Monthly.

This research-level journal publishes original articles, short communications, and reviews that contribute to the following fields of medicinal plant research and application: phytochemistry and chemistry of natural products, pharmacognosy, plant biochemistry, biology of medicinal plants, and pharmacology. The editors prefer that manuscripts be submitted in English but will also accept German and French articles. If the article is not in English, titles and abstracts are provided in English.

Each issue typically contains 10 to 12 research articles, a few short communications, and perhaps one review article. Occasionally, the Journal publishes abstracts of papers of meetings such as the International Research Congress on Natural Products as Medicinal Agents. The Journal is the official organ of the Gesellschaft für Arzneipflanzenflorschung.

118.   **Prevention: The Magazine for Better Health.** Emmaus, PA: Rodale Press (33 E. Minor St., Emmaus, PA 18049), 1950- . Monthly.

This popular magazine is similar to *Reader's Digest* in format. The issues contain articles on vitamins, minerals, proper diet and nutrition, "natural" foods, and "natural" medicine. Emphasis is on prevention of disease, which presumably can be achieved by following suggestions in the publication. Recipes for special dishes and use of herbs are included in articles. There are many advertisements. Features include letters to the editor, a column of questions and answers on food and health, and even a column on healthy pets.

This is one of the leading periodicals in the "health food" field. It is indexed in the *Readers' Guide to Periodical Literature*.

119.   **The Provender: Newsletter of the Northwest Provender Alliance.** Seattle, WA: Northwest Provender Alliance (1505 10th Ave., Seattle, WA 98122), 1978- . Bimonthly.

This publication is the newsletter of an organization of natural food stores, cooperatives, distributors, and producers. The aim of the organization is to promote regional self-reliance and better communication within the "alternative food system" in the Northwest. In addition to news of the organization and the natural foods industry, there are advertisements, letters to the editor, classified advertisements, and short items of practical help to those in the natural foods business.

120.   **The Provoker.** St. Catharines, Ontario: The Provoker (L2R 7C9, St. Catharines, Ontario, Canada), v.18, 1978- . Bimonthly.

Each issue of this publication, which looks like a newsletter, presents a few short articles on "health" foods and other "natural" remedies. There are sections on new books (with brief annotations), menus, recipes, letters to the editor, and many advertisements for books and products in the field.

The appeal is popular; no real results of research are reported. The letters published frequently are personal testimonials to the efficacy of some "natural" remedy. The following letter is typical: "Keep fighting your battle against quackery which hides under the guise of science, big business, government, medical associations, etc. The light of the world can't be hidden."

121.   **Qualitas Plantarum: Plant Foods for Human Nutrition.** The Hague: W. Junk (P. O. Box 13713, 2501 ES, The Hague, The Netherlands), 1952- . 4 times per year.

This scientific publication has had other titles. Volume 1 was called *Materia Vegetabiles*, and from 1953-1973 the title was *Qualitas Plantarum et Materia Vegetabiles*. It is the official organ of the Confoederation Internationales ad Qualitates Plantarum Edulium Perquirendas, and the Deutsche Gesellschaft für Qualitatsforschung (Pflanzliche Nahrungsmittel). It deals with the quality of food plants in terms of nutrition and health as influenced by genetics, ecology, plant nutrition, plant protection (pesticides and herbicides), growth regulators, management of soil and water supply, cooking, and processing. Also included are "topics of biochemistry, physiology, clinical and toxicological trials, and epidemiological surveys as far as plant food is concerned." Articles are in English, French, or German with summaries in English for articles in a foreign language.

Issues may present meeting papers and be devoted to single special topics. The role of plant foods in preventive medicine was recently covered.

122.   **Quarterly Journal of Crude Drug Research.** Lisse, Swets and Zeitlinger (P. O. Box 825, 2160 SZ, Lisse, The Netherlands), 1961- . Quarterly.

There has been an increasing interest of late in drugs of natural origin (as compared to synthetics). A number of successful ones have been introduced recently, and pharmaceutical industries are sometimes sending representatives to distant lands to explore for materials of possible value. Research Institutes also are searching for new crude materials of value in solving problems of health and disease. The editors of this journal feel there is a need for scientific and practical information on many plant and animal materials. They feature experimental studies and reviews of less well-known drugs because information on them so often has been scanty or lacking.

The Journal is devoted to the history; taxonomy; ecology; geographical distribution; morphology; histology; chemistry; methods of identification and determination; pharmacology; and local popular uses of plant and animal crude drugs.

Papers are accepted in English, French, German, or Spanish. However, of recent years nearly all have been in English. Book reviews are included.

123.   **Vegetarian Times.** New York: Vegetarian Life and Times, Inc. (41 East 42nd St., Suite 921, New York, NY 10017), 1974- . 10 times per year.

Each issue of this periodical contains several articles, news items, recipes for vegetarian and "natural" food dishes, advertisements, letters to the editor, and book reviews. Much of the material is not based on scientific evidence. For instance, an article was published about how laetrile, megavitamin therapy, and the switch to a vegetarian diet have given a young cancer victim a new lease on life.

More than vegetarianism is covered. "Natural" foods, holistic medicine, nutrition, and political matters have been treated in recent issues. Beginning with the December 1980 issue, a publication called *Well-Being* was consolidated with *Vegetarian Times*, and is included as an additional 24-page section. The *Well-Being* section presents articles on natural healing, herbs, gardening, alternative medicine, and "natural" food recipes as it did as a separate publication.

124.   **Vegetarian Voice.** Dolgeville, NY: North American Vegetarian Society (P. O. Box 72, Dolgeville, NY 13329), 1974- . Bimonthly.

This is a tabloid containing a variety of material, including short articles, vegetarian recipes, book reviews, news items, notices of meetings, lists of vegetarian restaurants and organizations, advertisements, announcements, and pictures.

125.   **Whole Foods: The Natural Foods Business Journal.** Berkeley, CA: Whole Foods Publishing Co. (2600 Eighth St., Berkeley, CA 94710), 1978- . Monthly.

This journal looks into the products, problems, and business practices of the natural foods industry. The aim of the industry is to sell foods that have undergone little processing and to fully disclose what goes into making the final product. No dietary philosophy is advocated, and exaggerated claims are seldom made for products.

Issues contain articles about food manufacturing processes, business practices (both retail and wholesale), advertising, growing food and herbs, new products, and product information. There are news columns and notices and many advertisements for products. Examples of recent articles include: how coffee is decaffeinated, organic food networks, business cycles, sweeteners, and the herb ginseng.

The July issue each year is a source directory which lists information of value to those in the health and natural food industry. It is a buyer's guide to manufacturers, distributors, and other health food suppliers. The product directory section includes sub-sections on foods, supplements and health aids, herbs, cosmetics, and accessories and store equipment. Also included are sections on industry services, an alphabetical address directory (manufacturers/distributors), geographical address directory (manufacturers/distributors), a trade name directory, and an advertisers' index.

126.   **Whole Life Times.** Newton, MA: Whole Life Times (132 Adams St., Suite 1, Newton, MA 02158), 1979- . Bimonthly.

This publication is a tabloid. Issues contain several articles on health and "natural" foods, many advertisements for "natural" food products, health devices, letters to the editor, and book reviews. Also included are lists of organizations and institutions supporting "holistic" and "natural" health, and "natural" food restaurants, distributors of health products, and the like.

127.   **The World Forum, Incorporating Health from Herbs.** London: H. H. Greaves, Ltd., 1864- . Quarterly.

This periodical, sponsored by the National Institute of Medical Herbalists, has served herbalists of Great Britain and Commonwealth countries since 1864. Information on herbal medicine and new herbals of interest to both professional herbalists and general readers is published.

PART II

Source Material by Subject Area

There are many interesting and beautiful books listed in this section on herb-als, and a great many have at least some reference value, although claims made for the medicinal properties of the herbs often tend to be exaggerated and based on myth and legend only. The more scientific works dealing with herbal plants are listed in chapter 11, "Medicinal Plants and their Constituents," and works dealing with folk medicines of various cultures and times are listed in chapter 9. Many of the latter are ethnobotan-ical studies of high quality.

As can be seen from perusing the materials listed, most information about herbs comes from old sources; virtually every work contains at least some history, leg-end, and lore. Medicinal properties are mentioned, but accurate scientific information (botanical, chemical, and pharmacological) is often lacking. There is a prevailing trend to make reprinted early books available, and a number are listed. Indeed, some are very old, such as the Culpeper, Dioscorides, and Gerard works which are classics of many centuries ago. Others, such as Grieve's *Modern Herbal*, originated perhaps 50 years ago. Curiously, most of the newer herbals are similar to early ones: there is a desire among modern herbalists to revive and imitate the early simpler times.

An outstanding feature of the traditional herbal is the art work. A great many are beautifully done. The early ones, particularly, had fine drawings and paintings as illustrations, such as the hand-painted watercolors of the Culpeper work. Recent ones often include fine color photographs.

The greatest contribution these books make, perhaps, lies in the artistic and historical spheres, although modern scientists are interested in them because suggestions about possible uses for plant substances can often be obtained from them.

* * * * *

128.   **The Bach Flower Remedies.** Including: **Heal Thyself** by Edward Bach, **The Twelve Healers** by Edward Bach, and **The Bach Remedies Repertory** by F. J. Wheeler. New Canaan, CT: Keats Publishing Co., 1979. 149p. index. $6.95. LC 79-87679. ISBN 0-87983-192-8; 0-87983-193-6pa.

Edward Bach, a homeopathic physician who died in 1936, developed a branch of herbal medicine which employed only the flowers and included no poisonous ones. He used the flower remedies to relieve mental distress.

This book contains a publisher's introduction, an interview with a physician about Dr. Bach's remedies, and the three previously published works named in the title above. *Heal Thyself* is an "explanation of the real cause and cure of disease." Bach suggests that patients seek within themselves for the origin of their maladies so they can assist in their own healing. *The Twelve Healers and Other Remedies* presents a listing of 38 plants placed under these headings: for fear, for uncertainty, for insufficient interest in present circumstances, for loneliness, or those over-sensitive to influences and ideas, for despondency or despair, and for over-care for welfare of others. No recipes or methods of preparation for remedies are included. For those who wish to treat themselves, stock bottles of the 38 remedies may be obtained from the Dr. Bach Centre in England. A few drops of the flower remedy is put in water, milk, or brandy and taken as required. *The Bach Remedy Repertory* lists conditions (such as anxiety, depression, inadequacy, insanity, anticipation, etc.) and the proper Bach remedy is indicated.

This is obviously an unusual book.

129.   Baïracli-Levy, Juliette de. **Common Herbs for Natural Health.** Illustrated by Heather Wood. New York: Schocken Books, 1974. 200p. illus. index. $2.75pa. LC 73-91335. ISBN 0-8052-0436-9.

This book was originally published in England as *The Illustrated Herbal Handbook.* The author comments that the twentieth century has seen a universal revival of and interest in herbal medicine. She has included some new medicinal herbs and herbal treatments of her own discovery and some unpublished ones collected on her travels.

Contents of the book is as follows: 1) Introductory; 2) Gathering; preparing and preserving herbs; 3) Herbal materia medica; 4) Recipes (cosmetic, medicinal, culinary and other); 5) Herbs applied to garden and orchard; and 6) Conclusion. Chapter 3, which makes up the bulk of the book, presents the herbs alphabetically by common name. Over 200 are included with their uses, dosage, habitat, and description. Scientific names are given, and there are a few line drawings of the plants.

130.   Bethel, May. **The Healing Power of Herbs.** 1972 ed. North Hollywood, CA: Wilshire Book Co. (12015 Sherman Rd., North Hollywood, CA 91605), 1972. 160p. $3.00pa.

The author of this small book believes that herbs rather than chemical wonder drugs should be used for treating disease because "no drug is ever free from side-effects." Statements of this kind are frequently found in herb books; the authors evidently do not realize that plant constituents are chemicals also and are as prone to producing side effects as any other chemical. This book is full of other statements which are untrue or at least misleading. For instance, after the remark that "large amounts of herb teas can be toxic and dangerous" (which is true), it is said that "no more so though than being gluttonous in eating foods of any kind" (which is nonsense). Some curious mixtures of old and new remedies are mentioned, for example, "B-12 injection is excellent for relief of neuralgia. Hot catnip tea is also good."

Most of the chapters are short. Titles are as follows: 1) A History of Herbalism; 2) What Herbs Can Do; 3) Doctor or Drug Induced Disease; 4) Herbal Treatment of Disease; 5) How the Glands Work; 6) Your White Bloodstream; 7) Refreshing Sleep Without Drugs; 8) Female Disorders; 9) Pregnancy and Delivery; 10) Babies and Their Care; 11) The Care of Older Children; 12) Beauty Secrets; 13) Your Crowning Glory; 14) The Art of Perfumery; 15) Herbal Beverages; 16) Help for the Smoker; 17) Herbs and Their Properties; 18) Medical Terms; 19) When and How to Gather Herbs; 20) Cooking with Herbs; 21) Plant a Herb Garden; and 22) Miscellaneous.

There is little of value in the book; the herbs mentioned are better treated in other works.

131.   Bianchini, Francesco, and Francesco Corbetti. **Health Plants of the World**: **Atlas of Medicinal Plants**. Illustrations by Marilena Pistoia; English adaptation by M. A. Dejey. New York: Newsweek Books, 1977. 242p. illus. (col.) bibliog. index. $19.95. LC 76-46692. ISBN 0-88225-250-X.

This is a beautiful book with 82 fine-colored full-page illustrations of herbal plants. The authors point out that herbal medicine for some time has been neglected in favor of synthetic drugs (many of them good), but that herbs have never been completely abandoned in Central Europe and the northern countries, and the old methods of healing are now being revived. Although the aim of the book is to broaden knowledge about medicinal treatments, "the doctor has to be consulted in cases of illness," the authors state. The suggestion is made, however, that with some guidance some plants may prevent more mundane illnesses.

The plants are grouped in separate sections, according to areas of use, as follows: digestive system, cardiovascular system, respiratory system, nervous system, genitourinary system, endocrine system, skin, and pesticide. Information given in the main body of the work includes description, chemical action, uses, history, scientific name, common names, and references to classical herbals. In addition, the role of herbs in mythology, sorcery, and in the kitchen is discussed. Most of the scientific information is found in an appended section. Other appendices include a botanical and a pharmacological glossary.

The work has been criticized because the remedies suggested are Old World, out of date, and some may be dangerous.

132.   Blunt, Wilfrid, and Sandra Raphael. **The Illustrated Herbal**. New York: Thames and Hudson, Inc. (500 Fifth Ave., New York, NY 10036), 1979. 191p. illus. (part col.). bibliog. index. $24.95. LC 79-84867. ISBN 0-500-01226-1.

This beautiful book is different from most recently published herbals. It is a careful biographical and bibliographical survey of herbalists and herbals with some of the best illustrations reproduced from early classics. There are 64 color plates and about 80 black and white manuscript illustrations, woodcuts, and engravings. Each is accompanied by the authors' descriptive, explanatory, and historical notes about the works. Included are stories of some of the documents, especially the early manuscripts, and their progression from the hands of collectors to the libraries where they are now found.

The book is divided into three sections. Section I, The Manuscript Herbals, contains the following chapters: 1) The First Herbalists; 2) The Anglo-Saxon Herbals; 3) The Anglo-Norman Herbals; and 4) The Rebirth of Naturalism. Section II, The Woodcut Herbals, includes these chapters: 1) Humble Beginnings; 2) The Golden Age; 3) The Herbal in Italy, Portugal and Spain; 4) The Herbal in the Low Countries, Switzerland and France; and 5) The Herbal in England. Section III is on The Metal-Engraved Herbals. In addition to the biographical and bibliographical details provided by the book, it also shows the evolution of the art and science of herbal production. It is a publication of high quality in every respect.

133.   Boxer, Arabella, and Philippa Back. **The Herb Book**. London: Octopus/ Mayflower, 1980. 224p. illus. (part col.). index. $19.95; $8.95pa. LC 79-22027. ISBN 0-7064-0991-4; 0-7064-1246-Xpa.

This illustrated guide to herbs is beautiful. It covers the history of herbs, the herb garden, identification and cultivation of 50 popular herbs, medicinal herbs, herbs for beauty and perfumery, and cooking with herbs. In addition, appended materials include a chart of herbs and their uses, a directory of plant names, and a list of herb suppliers in the United Kingdom, United States, Canada, Australia, and New Zealand.

The longest (more than half), and perhaps best, part of the book is on cooking with herbs. More than 275 recipes are provided, and they appear to be delectable. Measurements are given in both metric/imperial and American. Medicinal and cosmetic products described are not so appealing despite attractive photographs.

134.   Buchman, Dian Dincin. **Dian Dincin Buchman's Herbal Medicine: the Natural Way to Get Well and Stay Well.** New York: David McKay, 1979. 313p. illus. index. $12.95; $7.95pa. LC 79-17005. ISBN 0-679-51086-X; 0-679-51081-8pa.

This work is divided into four sections. The first is a listing of approximately 100 herbs and includes general usage information, remarks about harvesting, and historical data. This section is arranged in two separate alphabetical lists, the first being the author's favorite 20 or so herbs, the second being other popular and useful herbs.

The second section of the book is a listing of diseases and suggested herbal treatment. Specific preparations and dosages are given. The third section is a detailed discussion of how to make medicinal preparations using these herbs. The fourth section is a directory of sources and includes listings of seed dealers, herb societies, films about herbs, and a short list of herbal gardens.

The book includes ample information to serve as a home medical guide to using herbs should one be inclined to seek such guidance.

135.   Clarkson, Rosetta E. **Herbs, Their Culture and Uses.** New York: Macmillan Co., 1942. 226p. illus. index. $6.95. ISBN 0-02-526020-0.

Included in this work are only herbs that have been "used in the home, in industry, or in medicine in recent years." Medicinal plants listed are mainly those officially recognized ones from the *United States* or *British Pharmacopeia* and the *National Formulary* (the editions current at the time the book was written). Vegetables and flowers have been excluded.

The following chapters are included: 1) Why Have Herbs in Your Garden?; 2) Herb Arrangements in the Garden; 3) Propagation of Herbs; 4) Outdoor Planting; 5) Unusual Herb Plantings; 6) The Culinary Garden; 7) Fragrant Herb Garden; 8) Indoor Herb Gardens; 9) Harvesting and Drying; 10) Herb Dyes; 11) Potpourri; 12) Herb Products; 13) Herb Vinegars; 14) The Uses of Herbs in Cooking; 15) Herb Teas and Beverages; 16) Marketing of Herbs; 17) Tabular Paragraphs on 101 Useful Herbs; and 18) Herb Tables.

Chapter 17, which takes up about one-third of the book, lists herbs alphabetically by common name. Included are synonyms, scientific name, propagation, nature of plant, culture, uses, and line drawings. The herb tables (chapter 18) include lists by common traits such as: plants that grow in shade, those useful for hedges, and those with colorful flowers.

136.   Coon, Nelson. **Using Plants for Healing: An American Herbal.** Illustrations by Kenneth Raniere. 2d ed. Emmanus, PA: Rodale Press, 1979. 272p. illus. bibliog. index. $9.95. LC 79-1302.   ISBN 0-87857-247-3.

This book is a revised edition of a popular title first published in 1963. The author is a horticulturist who has written widely on plants. Since many herbals either have worldwide coverage or are limited to Great Britain, Germany, Switzerland, or Mexico, this work was written to fill the gap for the United States, particularly east of the Rockies.

The author does not claim to have compiled an exhaustive work on herbs, but has listed 160 familiar plants with line drawings, details on where to find them, how to identify them, their use, and preparation. Each description is about a page in length. In addition, brief descriptions on 77 less well-known plants have been provided.

Other chapters cover background and history of medicinal plant use; remedies used by Europeans, Mexicans, Hawaiians, American Indians, pioneer Americans, the Shakers, and Americans today; and preparing plants for use. Also included is a glossary, a chapter on medicines in house and garden, and two appendices: How to protect yourself from poisonous plants; and A plant collector's calendar. Plants in the main section are arranged alphabetically by scientific name, but there is also an index of scientific names as well as a general one which lists common names and the conditions for which the herbal remedies may be used.

The author has been careful to include warnings about plants which may be harmful even though they have a traditional medicinal use.

137.　　Crockett, James Underwood, and Ogden Tanner. **Herbs.** Alexandria, VA: Time-Life Books, 1977. 160p. illus. (part col.). bibliog. index. $8.95pa. (Time-Life Encyclopedia of Gardening, v.13). LC 76-51513. ISBN 0-8094-2550-5.

This attractive work is well illustrated, including many color photographs, and is directed toward the home gardener who is a beginner in herb growing.

The book begins with a general discussion of herbs and herbal history, the various uses of herbs, and general garden design and construction. This is followed with a section on getting started. It covers planning the herbal bed, hints to save work, getting the right soil chemistry, and cultural methods. Next is a section on growing herbs indoors. Then there is a section on the methods of harvesting, storage and preservation of the different types of herbs. Included is an encyclopedia describing the characteristics, culture, and uses of 126 herbs. They are listed alphabetically by genus and are cross-referenced by English names. The book concludes with climate zone and frost date maps, a table of characteristics of the 126 herbs, a short bibliography, and an index.

138.　　Cullum, Elizabeth. **A Cottage Herbal.** North Pomfret, VT: David and Charles, 1975. 127p. illus. bibliog. index. $9.95. LC 75-10563. ISBN 0-7153-7108-8.

The author of this charming book was inspired to write it after acquiring a 400-year-old Tudor cottage in a country hamlet in Great Britain. She made a herb garden on the property, attempting to recapture earlier times.

The following chapters are presented: 1) Making a Herb Garden; 2) Harvesting and Drying; 3) Herbal Fancies; 4) Culinary Herbs; 5) Country Wines and Herbal Teas; 6) Natural Dyes from Herbs; 7) Medicinal Herbs; and 8) Herbs as Cosmetics. An appendix includes a Table of Flowering times for the plants.

139.　　Culpeper, Nicholas. **The Complete Herbal and English Physician.** New edition. London: Thomas Kelly, 1850. 398p. illus. (col.). index. (Several reprinted editions of the 1826 edition are available).

Culpeper's herbal was quite popular in its time. An unusual feature was that it emphasized the astrological significance of medicinal herbs, a matter about which Culpeper was frequently criticized.

Plants are listed alphabetically under common names, with a description, uses, habit, and time of harvest. In addition, there is the zodiac sign, and Culpeper lists the "temperament" of herbs (such as hot or cold) and the effect this has on the patient.

There are sections on gathering and drying herbs and on the preparation of the medicines. Folklore is included, and not all the cures are of plant origin.

The archaic English makes the herbal difficult to read. The illustrations are one of the nicest features of the book. The edition under review here contains beautiful hand-painted watercolors. The book is of historical and artistic value rather than practical.

140.   Dawson, Adele. **Health, Happiness, and the Pursuit of Herbs.** With drawings by Robin Rothman. Brattleboro, VT: Stephen Greene Press, 1980. 278p. illus. bibliog. index. $12.95; $7.95pa. LC 79-21182. ISBN 0-8289-0362-8; 0-8289-0363-8pa.

The first part of this work deals with the philosophy of using herbs for food and medicine. In addition, there are sections on the identification of herbal plants, where to gather or purchase them, and how to use them. A few herbalists are mentioned briefly, for example, Hippocrates, Pliny, Gerard, and Culpeper.

The main section of the book is a listing of about 70 herbal plants with monographs on each. They are divided into four groups: 1) Salute to spring; 2) Summer—gourmet gardening; 3) Autumn: battening down; and 4) Winter: season of tisanes. Discussions on the specific herbs include scientific and common names, family name, name of botanist who first described the species (usually Linnaeus), description of the plant, uses, history, quotations from other works, and sometimes recipes for medicines and dishes that use the herb. Line drawings are provided for most plants. Following the main section are short chapters on the armchair herbalist, the history of herbs, and the use of honey and vinegar. Appendices include an alphabetical list of herbs, vocabulary, a list of vitamins and their roles in nutrition, and commerical sources of herb seeds, plants, and botanicals.

141.   Dioscorides, Pedanius. **The Greek Herbal of Dioscorides; Illustrated by a Byzantine, A.D. 512; Englished by John Goodyer, A.D. 1655; Edited and First Printed, A.D. 1933, by Robert T. Gunther.** New York: Hafner Publishing Co., 1959. (Repr. of 1933 ed.). 701p. illus. index. $23.00. LC 59-7041. ISBN 0-02-843930-9.

Dioscorides of Anazarbus in Cilicia originally compiled this work in the first century A.D. The Greek text was a source of inspiration for herbalists for more than 15 centuries. John Goodyer, the great English botanist of Petersfield, wrote out the entire Greek text with an interlinear English translation between 1652 and 1655. Goodyer's work was not printed and went unnoticed for centuries. This present edition is largely an uncorrected edition of Goodyer's translation. The editor says the printing is a "reproduction of his style, that it is a valuable historical document, and that it may still stimulate the curious to sift the indigenous from the exotic, and to discover the sources of much fictitious matter." The 396 illustrations are old line drawings by a Byzantine artist.

The five sections (called books) of the work cover these subjects: 1) aromatics, oils, ointments, trees; 2) living creatures, milk and dairy produce, cereals and sharp herbs; 3) roots, juices, herbs; 4) herbs and roots; 5) vines and wines, metallic ores. In addition, there is an appendix, "Dr. Charles Daubeny's Identifications," which is a table linking the name given by Dioscorides to a modern botanical name, and providing an evaluation of the drawings of the plants. The indexes provided are: Saracen's Latin Index, reprinted from the 1598 edition, and a supplemental index.

142.   Dowden, Anne Ophelia. **This Noble Harvest: A Chronicle of Herbs.** Illustrated by the author. New York and Cleveland, OH: Collins, 1979. 80p. illus. (part col.). bibliog. index. $12.95. LC 79-12021. ISBN 0-529-05548-1.

The author of this work is a well-known botanical illustrator, and attractive water-color pictures of herbal plants are the most outstanding feature of the book. A few wood cuts from ancient herbals are also included. The text material is simple and direct, suitable for young people, with history emphasized. A table of uses of herbs in cooking is appended.

143.   Dugdale, Chester B. **A Modern American Herbal: Useful Herbaceous Plants.** Vol.2. New York: A. S. Barnes; London, Thomas Yoseloff, 1978. 220p. illus. bibliog. index. $20.00. LC 71-86305. ISBN 0-498-01908-X.

Plants considered in this volume are treated in two sections, monocots and dicots. The former are subdivided into grasses, other grass-like plants, and wildflowers which are arranged by families. The dicots are arranged by leaf shape and size. The common and scientific names of the plant and its family are given for each species. Also included is a description to aid in identification, habitat, uses, and an intricate leaf print.

The comprehensive index includes scientific and common names. It also provides other information, particularly on uses, including edibility, medicinal value, dye use, protective covers, food for wildlife, and usable fibers. In addition, toxicity data is provided. The book also includes an index of leaf shapes, a short glossary, and a bibliography. The work is based on a collection of leaf prints, hence the emphasis on this manner of identification.

144.   **The Early American Life Handbook of Herbs: How to Plant a Colonial Herb Garden, Plus Age-Old Ideas for Cookery, Medicinals, and Fragrance.** From the editors of Early American Life, editor, Deborah B. Halverson. Gettysburg, PA: Early American Society, 1979. 48p. illus. LC 79-129753. (Available to new subscribers of Early American Life).

A concise work, this handbook presents descriptions and line drawings of about 60 herbs with comments on their culture, uses, and preservation. Topics covered include herb garden design, recipes containing herbs and cooking hints, herb lore, a list of suppliers of herbal plants and seeds, and a list of public gardens with descriptions. Most of the gardens are maintained by members of the Herb Society of America.

145.   Farwell, Edith Foster. **A Book of Herbs: How to Grow Herbs and Use Them for Seasoning, Fragrance, Decoration and as Natural Cures for Common Ailments.** Rev. ed. Piermont, NY: White Pine Press, 1979. 189p. illus. $6.95pa. LC 79-22580. ISBN 0-935720-01-4.

A revised edition of a widely sold book called *Have Fun With Herbs*, this work contains an assortment of materials. The foreword, by M. C. Goldman, executive editor of *Organic Gardening* magazine, encourages the reader to grow herbs for seasoning and medicine. A few of the chapters and some of the recipes were contributed by individuals other than Farwell.

Contents of the book is as follows: 1) American herbalists (biographical sketches of 6 herb growers); 2) Growing (includes a design for an herb garden); 3) Four herbs for the beginner (sweet and bush basil, chervil, sweet marjoram, and thyme); 4) Herbs to grow in the shade; 5) A companionate guide (lists herbs and indicates the plants they may best grow near); 6) Herbs for decoration; 7) The fragrant herbs; 8) The

Williamsburg gardens; 9) Herbal remedies (only a few are listed, and warnings are given about the dangers involved in treating oneself); 10) Substituting herbs for salt; 11) Recipes (the longest section, nicely done); 12) Encyclopedia of herbs (also a long section; lists 300 common herbs with Latin root-name origins, descriptions of uses, characteristics, and suggestions on growing); and 13) Directory (lists a few associations and a number of places to buy herbs and seeds).

For the most part, this is a good collection of material.

146.   Foster, Gertrude. **Herbs for Every Garden.** Rev. ed. New York: E. P. Dutton and Co., 1973. illus. bibliog. index. (A Sunrise Book). $7.50. LC 66-11558. ISBN 0-87690-098-8.

The author of this book, editor of *The Herb Grower Magazine*, (see entry 100) tries through this work to share her love of herbs with others. Her own garden of over 300 herbs has provided much of the material. The book begins with a general discussion of herbs and their uses. Included are sections on soils for herb beds, annuals and biennials grown from seed, perennials, herbs for the vegetable garden, plants for in and around the house, the harvest, and special uses of the plants. The latter includes herbs used in pomander balls, nosegays, and herb pillows. A method of implanting the outline of large-leaved herbs in concrete squares for paving is described. A few recipes are provided throughout the book.

The descriptive sections present the herbs alphabetically by common name. Included are scientific name, height, leaf and blossom, culture, habitat, uses, and other comments.

147.   Freeman, Margaret B. **Herbs for the Mediaeval Household, for Cooking, Healing and Divers Uses.** New York: Metropolitan Museum of Art, 1943. 48p. illus. index. $4.95. LC 43-18177. ISBN 0-87099-067-5.

This handsome, artistic work is printed in 12-point cloister old style type with headings set in Goudy text. The illustrations are from medieval works and include woodcuts. The author begins with an introduction to early sources used in compiling the book. True to its title, there are sections on 1) Herbs for cooking; 2) Herbs for healing; 3) Herbs for poisoning pests; and 4) Sweet smelling herbs.

Entries within each section are arranged alphabetically by common name. Included in each entry is the scientific name of the plant, uses mentioned in specific medieval sources, present uses, and a medieval illustration. There are indexes by common scientific names.

148.   Frost, Doris Thain. **Herbs for Flavor, Fragrance, Fun: In Gardens, Pots, in Shade, in Sun.** Washington, DC: U.S. Department of Agriculture (Available from the U. S. National Arboretum, 24th and R. Streets, N. E., Washington, DC20002), 1977. Reproduced from the **1977 Yearbook of Agriculture.** 7p. illus. (U.S. D. A. Publication No. YS-77-1). Free.

This pamphlet is a concise introduction to 17 of the most popular and available herbs. All can be home-grown throughout the United States.

After about two pages of introductory remarks about propagation, harvesting, and preserving, each of the 17 herbs is discussed in some detail. Each discussion includes remarks about culinary uses, but medicinal uses are not mentioned. A few recipes are included.

The booklet can serve as an introductory guide for the cook and herb grower.

149.   Garland, Sarah. **The Complete Book of Herbs and Spices.** New York: Viking Press, 1979. 288p. illus. (part col.). bibliog. index. (A Studio Book). $25.00. LC 78-27036. ISBN 0-670-36866-0.

A comprehensive guide to herbs and spices, this handsome, large book describes over 300 plants. It is illustrated with beautiful water colors, drawings, and photographs. Also included are more than 200 recipes from the author's own collection. In addition to foods, they include mixtures to repel insects, herbs for washing and polishing, pomanders, directions for incense and candle making, herbal dyes, preparations for skin care and hair, and treatments for coughs, colds, fevers, indigestion, and first aid.

The work is in several sections: 1) History and tradition; 2) A modern herbal (listing of herbs and spices); 3) The herb garden; 4) Cooking with herbs and spices; 5) Household herbs and spices; 6) Cosmetic herbs; and 7) Herbs for health. Section 2 is the longest. Plants are listed alphabetically by scientific name. Also included are common names and plant family name, closely related plants, habitat, methods of cultivation, harvesting and storage instructions, uses, historical references, myths, and legendary powers. Poisonous herbs are grouped together at the end of the section.

The author of the book lives in England, but a great many of the plants listed grow in the United States.

150.   Gerard, John. **The Herbal or General History of Plants.** The 1633 edition revised and enlarged by Thomas Johnson. London: Adam Islip Joice Norton and Richard Whitakers, 1633; repr. New York: Dover, 1975. 1678p. illus. index. $50.00. LC 74-18718. ISBN 0-486-23147-X.

This work, which is a republication of the famous 1633 edition entitled *The Herball or General Historie of Plantes*, is often considered the bible of English herbalists. Even though most of the illustrations and text of Gerard's *Herball* were borrowed from earlier works, it was popular and respected in England at that time, and most modern English herbals are derived from it.

The work was first published in 1597. Thomas Johnson, considered a more competent scholar and botanist than Gerard, corrected errors and added some newer material for this 1633 edition. This reproduction contains the fine woodcuts and Elizabethan prose of the original. About 2,850 plants are described and about 2,700 illustrations are included. Folklore and naturalistic descriptions of the time are included.

The body of the work is divided into three parts: 1) grasses, rushes, grains, reeds, irises, and bulbs; 2) food plants, medicinal plants, and sweet-smelling plants; and 3) roses, trees, shrubs, bushes, fruit-bearing plants, heaths, mosses, and fungi. Each plant is illustrated, and Latin and English names and text are provided. The text contains a physical description, habit (often its English locations), times of bloom, sowing, etc., synonyms, traditional medical theory of its "temperaments" or "humors," and "virtues." Following the main text are an index of Latin names, glossary/concordance of Latin names, index of English names, glossary of little-used English names, and an index of "virtues" (uses) and properties of the plants.

Original editions of this work are worth perhaps $750.00. It is of note also that a reprinted edition of the 1597 edition of Gerard is available (from Walter J. Johnson, in two volumes, for about $215.00).

151.   Gordon, Lesley. **A Country Herbal.** New York: Mayflower Books, 1980. 208p. illus. (part col.). bibliog. index. $19.95. LC 80-13531. ISBN 0-8317-4446-4.

The author says this book contains "a little history, a little folklore, some facts about cosmetics, the making of perfumes, the art of dyeing, a few hints about herb-growing."

The book lists alphabetically by common name over 130 herbs and spices. Some are common, some rare; some are poisonous, and some are useful. The illustrations are beautiful, many in color, and many have been taken from rare and ancient herbals. Information on each plant usually includes scientific name; zodiac sign involved; description; medicinal, household, and cosmetic uses; cultivation; history; supernatural properties; and recipes making use of the plant. Appended materials include a table of metric conversions for cooks, a list of dyers' plants, herbs and spices used in perfumery and cosmetics throughout the ages, a herb calendar, a list of herbal teas or tisanes, herbs and spices used in modern cookery or wines, and a list of bee-plants.

152. Grieve, Mrs. M. **A Modern Herbal: The Medicinal, Culinary, Cosmetic and Economic Properties, Cultivation and Folk-Lore of Herbs, Grasses, Fungi, Shrubs and Trees with all their Modern Scientific Uses.** With an Introduction by the editor, Mrs. C. F. Leyel. New York: Dover Publications, Inc., 1971. 2v. illus. bibliog. index. $11.00pa. LC 72-169784. ISBN 0-486-22798-7; 0-486-22799-5. (A republication of the work originally published by Harcourt, Brace and Co. in 1931).

This is a comprehensive work, containing nearly 900 pages, 96 plates, and 161 illustrations of plants. More than 800 varieties of plants have been included. Material is arranged alphabetically under the most familiar name of the plants, but an index of "country names" has been supplied. A large amount of information is usually provided on each plant, such as: scientific name; synonymous names; part used; habitat; description; chemical constituents; medicinal action and uses; dosage; antidotes; methods of cultivation; preparation of extracts and tinctures; economic, cosmetic, and other properties. In addition, recipes for making ointments, lotions, sauces, wines and fruit brandies, jams, tonics, and liniments are given.

It is noteworthy that much folklore has been included. The work will appeal to flower-lovers and gardeners, and is one of the classic "modern" herbals although it is 50 years old.

153. Hall, Dorothy. **The Book of Herbs.** Illustrated by Astra Lacis. New York: Charles Scribner's Sons, 1972. 212p. illus. bibliog. index. $7.95. LC 74-3666. ISBN 0-684-13822-0.

Emphasis in this book is on how to use and enjoy herbs with herb gardening also covered. The author is a commercial grower of herbs. The first 42 pages contain chapters on why herbs should be grown, general information on growing them, and soil fertility. The remainder of the book discusses 40 common herbs individually. The approach is popular. A little background is presented, then a description, information on growing, uses, presumed medicinal effects, and three or four recipes for using the herb. A pretty, delicate line drawing is included for each plant.

The presentation is nicely done, although there are perhaps too many unsubstantiated claims for medicinal value of herbs. For example, the author states, "Horseradish is very effective in the treatment of sinus and antrum congestion," and "Southernwood tea is also prescribed when people are convalescing from the flu; it helps combat that bodily weakness and pains in the limbs suffered with this wretched illness." These claims are not presented as folklore, but as facts.

154.   Harris, Ben Charles. **Make Use of Your Garden Plants.** Barre, MA: Barre
Publishers; distr. Crown Publishers, 1978. 224p. illus. bibliog. index. $8.95. LC 77-
17894. ISBN 0-517-53198-4.

After a few introductory pages on planning a garden, poisonous plants, and
harvesting and drying procedures, this book presents an alphabetical listing of 125 common plants. These plants are not all commonly considered "herbs"; many are trees,
flowers, and common shrubbery.

Each entry includes some historical information, a discussion of medicinal,
culinary, and cosmetic uses, and in most cases some interesting homespun philosophy.
Several entries include specific recipes, but most are fairly general about preparation
and dosages. A great many surprising uses are mentioned.

The index enhances the work because all of the plant uses mentioned in the
text are included there. This is a good basic herbal with an easy, readable style.

155.   Herb Society of America. **Herbs for Use and for Delight.** An Anthology from
The Herbarist selected and with an introduction by Daniel J. Foley. New York: Dover
Publications, 1974. 324p. illus. bibliog. $3.50pa. LC 74-80287. ISBN 0-486-23104-
6.

Collected here are 56 selections from *The Herbarist* (see entry 103), an outstanding journal of the herb field published by the Herb Society of America. Articles
were chosen from issues published from 1935 to 1971.

The introduction to the book provides information on the founding and history of the Society. The author says he has endeavored to present in the volume a
generous sampling of articles—many containing information not usually found in popular books on herbs. Herb lore is related, and the delights and pleasures of growing,
using, and enjoying the plants is expressed.

Following are titles of the selections: 1) Nature's Bags of Scent; 2) The Pronunciation of Herb; 3) The Modern Herb; 4) Angelica Archangelica; 5) Artemisias;
6) Seven Basils; 7) Chamomile; 8) Those Herbs Called Chervils; 9) Comfrey—The Cin-
derella of Plants; 10) "Righte Dittany"; 11) Dittany Redivivus; 12) On Fennel—Only
Slightly Botanical; 13) Alchemilla—Lady's Mantle; 14) In Quest of Lavenders; 15) Lemon Verbena; 16) Lovage; 17) Notes on the Marjorams; 18) Herb of Honor (marjoram);
19) A Study of Mints; 20) Mints and Microscopes; 21) Some Common Mints and Their
Hybrids; 22) Calendula Officinalis; 23) The Way of the Poet's Marigold; 24) Rosemary—
the Herb of Remembrance; 25) Variety in Rosemary; 26) In Praise of Sage; 27) Notes
on a Few Savories; 28) The Tarragons, Cultivated and Wild; 29) Thymus; 30) The
Thymes; 31) Herb Gardens, 1960 Notes on Design; 32) Color in the Herb Garden; 33)
Herbs in the Rock Garden; 34) Herbs in Knots and Laces; 35) Herb Symbiosis—Companion Plants; 36) The Significance of Botanical Pesticides; 37) Herbs of the Mediter-
ranean; 38) A List for an Old English Wort Garden; 39) Some Herbs from the Old
World and the New; 40) The Tussie Mussie, an Herbal Bouquet; 41) Pot-pourri Album;
42) Tastes in Tea; 43) Some Notes upon the Use of Herbs in Norwegian Households;
44) Dyeing with Herbs; 45) Indigo, the True Blue; 46) Early American Dyeing; 47) In
Praise of Herbals; 48) Flowers and Perfume; 49) The 17th Century Still-Room; 50)
Herbs for My Lady's Toilet; 51) "Resembling a Citron Pill"; 52) Scented Geraniums;
53) Our Oldest Garden Roses; 54) Spice Caravans; 55) Shien—Some Noteworthy Edible
Herbs of China; and 56) Wreaths and Garlands.

This is a nice, well-selected collection.

156.   **An Herbal (1525).** Edited and transcribed into modern English with an introduction by Sanford V. Larkey and Thomas Pyles. Delmar, NY: Scholars' Facsimiles
and Reprints, Inc., 1978 (repr. of 1941 edition). 86p. index. $20.00. LC 42-7657.
ISBN 0-8201-1197-X.

    This work, which the editors refer to as *Banckes's Herbal*, contains an intro-
duction, a facsimile reprint of the 1525 edition (reproduced from the copy in the
British Museum), a modernized version of the herbal, and an index of herbs and plants
not given in chapter headings but which are mentioned in the text. The original work
was a quarto volume from the press of Richard Banckes, a London printer.

    The editors believe the work will be "of interest to the amateur of flowers as
well as to the herbalist, the botanist, the antiquarian, and the medical historian; its
manner, quaint, old fashioned, yet racy and vigorous, should guarantee it an even wider
appeal." It was popular in its day; there were at least 15 editions that followed through
1560. The material is believed to have been compiled from several earlier English herbals, with little new or original information.

    Herbs are listed alphabetically and described in a paragraph or two with other
names, habitat, and uses indicated. There are 207 entries. The following is an example
from the modernized version under *Altea*: "This herb is called hollyhock or the wild
mallow. The virtue of the herb is thus. Take and stamp it and fry it with sheep's tal-
low, and make a plaster, and lay it to a podagre (gouty) man, and it shall help him
within three days... This herb groweth in gardens and in moist places."

    The work is more medical than botanical, and there are no illustrations. The
information on each herb contains much medieval superstition and medical folklore.

157.   **Herbarium Apulei Platonica,** 1481 (Vol.1); **Herbolario Volgare,** 1522 (Vol.2).
Facsimile reprints with introductions by Erminio Caprotti and William T. Stearn.
Milan, Edizioni Il Polifilo, 1979. 2v. illus. bibliog. index. (Libri Rari, Collezione de
ristampe con nuovi apparati, III.). About $90.00.

    Two well-known and rare ancient herbals are reprinted here in facsimile. The
first volume, *Herbarium Apulei Platonica*, published in Rome in 1481, was probably
the earliest illustrated herbal ever printed. It is illustrated with crude woodcuts. The
second volume, *Herbolario Volgare*, published in Venice in 1522, was the first herbal
printed in Italian. Its woodcuts are of better quality than those in the earlier work.
The herbals describe the plants and provide a list of their virtues and the diseases they
can presumably cure. Recipes for medicines prepared from the herbs are included.
Supposed magical qualities of the plants are mentioned in some instances.

    Caprotti's and Stearn's introductory essays are in English as well as Italian,
making it possible for those unfamiliar with Latin and Italian to enjoy the herbals.
Also included are tables and indexes for the identification of the plants under their
scientific and corresponding Italian and English names. The books are excellent examples of fine printing.

158.   **Herbarium: Natural Remedies from a Medieval Manuscript.** Texts by Adalberto
Pazzini and Emma Pirani; original captions by Ububchasym de Baldach. New York;
Rizzoli International Publications, 1980. 54 leaves. illus. (col.). $12.50pa. LC 79-
93004. ISBN 0-8478-0305-8.

    This is more an "art" book than a practical guide to herbal remedies. It is
made up primarily of 47 attractive full-page colored plates taken from fourteen-and
fifteenth-century manuscript illustrations in the iconographic tradition. A number
show human figures harvesting the plant illustrated.

Descriptions that accompany the illustrations are taken from Latin captions of Ububchasym de Baldach in the Casanatense manuscript and from notes found in other late medieval herbaria. Much of the terminology may be unfamiliar. Such terms as "hot and moist in the first degree" and "inflates the humours" are frequently found. For each plant or herb shown, there are brief comments about when to use it, how it is used, its benefits, its harmful effects, and how such effects can be prevented. All plants mentioned are common.

The introduction contains mostly bibliographical information about the manuscripts used in compiling the book, but it also contains useful explanatory material about the terminology used in the descriptions. The work is of interest mainly for its artistic and historical value.

159.   Hermann, Matthias. **Herbs and Medicinal Flowers.** Engravings by Redouté, Daffinger and several artists; translated by Grace Jackman. New York: Galahad Books, 1973. 128p. illus. (col.). index. $12.50.

The most outstanding feature of this guide is the beautifully printed color illustrations of about 200 medicinal plants.

An introduction of two pages outlines the history of herbalism and presents a short list of diseases and conditions with the plants useful for their treatment. Two indexes follow, one by common name of the plant and one by botanical name. The remainder of the book consists of fine illustrations, arranged by botanical name, and short paragraphs giving uses of each plant. Little other information is provided. References to other herbals are made in the text, particularly to early ones, but no bibliography is provided.

The book can be highly recommended for its illustrations that would be useful in identifying medicinal plants.

160.   Hewlett-Parsons, J. **Herbs, Health and Healing.** London: Thorsons Publishers Ltd., 1968. 96p. (The Health and Harmony Series). ISBN 0-7225-0153-6.

The format of this book is different from most of its kind. Herbs are not listed with their uses, but rather they are dealt with in their relationship to the various systems in the human body and in their application to the treatment of various diseases. The author does not believe in the use of drugs extracted from plants and purified, but thinks the whole plant should be used.

Chapter headings are: 1) The Circulatory System; 2) Diseases of the Digestive System; 3) Diseases of the Skin; 4) Diseases of the Respiratory System; 5) Diseases of the Nervous System; 6) Diseases of the Liver and Gallbladder; 7) Diseases of the Urinary System; 8) Women's Complaints; and 9) Some Useful Information. Each chapter lists specific diseases and gives instructions for preparing herbal remedies for treatment.

161.   Huson, Paul. **Mastering Herbalism: A Practical Guide.** Illustrated by the author. New York: Stein and Day, 1974. 371p. illus. bibliog. index. $4.95pa. LC 73-90704. ISBN 0-8128-1847-4.

Virtually all aspects of herbalism are covered in this well-organized guide. The author asks in his foreword what herb mystique is; what can one do with herbal plants? He answers as follows: "Well, you can eat them and brew them into health-giving teas, or bathe in them and smoke them, or pound them up and plaster them all over your face and body; or you can grow them and dry them and perfume yourself and your friends with them; or you can wash your hair in them. More than that, you can follow age-old traditions and if you are talented in that direction, even cast spells with them. And last, but by no means least, you can live to a ripe old age by means of them."

Huson takes up these aspects of the subject, and, in addition, includes chapters on growing the plants and where to buy them. Also included are a glossary and appendices as follows: A) Planting and harvesting by the moon; B) Weights and measures; C) Herbs as nutritional sources; and D) A Christianized conjuration of the herb valerian.

A great deal of history and folklore and many recipes, cultivation tips, and remedies are presented in the book. It is all fascinating to read. The claims for the wonder-working, of course, should not be taken seriously.

162.   Hutchens, Alma R. **Indian Herbalogy of North America.** N. G. Tretchikoff, Herbalist, general plan and direction; Natalie K. Tretchikoff, Russian material and bibliography. 5th ed. Windsor, Ontario, Canada: Merco (620 Wyandotte East, Windsor 14, Ontario, Canada), 1974. 382p. illus. bibliog. index. $10.95.

This is a study of herbal medicine used by American Indians in the United States and Canada. Anglo-American, Russian, and Oriental literature was studied to produce this work.

The book begins with an introductory section which includes discussions of the following: general remarks; sources and bibliography; language barrier for research; aborigines of America; from the old world to the new; daily life and culture; foods from the mother earth; health and sickness; first Americans were their own physicians; Indian healer; Indian herbs for the glands; Samuel Thomson and white man's nature healer; civilization versus culture; empirism and dynamics of herbalogy; herbalogy abroad; literature abroad; and conclusion.

The main section of the book consists of 318 pages of monographs, each a page or two in length, on various herbs. Arrangement is alphabetical by common name. Information provided is as follows: scientific name, other common names, features, part of plant used, solvent, bodily influence, uses, dose, and external use (if any). Line drawings are provided for most plants. The bibliography is exceptional. Works listed are completely described, even including size, and an annotation is given for each. Materials are listed under these headings: general and reference publications, herbalogy, Russian publications, and periodicals. A few of the latter are North American native people's titles.

The author and her co-workers have done a careful study of the literature on Indian herbalogy. There is a good deal of digression, though, into the medical and health field that is not based on any scientific evidence.

163.   Hylton, William H., ed. **The Rodale Herb Book: How to Use, Grow, and Buy Nature's Miracle Plants.** With chapters by Nelson Coon, Louise Hyde, Bonnie Fisher, Marion Wilbur, Barbara Foust, and Heinz Grotzke. Emmaus, PA: Rodale Press Book Division, 1974. 653p. illus. bibliog. index. (An Organic Gardening and Farming Book). $12.95. LC 73-18902. ISBN 0-87857-076-4.

This is a rather comprehensive encyclopedic work on herbs, covering their identification, uses, lore, mystique, history, growing, and cooking. Amateurs and those already familiar with the plants will find it of value.

The book begins with short sketches on each of the contributors. Chapter headings are: 1) Herbal Beginnings; 2) The Healing Herbs; 3) The Culinary Herbs (includes a number of recipes); 4) The Aromatic Herbs (includes perfume essences); 5) The Colorful Herbs (on dyeing); 6) Cultivating the Herbs; 7) The Companionable Herbs (plants for pest control); 8) Landscaping with Herbs.

About half the book is taken up by appendices, which include an herbal encyclopedia, a glossary, a bibliography and a list of sources for buying herbal plants, seeds, and related materials. In the encyclopedia section, more than 150 herbs are listed.

Each monograph includes common names, scientific name, family name, description, propagation, history, uses, preparation for use, and other interesting miscellaneous information.

This is a nice compilation, well written and with fewer extravagant claims than are found in many herb books. Illustrations, mostly photographs, are an added attraction.

164. **The Illustrated Earth Garden Herbal.** Text and illustrations gathered from ancient sources and the classic herbals by Keith Vincent Smith. London: Elm Tree Books, 1979. 157p. illus. bibliog. index. £4.95. ISBN 0-241-10094-1.

Originally published in West Melbourne, Australia in 1978, this work was compiled by a journalist interested in herb gardening. His book, which is called an herbal companion, is a historical account by ancient and more recent herbalists, of about 40 herbs. Included are their uses, "virtues," and illustrations with recipes for preparing the herbs for use.

The book is attractive and has been compiled with care.

165. Kamm, Minnie Watson. **Old-Time Herbs for Northern Gardens.** Boston, MA: Little, Brown, 1938; repr. New York: Dover Publications, 1971. 256p. illus. index. $3.00pa. LC 79-143677. ISBN 0-486-22695-6.

After an introductory chapter regarding the history, cultivation, and use of herbs, this book presents discussions of individual herbs grouped together by family. Twenty-four families are included. Also provided is a list of herbs according to their uses as condiments, medicinals, perfumes, or dyes. There are indexes to the herbs mentioned in the text by Latin and by English names. A number of photographs and many line drawings of plants are included.

Material is nicely presented with charm. Emphasis is on historical uses of the plants, and extravagant claims are not made for them as medicinals. Passages of poetry and quotations from classical works are interspersed throughout.

166. Keller, Mitzie Stuart. **Mysterious Herbs and Roots: Ancient Secrets for Beautie, Health, Magick, Prevention and Youth.** Culver City, CA: Peace Press (3828 Willat Ave., Culver City, CA 90230), 1978. 402p. illus. bibliog. index. LC 78-62301. ISBN 0-915238-25-X.

This is a collection of historical material and lore regarding 27 herbs and roots, illustrated with reproductions of woodcuts from fifteenth- and sixteenth-century herbals and a few engravings from more modern works. Recipes for dishes and cosmetic preparations are included throughout, as are instructions for preparing a few medicines.

Contents of the book is as follows: 1) Asparagus; 2) Basil; 3) Bay leaf; 4) Beans; 5) Beets; 6) Brussels sprouts; 7) Cabbage; 8) Caraway seeds; 9) Celery; 10) Chervil; 11) Cucumber; 12) Dill; 13) Garlic, chives, leeks and onions; 14) Ginger; 15) Marjoram, oregano; 16) Mint; 17) Parsley; 18) Rosemary; 19) Sage; 20) Savory; 21) Tarragon; 22) Thyme; 23) Watercress; 24) Herbs in cooking; 25) Beauty diet; and 26) Planting, Harvesting and Preserving.

167. Krutch, Joseph Wood. **Herbal.** New York: a Balance House book published by G. P. Putnam's Sons, 1965. 255p. illus. bibliog. index. LC 65-20676.

This is a fine edition of a delightful book. The author, a distinguished naturalist and scholar, examines classical herbals and the theories and discoveries of herbalists from ancient to recent times. An introductory section presents suitable classical quotations and a discussion of such matters as the Doctrine of Signatures, herbs and astrology, herbs and modern drugs, herbals and gardening, and herbs in cookery.

The main value of the book, however, lies in its artistic and historical contribution. The bulk of the book is made up of plant descriptions and illustrations. About 100 herbs and six creatures are illustrated full-page, (quarto size), taken from the woodcuts in Pierandrea Mattrioli's large folio volume *Commentaries on the Six Books of Dioscorides*, issued in Prague in 1563 and Venice in 1565. Illustrations are very fine and well-reproduced in this edition. On the page facing each illustration is a descriptive monograph containing material from the classical herbals listed in the bibliography.

The tone of the work is best illustrated by this passage from it: "Perhaps the chief charm of the Herbalists (and certainly the one this book would like especially to suggest) is just that they are more likely than the modern scientist to impart a sense of beauty and wonder—both of which the scientist may feel, but considers it no part of his function to communicate."

168.   Law, Donald. **Herbs for Cooking and for Healing.** North Hollywood, CA: Wilshire Book Co., 1972. 104p. illus. $2.00pa. LC 72-451196. ISBN 0-572007-02-7.

This book is divided into two sections, the first consists of several short chapters on identifying and collecting herbs, preserving and drying techniques, first aid using common kitchen ingredients, cooking with herbs, and recipes for herbal treatments.

The "recipes" are general directions for preparing ointments and decoctions, using an herb or herbs appropriate for treating the malady. There are lists of diseases and complaints, giving the herbs used for treatment, without specific recipes and dosages included. The latter half of the book is an alphabetical listing of herbs by common name. Each entry provides general information about habitat, use, and which part of the plant is used. The book contains a lot of general information.

169.   Law, Donald. **Herbs for Health and Flavor.** New York: St. Martin's Press, 1975. 62p. illus. (col.). $5.95. LC 76-22931.

As the title suggests, this book tells how to use herbs for food flavoring and in simple medicines. After a brief introduction, there are sections on sandwiches; omelettes, soups and biscuits; salads; and garnishing and flavor. An "Index of Illnesses, with herbs whose healing virtues can bring relief," follows, along with a page on preparing herbs for medicinal use. The main part of the book consists of a list of herbal plants, arranged alphabetically by common name. Each is pictured with an attractive colored illustration. Information about each herb is given, including Latin name, description, use in food and/or medicine, historical uses, and how to prepare various concoctions.

Many of the recipes sound appetizing, but medicines suggested are of doubtful value. It is not true, either, that herbs do not have harmful side effects, as the introduction states; many contain toxic substances. The author says, however, that he has taken care to mention only safe herbs, and, for the most part, this is true.

170.   **Leaves From Gerard's Herball.** Arranged for garden lovers by Marcus Woodward with 130 illustrations after the original woodcuts. Boston, MA: Houghton Mifflin Co., 1931; repr. New York: Dover Publications, 1969. 305p. illus. index. $3.50pa. LC 79-82793. ISBN 486-22343-4.

This work is based on the famous English *Herball or General Historie of Plantes* by John Gerard, originally published in 1597 (see entry 150). Passages characteristic of Gerard's work are presented (in Early Modern English), but the entire book has been rearranged to form a "garden Calendar" with plants grouped according to time of flowering or special appeal. Each entry includes a description of the plant; habitat; and medicinal, culinary, and cosmetic uses. Medicinal uses are emphasized, but specific recipes and formulations are not given. The flowers and shrubs discussed are favorites today as they were in Gerard's time. Included are sections on nettles, lilies, potatoes, tobacco, poppies, sunflowers, peach trees, onions, sage, lavendar, lettuce, violets, and many other plants.

A section of notes has been provided and also a table of "sundry vertues" (really an index of ailments with appropriate page numbers given for referral to the text). There is also an alphabetical index of plant names.

171.   Leek, Sybil. **Sybil Leek's Book of Herbs.** New York: Cornerstone Library (Simon & Schuster), 1973. 199p. illus. index. $3.95pa. ISBN 346-12435-2.

Presented here are 13 chapters on the world of herbs, with the emphasis on background and history. Over one-fourth of the book pertains to historical aspects of the plants, including one unique chapter containing biographies of well-known herbalists.

Other chapters discuss legends and myths; perfumes, potpourris and sachets; beauty aids; and culinary uses of herbs. The latter includes general culinary information on the most popular herbs, but specific recipes are not given. Medicinal uses of herbs are not usually considered. One chapter calls for more investigation and research into Chinese and American Indian uses of herbs, especially in diet and medicine. The author maintains that there are valuable secrets which have not yet been discovered by modern man.

Leek claims to be a witch and a member of a family that has practiced witchcraft for 800 years. The book is probably most valuable for its folklore.

172.   Lehner, Ernst, and Johanna Lehner. **Folklore and Odysseys of Food and Medicinal Plants.** New York: Tudor Publishing Co., 1962. 128p. illus. index. LC 61-12333.

The authors of this attractive work tell of the voyages, expeditions, intrigues, and wars it took to bring the plants of daily use to us. Most of the grains, vegetables, herbs, fruits, spices, and stimulants used today originated hundreds, or even thousands, of years ago. The curious and little-known facts about them are presented with about 200 illustrations taken from old classic herbals and rare manuscripts.

Material is arranged under these headings: 1) The Cereals; 2) The Stimulants; 3) The Odysseys of Plants; 4) The Physic Garden; and 5) Culinary Herbs. A list of illustrations has been provided, indicating the original source (no bibliography as such is included).

The book is of special interest to artists, folklorists, and collectors interested in herbs.

173.   Leyel, Mrs. C. F. (Hilda). **Culpeper's English Physician and Complete Herbal.** Arranged for use as a first aid herbal. 1972 edition. North Hollywood, CA: Wilshire Book Co. (12015 Sherman Rd., North Hollywood, CA 91605). 1971. 128p. illus. index. $2.00pa. ISBN 0-87980-025-9.

The compiler of this work has taken descriptions of about 120 herbs from Nicholas Culpeper's classic work, *English Physician and Complete Herbal* (see entry 139) and, in addition, has provided paragraphs on modern uses. She says, however, that most herbs described by Culpeper are used by herbalists today for the same purposes. An introductory chapter presents a brief biography of Culpeper, who lived from 1616 until 1654. His herbal was widely used for over 200 years.

Herbs listed are arranged alphabetically by common name. Included is a drawing of the plant, the botanical name, natural order name, description, habitat, former uses (Culpeper's), and modern uses. Culpeper's contributions include statements that the plants are under the domination of various planets, the sun, or the moon. There is a botanical and a clinical index.

The book is interesting as a curiosity, but the information given on uses, both the former and the modern, should not be relied upon without caution and further authority. Other works do not mention pears as being an antidote to poisonous mushrooms, nor do they say lily of the valley is not poisonous. The latter is usually considered a toxic plant.

174.   Loewenfeld, Claire, and Philippa Back. **The Complete Book of Herbs and Spices.** 2d rev. ed. Newton Abbott: David and Charles, 1978. 319p. illus. (part col.). bibliog. index. $19.95. LC 78-321443. ISBN 0-7153-7656-X.

First published in 1974, this edition of the book is almost identical to the first, except for the addition of some fine color illustrations, including German herbal prints.

Spices and herbs of the world are covered, including their history and tradition; use of herbs and spices in health, cooking, and cosmetics; and the significance of wild herbs and spices. The second part of the book describes the plants in detail and includes information about botanical and common names, habitat, uses, recipes, and the like. There are good charts on the making of medicinal teas, the making of herb and spice mixtures for cooking, and the use of herbs as cosmetics.

175.   Lucas, Richard. **Common and Uncommon Uses of Herbs for Healthful Living.** West Nyack, NY: Parker Publishing Co., 1969; repr. New York: Arco Publishing Co., 1978. 238p. index. $1.65pa. LC 74-128898. ISBN 0-668-02396-1.

This is Lucas' second book, and it provides information on some herbal substances that were not included in the first book, *Nature's Medicines* (see entry 177). Much material comes from works of early modern herbalists (Gerard, Parkinson, and Culpeper) and from recent writings that are referred to in footnotes.

Contents of the book is as follows: 1) Elder: favorite all-time remedy; 2) Dandelion: the wayside healing wonder; 3) Golden healing oil from the olive tree; 4) Nettle: the versatile healing plant; 5) Sage: the heritage herb for good health; 6) The onion: bulb of valuable natural medicinals; 7) Healing plants from the sea (algae, kelp, carrageen) 8) Herbal health secrets of the American Indians; 9) Mistletoe: mystic herb of the Druids; 10) The humble parsley: a treasury of natural remedies; 11) Sassafras— "chief medicine" plant; 12) The "Green Hope" in the fight against cancer (the search for currative possibilities in herbs); 13) Variety of uses of rosemary; 14) How to use herbs for bathing and beauty benefits; 15) Herbs and their effect on the emotions; 16) Herbal smoking substitutes for tobacco; and 17) Roundup of miscellaneous herbs. A glossary of terms and a list of herb dealers and homeopathic pharmacies have been appended.

176.   Lucas, Richard. **The Magic of Herbs in Daily Living.** West Nyack, NY: Parker Publishing Co., 1972. 263p. index. $8.95. LC 72-6870. ISBN 0-13-544-981-2.

Extensive coverage of herbal remedies for a wide variety of health problems, along with treatments to help tone sex organs, lose weight, treat baldness, and explore the supernatural, are covered in this book.

Chapter headings are: 1) How to Use Herbs to Tone the Sex Organs; 2) How Herbs Can Help Restore Youthful Digestive Powers; 3) How Herbs can Strengthen Your Vision; 4) How Herbs Can Help Build Your Blood for a more Youthful Vitality; 5) Selected Herbs to Help Grow and Promote a Beautiful Head of Hair; 6) How Herbs Can Help Sharpen Your Memory; 7) Herbal Preparations to Help You Sleep; 8) Legendary Occult Powers of Herbs, 9) Herbal Preparations for the Relief of Headaches and Tensions; 10) How Herbs Can Help Ease Your Foot Trouble; 11) How Herbs Can Help Shed Unwanted Pounds; 12) How to Use Herbs for Youthful Skin and Complexion; 13) Secrets of Longevity Using Selected Herbs; and 14) Herbal Glamorizers for Daily Use in the Home. A short glossary and a list of herb dealers are included.

The book has merit when viewed as the history or folklore of herbs.

177.   Lucas, Richard. **Nature's Medicines: The Folklore, Romance, and Value of Herbal Remedies.** West Nyack, NY: Parker Publishing Co., 1966; repr. North Hollywood, CA: Melvin Powers Wilshire Book Co., 1977. 224p. index. $3.00pa. LC 66-17159. ISBN 0-87980-105-0.

This book is for the lay public, but the author hopes it will inspire physicians and scientific researchers to give more attention to healing agents from plants. The work discusses various herbal remedies used through the ages and then attempts to show that their use was, and still is, justified. Also folklore, romance, and history of herbs are covered. In addition, there is a chapter on mystical plants and their supposed properties.

Contents of the book is as follows: 1) Herbs: our ancient health secret; 2) How ancient herbs become modern medicines; 3) The bulb with miracle healing powers (garlic); 4) The wonder remedy of bygone days (sarsaparilla); 5) A magic herb of proven value (comfrey); 6) One of man's oldest herbal remedies (myrrh); 7) The magic of seeds; 8) The favorite of the Pharaohs (licorice); 9) Strange and mystic plants; 10) The medicine tree (papaya); 11) Citrus fruits; 12) The herb of the Cherokees (golden seal); 13) The intriguing herb that hides from man (ginseng); 14) The secret of perpetual youth; 15) Herbs that condition and beautify the hair; 16) Miscellaneous herbs; and 17) Conclusion. A list of place to purchase herbs and a glossary are appended.

The author concludes that we may be entering a botanical renaissance.

178.   Lust, Benedict. **About Herbs: Medicines from the Meadows.** Edited by P. C. Norris. Wellingborough, Northamptonshire, England: Thorsons Publishers Limited, 1961. 64p. illus. (About Series). $1.75pa. ISBN 0-7225-0074-2.

Herbs which are commonly used in medicine are discussed in this book. Those listed have been selected from the famous Sebastian Kneipp's herbal prescriptions. (Kneipp was well known for his hydrotherapy technique, i.e., "water cure.") Approximately 150 herbs are included in this listing.

Entries are alphabetical by common name, and each includes German, French, Spanish, and Latin names for the herb (and, in some cases, other foreign identifications). Each entry gives a brief note on origin, the maladies for which the herb is prescribed, and how it is used. A few illustrations (line drawings) have been included. Preparation and dosages are not very specific; therefore, it would be somewhat difficult to use this book as a practical home medical guide, although the introduction states the intent is to give directions for use of herbs. The most unique aspect in the book is the inclusion of plant names in other languages, although there is no index to them.

179.   Lust, John B. **The Herb Book.** New York: B. Lust Publications, 1974. 623p. illus. bibliog. $12.95. LC 74-75368. ISBN 0-87904-007-6.

This has been a very popular, rather comprehensive catalog of herbs. It has been reprinted a number of times and is available in paperback (Bantam Books) as well as in hard binding.

The presentation is in several parts, covering history; plants and their properties and applications to various ailments; a listing of medicinal plants with their botanical descriptions and uses; and methods of preparing various concoctions to be used for treatment. The plants are illustrated by 275 line drawings. There are remedies to sooth nerves, cure coughs, and stop nightmares, with case histories provided. Also included are instructions for dyeing fabrics, perfuming the bath, spicing foods, and freshening the breath.

A good deal of basic information is included in the book; it is especially intended for those new to the uses of herbs.

180.   Macleod, Dawn. **A Book of Herbs**. London: Gerald Duckworth and Co., 1968. 191p. illus. (part col.). bibliog. SBN 7156-0406-6.

Ancient lore and up-to-date practical information on how herbs are used in the modern world are discussed in this work. An introductory chapter on herbs is provided. Next comes the largest section of the book—an alphabetically arranged collection of short monographs (about one-half to one page in length) on individual plants, giving their histories, uses, and how to grow them. The remainder of the book includes discussions on the following: pomanders and clove oranges, pot-pourri, cooking with herbs, dyeing with plants, Indian herbs, and terms used by herbalists. In addition, there is a list of suppliers of herb plants, seeds, and prepared herbs, all located in the United Kingdom.

The book has attractive illustrations, some in color. It is interesting and serves well as a reference work.

181.   McNair, James K. **The World of Herbs and Spices**. San Francisco: Ortho Books, Chevron Chemical Co., 1978. 96p. illus. (col.). index. $3.95pa. LC 78-57892. ISBN 0-917102-72-X.

The beautiful, glossy, color photographs of this book catch the eye. It resembles a corporate annual report issued for the public. Despite a "commercial" appearance, good information has been provided.

The book is arranged in six sections. "Herban renewal" is a general overview of the subject, providing background and historical material and a discussion of why there has been renewed interest in herbs. "Utilitarian landscapes" is a discussion of the use of herbs as landscape materials and provides lists of plants used for specific landscape locations.

"Getting down to basics" tells how to grow and preserve herbs. "Herbs and spices for home gardens" gives details of habitat and characteristics of several different herbs. Each description includes a small color photograph of the plant. "Creative ways with herbs and spices" provides all kinds of food recipes as well as ideas for aromatics, cosmetics, fabric coloring, and decorative uses. A final section entitled "Illustrated guide to herbs and spices" includes color photographs of the dried forms of over 160 herbs and spices. Included are remarks about origin, scent, uses, and where grown.

An index, lists of sources of supply (including mail order), and a list of public gardens in the United States enhance the value of this work. The book covers a tremendous variety of information in a fairly short space while, at the same time, being very readable and attractive.

182.   Mausert, Otto. **Herbs for Health: A Guide to Health by Natural Means.** 2d ed. San Francisco, CA: The author, 1936. 200p. illus. (part col.). index.

Although a reprinted edition of this book does not seem to be available, it is the kind of work that reprint publishers are reissuing. The title page says it is "a concise treatise on medicinal herbs, their usefulness and correct combination in the treatment of diseases."

The book consists of sections on: 1) Symptoms and what they may mean; 2) Diseases, their symptoms and suggested remedies; 3) Formulas (remedies referred to in Section 2); 4) Materia medica index (a list of diseases with herbs listed which are used for treatment); and 5) Materia medica (herbs listed with uses and doses. German, French, and Spanish common names are included as well as scientific names for some plants).

183.   Mességué, Maurice. **Health Secrets of Plants and Herbs.** New York: William Morrow and Co., 1979. 336p. illus. (part col.). $17.95. LC 79-87534. ISBN 0-688-03549-3. (Translation of **Mon Herbier de Sante**).

The author states this is not a book to be read straight through, but is a reference work for everyday—a kind of home medical guide using herbal medicine. A number of color plates of selected herbs and many ink drawings make it an attractive work.

There is a short discussion about how various preparations are made and administered, but the largest part of the work is taken up by an alphabetical listing of 100 plants used for medicinal purposes. Each entry (approximately two to three pages) includes a black and white illustration, a brief discussion of the plant's history and the author's own experience with it, how and when to gather the plant, the possible preparations for use as a medicine, and the various therapeutic uses of the herb. Each entry is specific about preparation, dosages, and use.

Even though the author's contact with herbs was evidently mainly in France, most of the plants included are common in the United States or are at least readily available.

An alphabetical "index of complaints," with the author's specific therapeutic advice, makes this work a practical reference book too, particularly for people interested in finding a primitive remedy for something. A short glossary of medical terms completes the book.

184.   Meyer, Joseph. **The Herbalist.** Rev. and enl. ed. by Clarence Meyer. Glenwood, IL: Meyerbooks, (Available from Indiana Botanic Gardens, Hammond, IN 46325), 1960. 304p. illus. (part col.). index. $8.95.

Concise descriptions of over 500 medicinal herbs make up the first half of this book. Each description includes common names, medicinal part of the plant, therapeutic uses, and dosages. Many entries are illustrated by ink drawings, and another section of the book depicts over 250 of these plants in colored plates. Although the plates are colorful, they are of questionable quality for use as a field identification tool.

One section of the book presents listings of herbs by use, such as astringents, cathartics, diuretics, and sedatives. Other sections provide discussions and listings of teas, spices and flavors, cosmetics, wines and cordials, aromatics, dyes, botanical smoke mixtures, and botanical curios. All of these sections give recipes, advice, and all kinds of interesting and useful information. A good general index enhances the value of this book, which is one of the best choices for a basic herbal. It was first published in 1918 and has been regularly printed and revised since that time.

185.   Mitton, F., and V. Mitton. **Mitton's Practical Modern Herbal.** London: W. Foulsham and Co. Ltd., 1976. 134p. illus.   £2.95. ISBN 0-572-00901-1.

The authors of this book are international retail herbalists. The work is presented in two sections. About one-third of the book is taken up by a discussion of the therapeutic properties of herbs and ailments and their herbal medication. The second section is an encyclopedia of herbs. Arrangement is alphabetical by common name, and a line drawing is provided for most plants. Other information given includes scientific name, synonyms, habitat, appearance or description, therapeutic or culinary uses, traditional and/or reputed uses, and authors' comments that include warnings about toxic herbs.

186.   Monardes, Nicholas. **Joyfull Newes Out of the Newe Founde Worlde.** Written in Spanish by Nicholas Monardes, Physician of Seville, and Englished by John Frampton, Merchant, Anno 1577, with an Introduction by Stephen Gaselee. London: Constable and Co., New York, Alfred A. Knopf, 1925; repr. New York: AMS Press. 2v. illus. (Tudor Translations, Second Series, nos. 9-10). $30.00 the set. ISBN 0-404-51990-3.

This is another old book, available now in a reprinted edition.

At the time the original work was written, hitherto unknown medicines from the New World were becoming available and, although untried in Europe, they had the reputation of near magical potency. Monardes became so interested in them that he developed these volumes that provide a historical description of the medicines. The book became popular and appeared in several editions.

Monardes begins by describing certain gums, China-root, sarsaparilla, blood stone, pepper or pimiento, and other plant products. The second part includes descriptions of tobacco (at some length), sassafras, a certain kind of barley, "dragon's blood," ambergris, and, surprisingly, an armadillo. The third part is composed of descriptions of medicines of less importance, some extensions of those mentioned previously. Included are cinnamon, rhubarb, ginger, verbena, and balsams (already known in the Old World). There are also essays on materials of supposed special virtue, the Bezaar stone (a kidney stone from a goat), and the herb escuerçonera (presumed to be an antidote for poisons). The remainder of the work is taken up by discussions on subjects connected with health and medicine; the first is on iron and its virtues, the second on snow.

The work is a curiosity and of considerable historical interest; however, it is difficult to read because of the old (probably Middle English) spelling used.

187.   Morton, Julia F. **Herbs and Spices.** New York: Golden Press, a division of Western, 1976. 160p. illus. (col.). index. $5.95. LC 76-5918. ISBN 0-307-64364-0.

More than 370 plants used for flavoring and seasoning are presented in this work with concise botanical and horticultural notes provided. An outstanding feature of the book is the color illustrations included. The author is a botanist known for her works on medicinal and other economic plants.

188.   Moulten, LeArta. **Nature's Medicine Chest.** Provo, UT: BiWorld. 6 sets of cards. Sets 1-2, $3.50 each; sets 4-6, $4.50 each.

This collection of file cards contains 240 cards with photographs and 226 additional information cards. Color photographs of herbs appear on one side of the picture cards and, on the other side, there is information on how to identify, grow, gather, use, and store the herbs.

The picture cards feature useful roadside plants; spice herbs; trees, shrubs, berries, flowers, and roots used as medicinals; edible plants; and poisonous plants. The information cards cover a variety of topics such as beauty aids, perfumes, pesticides, wild herbs for food, domesticating wild plants, and a glossary of medicinal effects and the herbs which produce them.

189.   Muenscher, Walter Conrad, and Myron Arthur Rice. **Garden Spice and Wild Pot-Herbs: An American Herbal.** With illustrations cut on wood by Elfriede Abbe. Ithaca and London, Comstock Publishing Associates, a division of Cornell University Press (124 Roberts Place, Ithaca, NY 14850), 1978. 213p. illus. index. $6.95pa. LC 78-56899. ISBN 0-8014-9174-6.

This work is a recent edition of a book first published in 1955 that was a hand-set edition. A description of more than 250 common and a few exotic plants is provided, along with hints on how to recognize, grow, harvest and prepare them for use.

The authors comment that much of the information published on herbs emphasizes historical and legendary aspects and medicinal uses, but that accurate botanical information about the plants is often lacking. Also, many inaccuracies are reflected in catalogs and advertisements. An attempt is made here to provide correct botanical information.

The book is in four sections as follows: 1) Descriptions of the herbs; 2) Treatment of the herbs. Propagation and hardiness; harvesting, drying, and storing; 3) Wild pot-herbs; and 4) The classification and naming of plants; list of synonyms. In addition, a glossary and a section illustrating and describing seeds have been provided. The first section makes up about two-thirds of the book. Entries are arranged by families. Common features of each are described, and familiar members of the family are named. Each entry begins with the Latin name of the plant (updated according to *Hortus III*. See entry 34) followed by its most common English name. Other names, including those in French, German, and Italian, are also given. The first paragraph of each entry is a botanical description; then culinary and other uses are given, culture described, and natural distribution indicated. The third section (on wild pot-herbs) describes 16 herbs that taste good.

The book is enhanced by a special typeface and attractive woodcuts.

190.   Northcote, Lady Rosalind. **The Book of Herb Lore.** (Formerly titled: **The Book of Herbs**). New York: Dover Publications, Inc., 1971. 212p. illus. bibliog. index. $2.50pa. LC 75-143676. ISBN 0-486-22694-8.

This is an unabridged republication of the second edition of a work published in 1912 by John Lane: *The Bodley Head.* The book cites thousands of traditions and lore associated with herbs throughout history. In addition, there are descriptions of practical uses the ancients made of herbs.

Nearly every aspect of herbs and herb lore is covered as can be seen by the chapter headings: 1) Of the Chief Herbs Used in the Present Time; 2) Of Herbs Chiefly Used in the Past; 3) Of Herbs Used in Decorations, in Heraldry, and for Ornament and Perfumes; 4) Of the Growing of Herbs; 5) Of Herbs in Medicine; 6) Of Herbs and Magic; 7) Of Herbs and Beasts. An appendix provides a list of seeds and herbs for the kitchen.

A bibliography has been provided, and numerous literature references are made in the text. It would be difficult, though, to follow up on many of the references since only authors and titles are given with an occasional date; however, some of the references are to classic works.

191.   Null, Gary, and Steve Null. **Herbs for the Seventies.** New York: Dell Publishing Co., 1972. 256p. bibliog. index. $1.25pa. ISBN 0-440-13549-4.

This is an account of the uses of herbs presumed to be beneficial for healing, maintaining health, and beauty. The first chapter is a brief historical overview of the uses of herbs in ancient China, the Bible, ancient Egypt and Greece, and by the American Indians. Other chapters are as follows: 1) The Herb Way for the 70's; 2) The Nervines; 3) Alfalfa Is "People" Food; 4) The Lemon—Another of Nature's Treasures; 5) The Many Benefits of Licorice; 6) The Mistletoe Mystery; 7) Nettle—A Useless Weed or a Useful Plant?; 8) The Olive Tree—A Symbol of Peace; 9) Rosemary, Sage and Time; 10) The "Man-Shaped" Roots; 11) The Modest Onion; 12) Herbs as a Treatment for Poison Ivy; 13) Herbal Beauty; 14) The Second Stage to Beauty; 15) Herbs and the Feet; 16) More about Water and Disease; and 17) Hair Is Beauty.

The last chapter, "Definition of Medicinal Properties of Herbs," makes up about half the book. Herbs are listed alphabetically by common name with a brief paragraph on each. Other names for the plants are indicated with uses and virtues outlined. The bibliography lists mainly old works.

The authors come very close to rash exaggeration when discussing the value of herbs; however, in all fairness, the statements are often tempered by such phrases as "it has been used for," "reportedly it will," "doses taken have been said to," or "it has been known to."

192.   Page, Mary. **The Observer's Book of Herbs.** With illustrations by Norman Barber. London: F. Warne, 1980. 184p. illus. (part col.). bibliog. index. (Observer's Pocket Series). £1.50. ISBN 07232-1610-X.

A good deal of miscellaneous information about herbs is presented in this book. About a third of the contents is given to descriptions and colored illustrations of about 65 species of plants. Another third covers cultivation, culinary uses, and medicinal uses of herbs. Included are suggestions on how to lay out the herb garden, and historical information and lore is related. The last part of the book deals with cultivation and growing herbs in special places such as in tubs, window boxes, and lawns. In addition, instructions on preserving the herbs for home use are given.

193.   Parvati, Jeannine. **Hygieia: A Woman's Herbal.** Drawings by Tamara Slayton Glenn; calligraphy by Quill Cleaver. Distributed by Bookpeople (2940 7th St., Berkeley, CA 94710), 1978. 248p. illus. bibliog. index. (A Freestone Collective Book). $9.00pa. LC 78-67918. ISBN 0-913512-54-0.

This is indeed a most unusual book on herbs. The author of the work, a midwife, yoga teacher, feminist health counselor, astrologer, and mother, calls upon Hygieia, the Greek goddess of health, to give guidance in herbal remedies for feminine health. Parvati says she has written from a wholistic perspective on female sexuality and fertility.

About 300 herbs are mentioned in the book. Popular and scientific names are given for each, with history, myths, and folk tales about them included. In addition, the author has assembled herbal recipes. She makes no guarantees about the efficacy of the concoctions, but suggests reliance on intuition and mind-power, and states that herbs are psychic tools.

There are chapters on menstrual rituals; infertility; herbal birth control; anaphrodisiacs; aphrodisiacs; herbs for the mind (such as marijuana, ergot, LSD, and peyote); self-health; balancers and toners; pregnancy, childbirth, lactation; and the menopause. In addition, there is a glossary, a bibliography, and a large number of appendices. The latter take up about one-third of the book and are a motley assortment of materials, including poetry, dreams, meditations, stories, and letters. Much material evidently is contributed by friends and correspondents.

The book is a curious mixture of material. It is attractive in many respects and has some nice illustrations and decorations. The author is literate and educated. However, a great deal of the text makes little sense; some material is offensive, and claims do not appear to be based on scientific evidence (a point the author herself makes from time to time). Then why was the book written? Perhaps the best answer can be found in the statement that this work reportedly is "the first book of its kind to interweave the ancient practice of herbalism with the new women's consciousness and wholistic health." Despite the claims, this book adds no desirable dimension to the women's movement.

194.   Petulengro, Leon. **Herbs, Health and Astrology.** New Canaan, CT: Keats, 1977. 95p. illus. (Keats Living with Herbs Series, No.1). $2.50pa. LC 76-58769. ISBN 0-87983-140-0.

The arrangement of this little book is by astrological sign. Three or four herbs are listed under each sign, plus a concise statement of health problems and diseases associated with the sign. For each herb mentioned, there is a discussion of uses, habitat, and nutritional information. A few historical remarks are given, and several recipes, both culinary and medicinal, are included, many which were passed down to the author by his relatives. The book ends with one page of directions on how to dry herbs and a glossary of medical terms.

195.   Reppert, Bertha P. **A Heritage of Herbs.** Illustrated by Margaret S. Browne and Marjorie L. Reppert. Harrisburg, PA: Stackpole Books, 1976. 192p. illus. bibliog. index. $8.95. LC 76-8239. ISBN 0-8117-0796-2.

Included in this engaging work is material on the history of herbs, early herb gardening, and old recipes.

The first chapter discusses herbs colonists found in America. About 230 are listed alphabetically with brief information given. The second chapter, "Early American Gardens," contains, in addition to text, a chronological list of quotations from early book and periodicals about herbs. The Shakers are discussed. The next chapter describes and pictures several colonial herb gardens. A plan of the kitchen garden of Mount Vernon is included. Other garden discussed are the bee garden, the apothecary's garden, the dyer's garden, and the sentimental garden. The following chapter contains about 75 modernized antique recipes with discussions of the use of the rose, boxwood, and espaliers and topiaries. Recipes include such preparations as skin creams, cough syrups, salves, rinses for the hair, cologne, and teas, as well as foods. There is a chapter on today's public herb gardens in which a number are listed, by state and city, with brief information. The last chapter, "Garden Herbs at a Glance," lists about 85 useful herbal plants with statements on lifestyle (annual or perennial, etc.), how to plant, when and where to plant, harvesting, preservation, description, uses, and special notes.

The book is attractively illustrated with photographs of gardens and line-drawings of the plants described.

196.   Riggs, Carol. **Herbs, Leaves of Magic.** Illustrated by Betsy Rodgers-Knox. Boulder, CO: Sycamore Island Books, 1979. 199p. illus. (part col.). $7.95pa. LC 78-27503. ISBN 0-87364-153-1.

The underlying view taken by the author of this book is that herbs hold a unique place in nature—to enrich our lives with their flavors, fragrances, and foliages. The presentation helps the reader make the most of herbs as ornamentals and in enhancing foods. The book begins with herbal history, takes up planting an herb garden, provides information on harvesting and preserving the crop, and ends with information on how to use herbs at the table.

197.   Rose, Jeanne. **Herbs and Things: Jeanne Rose's Herbal.** New York: Grosset and Dunlap, 1973. 323p. illus. bibliog. index. $5.95pa. LC 70-145729. ISBN 0-448-01139-5.

This book contains three sections—Directions, Recipes, and Secrets. The Directions section, which makes up about one-third of the book, provides information on almost every aspect of herbalism. There is a "materia medica" included as well as a directory of sources for herb plants and seeds. Also, miscellaneous information on cosmetic and culinary uses of herbs is found throughout the section along with historical remarks. The second and largest section is a discussion of diseases and other medical complaints with suggested herbal treatment for each. Exact preparations and dosages are given. The third section includes information about astrological signs and their relation to various plants, a "language of flowers," and "forbidden secrets." Discussed, among other things, is how to summon evil spirits.

A comprehensive bibliography is included.

198.   Rufinus. **The Herbal of Rufinus.** Edited from the Unique Manuscript by Lynn Thorndike, assisted by Francis S. Benjamin, Jr. Chicago: University of Chicago Press, 1946. 476p. index.

This is a publication of the late thirteenth-century manuscript work of Rufinus on herbs. There was only one known existing manuscript of it at the time of this edition. The work, which is in Latin, was prepared from a photostatic copy of the original, which was housed in the Laurentian Library at Florence. Even though Rufinus's work was not well known to scholars and historians of botany, the editor felt it would enrich our knowledge of medieval botany and medicine.

Much of Rufinus's work is based on that of other authorities such as Dioscorides. About one-fifth of the text is by Rufinus himself. Most of the work deals with herbs and vegetable products, but there is some coverage of animal products and minerals. The following indexes are provided: I) Herbs and other simples and some compound medicines; II) Diseases and parts of the body affected; III) Measures, instruments, and utensils; IV) Names of persons and titles of anonymous works; and V) Names of places.

199.   Rutherford, Meg. **A Pattern of Herbs: Herbs for Goodness, Food and Health and How to Identify and Grow Them.** With medical notes by Ann Warren-Davis. New York: Doubleday and Co., Inc., 1976. 157p. illus. bibliog. index. (Dolphin Books). $2.95pa. LC 74-18848. ISBN 0-385-07065-9.

This book is intended for those who have difficulty in identifying herbs. The drawings, done by the author in what is referred to as a neo-Victorian style, should assist the beginner. Smaller plant details have been omitted in order not to obscure the shape of the plant, and silhouette drawings are often provided.

Preliminary material in the book includes an index of herbs, an introduction, sections on herbal medicine and medicinal uses, and a list of medical terms. The main part of the work presents herbs divided into these sections: 1) Herbs from various families; 2) Daisy family; 3) Two-lipped flowers; and 4) Umbelliferae. About 50 plants are discussed, with the following given about each: names, description, habitat and cultivation, kitchen uses, and recipes. The work concludes with a "kitchen summary" that lists common foods and herbs that complement them.

200.   Sanecki, Kay N. **The Complete Book of Herbs.** Advisory editor, Gertrude B. Foster; drawings by Edward Russell. New York: Macmillan, 1974. 247p. illus. (part col.). bibliog. index. $9.95. LC 73-2123.

Although this book covers many topics relating to herbs, the actual number of plants included is rather small, being limited to plants that die at the end of the growing season and that have medicinal, savory, or aromatic qualities. Information provided seems to be accurate and interesting, and includes gardening, cookery (with recipes), medical botany, and biographical material on herbalists and collectors.

The plants are arranged alphabetically by common name, and each is described with history, uses, cultivation, and a fine line drawing. Some color plates are included.

201.   Schaeffer, Elizabeth. **Dandelion, Pokeweed, and Goosefoot: How the Early Settlers Used Plants for Food, Medicine, and in the Home.** Reading, MA: Addison-Wesley, 1972. 94p. illus. bibliog. index. $5.95pa. LC 79-17852. ISBN 0-201-09306-5.

This small, attractive book is divided into three parts. Part 1 is brief but contains a good general discussion of herbal terminology, including problems of Latin names and of a meaningful definition of an "herb." Some historical information is also included in this section. Part 2 makes up most of the book and is itself divided into three parts by category of plants: those found in woodlands, pasturelands, and swamplands. Plants are discussed as to their medicinal, food, and household values. Information on habitat and description is included, but specific recipes, dosages, preparation, and harvesting information is usually lacking. Most of the entries are illustrated by ink drawings. Part 3 is a concise discussion of making your own garden, collecting and drying herbs, general hints on making teas and salads, and how to dye cloth using selected plants.

The book is interestingly written but is not very detailed.

202.   Silverman, Maida. **A City Herbal: A Guide to the Lore, Legend, and Usefulness of 34 Plants That Grow Wild in the City.** New York: Albert A. Knopf, 1977. 181p. illus. bibliog. index. $10.00; $5.95pa. LC 76-47930. ISBN 0-394-498526; ISBN 0-394-73297-9pa.

The author tries in this attractive book to foster an appreciation for common herbs ("weeds" to many individuals) growing wild in large cities such as New York, where she lives.

After a short introduction, the plants are listed alphabetically by common name. Each monograph runs several pages, and included with each is a line drawing of the plant done by the author. The following information is usually given for each plant: scientific name; folknames; location; botanical description; historical lore, legends, and uses; and additional suggested uses. Recipes are sometimes included for breads, salads, seasonings, teas, dyes, and cosmetics. Supplementary materials include an appendix on Dyeing with Natural Plant Materials and a glossary.

203.   Simmons, Adelma Grenier. **The Illustrated Herbal Handbook.** New York: Hawthorn Books Inc., 1972. 124p. illus. index. $2.95pa. LC 75-182819. ISBN 0-8015-3960-9.

The one and only section of this book is made up of a listing of herbs arranged by horticultural name. A short index provides one or two common names for each plant.

Each entry includes brief historical information, a description of the plant, uses, culture, and an illustration. Uses are mainly culinary, but occasionally medicinal and cosmetic uses are included. Several known varieties of a particular plant are given in certain cases, for instance, the geranium. A brief description is included for each of these special varieties.

Specific recipes are not provided in the book. However, the sections on culture with each entry are comprehensive enough to be useful.

204.   Smith, William. **Wonders in Weeds.** Bradford, England: Health Science Press, 1977. 187p. illus. $10.00 ISBN 0-85032151-4.

Detailed discussions of 56 common herbs make up this book. Those familiar with herbs will recognize most of the plants. Each description is two to three pages in length and includes information about natural habitat, cultivation and uses, modern medicinal and culinary uses, and how the plant may be identified. Arrangement is alphabetical by common name. Most plants are illustrated by ink drawings.

The book also contains a short section on how to prepare herbal remedies, a glossary of botanical names, a glossary of medical terms, a therapeutic index which lists herbs and indicates medical problems that can be treated by each, and, in addition, another index listing complaints and disorders with herbal remedies suggested. The book provides a good deal of basic and interesting information. However, like many other herb books it is extremely biased against conventional medicine. The author states in the foreword, "It cannot be emphasized too highly that herbal medicine is 'safe medicine', a claim that cannot be applied to orthodox remedies." This is absolutely untrue; many medicinal plants, including some listed in the book, are toxic.

205.   Spoerke, David G., Jr. **Herbal Medications.** Santa Barbara, CA: Woodbridge Press Publishing Co. (P. O. Box 6189, Santa Barbara, CA 93111), 1980. 192p. illus. (col.). bibliog. index. $5.95pa. LC 80-17551. ISBN 0-912800-72-8.

Putting herbal medicines in proper perspective is the goal of the author of this work, a professor of clinical pharmacy at the University of Utah and managing director of the Intermountain Regional Poison Control Center. Spoerke points out that a growing number of individuals believe herbal medicines are the only true means of obtaining "natural" health. Likewise, he says, there are those who believe all herbal medication is quackery and that the only safe, effective drugs are those produced by pharmaceutical companies. The truth lies somewhere between these views, the author claims.

Many herbs have had little pharmacologic testing, Spoerke reports, and precise information about them is lacking. One of the aims of this book is to clarify some of the claims made for various herbs. Many herbs are harmful despite the widespread belief to the contrary, the author states. The quantity of the active constituents of a plant may be quite variable, for instance.

The book presents monographs of about a page on more than 200 medicinal herbs, arranged alphabetically by common name. Information provided includes scientific name, synonymous names, known principles, mode of action, alleged uses, toxicity, comments, and references to literature. Also included is a glossary of terms.

Spoerke has made a noteworthy attempt to present information based on scientific evidence. If there is no basis in fact to be found for claims made for various herbs, or if adverse effects have been reported, he has so stated.

206.   Stobart, Tom. **The International Wine and Food Society's Guide to Herbs, Spices, and Flavorings.** New York: McGraw-Hill, 1973. 261p. illus. (part col.). index. $9.95. LC 72-3583. SBN 07-061565-9.

The first part of this book covers the history of herbs, spices, and flavoring; the importance of flavorings; synthetic and harmful flavorings; and herb growing. The second part lists alphabetically about 400 herbs, spices, and flavorings. French, German, Italian, and Spanish translated names are given for some entry words; botanical and family names are always indicated. The book includes some color plates and nice line drawings.

207.   Thomson, William A. R. **Herbs That Heal.** New York: Scribner's, 1976. 184p. illus. bibliog. index. $4.95pa. LC 77-72361. ISBN 0-684-14913-3.

This book is not a listing of herbs or diseases as most herbals are, but is a discussion of the part that herbs can play in modern medicine. Herbs still have value in modern medicine, the author states, and more research needs to be done to further utilize nature. The author is a British physician.

There are 10 chapters that discuss the usefulness of various herbs and plants in relation to nourishment of the body, soothing the body, cancer, heart disease, blood clotting, colds, and fertility. Other topics included are Oriental medicine; the value of licorice root; and a discussion of ergot, a cereal fungus used in modern medicine (the substance from which LSD is made). Each discussion includes considerable historical information, several case histories, and general information on dietary matters. Even though there are general references to scientific studies, such literature is not specifically cited. The bibliography includes mostly medical histories and herbals.

208.   Tierra, Michael. **The Way of Herbs.** Edited and supplemented by Subhuti Dharmananda. Santa Cruz, CA: Unity Press, 1980. 216p. illus. bibliog. index. $6.95pa. LC 12190. ISBN 0-913300-43-8.

Eastern, European, and American Indian herbal medicine traditions are blended in this book. The author is evidently a practicing herbalist, a certified acupuncturist, and holds a naturopathic degree. The editor is an herbalist with an imposing background in biochemistry, physiology, and practical pharmacology, and holds a Ph.D. degree.

Chapter headings and contents of the book are as follows: 1) Balance: The Key to Health; 2) Theory of Using Herbs; 3) Herbal Therapies (Traditional methods of herbal therapy described. Among these are stimulation, tranquilization, blood purification, and tonification); 4) Methods of Application (Details are provided for the proper method of making teas, tinctures, liniments, salves, pills, etc.); 5) Herbal Propertics (Types of drugs, such as analgesics, antacids, etc., are listed with definitions and examples); 6) Diagnosis and Treatment (A system is presented based on Chinese Yin/Yang theory); 7) A Balanced Diet; 8) Kitchen Medicines (Lists spices commonly used in foods with comments about their supposed medicinal qualities); 9) Herbs to Know (Provides descriptions and uses for 80 common Western herbs and 18 important Chinese herbs. Includes common and botanical names, part of plant used, systems of the body affected by the herb, properties, methods of preparation, and dosage); 10) Obtaining and Storing Herbs; 11) Making an Herbal Formula (Presents about 25 herb formulas such as tonics for the liver and kidneys, an eyewash, a heartburn formula, an all-purpose liniment, and a sleep formula); 12) Treatments for Specific Ailments (Formulas for a variety of problems such as arthritis, fevers, hemorrhoids, overweight, skin problems, burns, headaches, and weakness); and 13) Cautionary Notes on Herb Use (Potential hazards are stated, including irritating effects of essential oils, possible overdose, and cumulative effects of herbs).

There are three appendices as follows: 1) Traveler's first aid (A chart showing ingredients for a first aid kit. Includes treatments for such problems as sunburn, diarrhea, poison ivy, and wounds); 2) Where to buy herbs (Includes addresses of sources);

and 3) East-West master course in herbology (A notice about a correspondence course the author has prepared).

209.   Tobe, John H. **Proven Herbal Remedies.** With a section on General Rules for Gathering and Preserving Herbs by Thomas Green. St. Catharines, Ontario: Provoker Press, 1969. 303p. bibliog. index. (Also Pyramid Press, 1973. $1.50pa. ISBN 0-515-0329-5).

The main section of this book is an alphabetical listing of ailments with an herbal plant named to be used for that condition. Provided with each entry is scientific name, common name, where found, part used, action, dissertation (comments), method of preparation, and dosage. Quotations from well-known and classic herbals are used often. The entries are about one-third to a half-page in length.

Other short sections are as follows: 1) Herbal compounds; 2) Herbs used in cancer; 3) Guide to therapeutic action; 4) Forms of botanical medicinal preparations; 5) Definitions of herbal medical terms; 6) Common doses and equivalents; 7) Abbreviations for weights and measures; 8) Table of weights and measures; 9) Vitamins and their botanic sources; 10) Herbal teas; 11) Gather your own herbs. The bibliography contains incomplete references to some ancient (beginning with the Bible) and some modern works. Indexes are by common name, botanical name, and ailments and uses.

210.   Twitchell, Paul. **Herbs: The Magic Healers.** New York: Lancer Books, 1971. 189p. $1.95pa.

The author of this book is called a modern living master of the ancient order ECKANKAR, a group who believed in soul travel and who realized that healthy bodies aided in developing the concentration needed to reach the supreme diety. The masters of ECKANKAR were evidently proponents of "natural organic" foods and used herbs for their "magic" curative powers.

The book presents, in narrative form, information about the ancient and modern uses of various herbs, with background and historical information stressed. A good deal of superstition seems to be involved. There are no literature references included. It is difficult to find information on any one herb because there is no index, and little classification is attempted.

Following are chapter titles: 1) Herbs, The Ancient Way to Physical and Spiritual Well-Being; 2) The Restoration of Spiritual Health through Herbs; 3) The Herbs that Give Life for the Vital Powers; 4) The Magic of the Wonder Herbs; 5) The Life-Giving Properties of Seeds; 6) Herbs and Karmic Conditions of Man; 7) The Sacred Herb of the Ancient Mystics; 8) The Strange and Curious Herbs that Bring Health; 9) Herbs and the Wheel of the ECK-Vidya; 10) The Sacred Herb of the ECK Masters for Longevity; 11) Health Secrets of the ACK Adepts; and 12) Health as an Aid in Spiritual Growth.

211.   Weiner, Michael A. **Weiner's Herbal: The Guide to Herb Medicine.** With Janet Weiner; and with recent chemical and pharmacological findings by Norman R. Farnsworth. New York: Stein and Day, 1980. 224p. illus. bibliog. index. $18.95; $6.95pa. LC 78-26616. ISBN 0-8128-2586-1; 0-8128-6023-3pa.

Because the practice of herbal medicine goes back many thousands of years, a great deal of folklore has grown up around it. The introduction to this book rightly points out that many herbal remedies do not work, and that no ailment should be treated herbally for a long period of time. A physician should be consulted instead.

The main part of the presentation consists of monographs on herbal plants, arranged alphabetically by common name. For each is given a botanical description, medicinal uses with history and folklore, and usual dose. Warnings about side effects and overdoses are provided. A noted pharmacognosit, Norman R. Farnsworth, has provided recent chemical and pharmacological findings. There are indexes by Latin name, common name, and medicinal use.

212.   Yemm, J. R., ed. **The Medical Herbalist.** 1977 edition. North Hollywood, CA: Wilshire Book Co. (12015 Sherman Road, North Hollywood, CA 91605), 1976. 231p. illus. $3.00pa. ISBN 0-87980-309-6.
        This book is a collection of articles written by several authors, including a person identified simply as "Aunt Jennie." Although no indication is given of the source or date of the material, it seems to be a selection of articles from *The Medical Herbalist*, a periodical published in England in the 1930s. By chance it was found that the publication is a virtually exact reprint of a book published in the 1930s containing articles from Volume XI (about 1935-37) of the periodical (published by the National Association of Medical Herbalists of Great Britain, Ltd.).
        The articles are on a variety of subjects, but most discuss the use of herbs for therapeutic purposes; several address the value of good nutrition and diet, while others attack modern medicine. Herbal preparations (formulas or recipes) are found throughout the book. Included are concoctions for treating every ailment from a simple sore throat to cancer. Treatments for cancer include herbal preparations for purifying the blood as well as external poultices. Several historical sketches are scattered throughout the publication.

6
HERB GROWING

A number of practical works covering the techniques of herb growing, both in and out of doors, are included here. Also included are books that discuss the plan and design of herb gardens, describe some famous gardens of the past and today, and emphasize appreciation of gardening. Some individuals feel that culture of herbs should be more for enjoyment than for any practical use.

In addition, there are several works on growing illegal hallucinogenic plants (often described as "herbs") such as marijuana, psilocybin mushrooms, and peyote cacti.

* * * * *

213.   Back, Philippa. **Choosing, Planting, and Cultivating Herbs.** New Canaan, CT: Keats Publication, 1977. 93p. illus. bibliog. (Keats Living with Herbs Series, No.2). $2.50pa. LC 76-58770. ISBN 0-87983-149-9.

As the title indicates, the emphasis of this small book is on cultivation, maintenance, and marketing of herbs. There is very little historical and medicinal information. It contains seven chapters as follows: 1) Choosing the Best Herbs for Different Purposes; 2) Planning a Garden; 3) Alphabetical Listing of Herbs with Notes on Cultivation; 4) General Cultivation of Garden Plants and Herbs; 5) Harvesting and Drying Herbs; 6) Marketing Techniques; and 7) Alphabetical Listing of Herbs with Notes on Their Various Ues. The last chapter covers 36 herbs.

The book is a concise introduction to an important aspect of herbalism.

214.   Birdseye, Clarence, and Eleanor G. Birdseye. **Growing Woodland Plants.** New York: Oxford University Press, 1951; repr. New York: Dover Publications, Inc., 1972. 223p. illus. bibliog. index. $2.75pa. LC 72-87872. ISBN 0-486-20661-0.

Cultivation of woodland plants, many of which are becoming quite scarce, is encouraged in this book. Suitable for both novices and experienced gardeners, information is included on over 200 wildflowers and ferns native to the United States, particularly north of Virginia and east of Montana. For each plant is given: common and scientific names, description, illustrations (line drawings), blossoming time, habitat, range, cultural requirements, and propagation directions.

The work is in two parts. The first 54 pages present the following chapters: 1) Woodland Conditions; 2) Making Synthetic Soil; 3) Stepping Stones, Paths, and Groundlitter; 4) Making the Woodsgarden; 5) Collecting Wildflowers; 6) Care of Woodsgardens; 7) Shade-houses; 8) Propagation; 9) Using Surplus Plants; and 10) Indoor Forcing. The second section presents descriptions of plants. Uses and myths regarding them have been included. Also provided are a table of soil reaction requirements for plants (preferred pH) and a glossary.

The authors do not consider themselves authorities on horticulture and have written in lay language. The material seems to be scientifically correct, however, as a number of recognized authorities were consulted about the book. Information presented should prove valuable to herb gardeners interested in woodland plants.

215.   Brimer, John Burton. **Growing Herbs in Pots.** New York: Fireside Books (Simon and Schuster), 1976. 206p. illus. index. $3.95pa. ISBN 0-671-24207-5.

The first half of this book is a discussion of 11 popular herbs with cultivation instructions, references to general types of culinary recipes for the specific herb, some historical information, and remarks on uses other than culinary. Twelve other herbs are also listed with brief remarks about their uses. Other chapters in the first half of the book cover instructions for planting and care of plants, discussions of light and water needs, and preservation of harvested herbs. The second half of the book is made up of recipes arranged under broad headings such as sauces, meats, and butters, to name a few. There is both a recipe and a general index.

The emphasis of the book is on culinary uses of popular herbs and how to grow them in limited space such as indoors.

216.   Clarkson, Rosetta E. **Green Enchantment: The Magic Spell of Gardens.** Illustrations from early gardening books and herbals. New York: Macmillan, 1940; repr. New York: Dover, 1972. 328p. illus. index. $3.00pa. ISBN 0-486-22869-X. (Reprinted ed. has title **The Golden Age of Herbs and Herbalists**).

The author intends through this work to recapture the mystery and lure of gardens and to recount tales and legends surrounding the plants. Although the book contains no formal bibliography, many references are made to early works, and there is an index to the books and authors mentioned. The fine illustrations included are all from such books. In addition, the author has provided many quotations from classics, both literary and herbal.

Following are chapter headings: 1) In a Monstery Garden; 2) The Golden Age of Herbalists; 3) Beginnings of the Flower Garden; 4) Herbs of Beauty; 5) Some Creeping Thymes and Fragrant Mints; 6) Old-Time Favorites; 7) Scented Geraniums; 8) The Tooth of Saturn; 9) Early Gardening Tools; 10) Flowers in Food; 11) Flowers in Medicine; 12) A Prelude to Salads; 13) The Witches' Garden; 14) Herbs that Never Were; 15) The Modern Role of Ancient Herbs; and 16) Garden Designs.

The book is nicely done in every way.

217.   Clarkson, Rosetta E. **Herbs and Savory Seeds.** New York: Macmillan, 1939; repr. New York: Dover, 1972. 369p. illus. index. $3.00pa. ISBN 0-486-22728-6. (Original title: **Magic Gardens: a Modern Chronicle of Herbs and Savory Seeds**).

The author states this work is not meant to be just about herbs, but is intended also "to be rather a foundation book for any gardener and still of interest to the general reader who likes the thought of a garden or who loves to dream of the gardens of long ago." Illustrations have been taken from the "old herbals and ancient gardening books."

The main emphasis is on herbs, their culture, harvesting, and uses. Plants covered are not only the ones grown for medicinal qualities, but also include those used for fragrance, flavor, and beauty. Construction of herb gardens is discussed and illustrations included. Garden designs are taken from ancient gardens and contain walls and wattles, knots and parterres, and mazes and labyrinths.

There is no separate bibliography or list of references in the work; instead a large number of old works are described and quoted in the text. There is a special index to these books by author and title. The last chapter is a list of "noteworthy herbs" that includes botanical names and descriptions. Tables of the following are also presented: 1) Herbs for fragrance; 2) Culinary herbs for foliage; 3) Culinary herbs for savory seeds; 4) Herbs of legendary or historic interest; 5) Stately herbs; 6) Colorful herbs; 7) Doctrine of signatures; 8) Herb teas; and 9) Language of the herbs.

218. **The Compleat Psilocybin Mushroom Cultivator's Bible.** 2d ed. Miami, FL: Hongero Press, 1976. 71p. illus. (part col.). bibliog. $5.00pa.

This booklet offers complete growing directions for cultivating psilocybin mushrooms, a hallucinogenic plant. In addition, instructions are given on preserving and using the crop. Also included is a field guide section of all North American species and a color identification section of plates.

Following are chapter headings: 1) Psilocybin and Psilocin; 2) In the Field; 3) Spore Printing; 4) Growing Mycelium; 5) Growing Spawn; 6) Casing Grain Jars; 7) Cultivating in Beds; 8) Pests of Mushroom Beds; 9) Preserving; and 10) Ingestion.

219. Drake, Bill. **The Cultivator's Handbook of Marijuana.** Rev. and expanded ed. Berkeley, CA: Wingbow Press; dist. Bookpeople (2940 Seventh St., Berkeley, CA 94710), 1979. 223p. illus. bibliog. index. $8.95. ISBN 914728-31-8.

Complete information on how to grow and cultivate the marijuana plant is presented here, with photographs, charts, maps, and diagrams. The book covers identification of male and female plants (females yield the more potent substances), choosing a site for planting, chemical makeup of the soil, pruning, grafting, light, seed selection, transplanting, and water and atmospheric requirements. In addition, harvesting and curing are discussed. The book also contains a chapter on the history of the use of the marijuana plant, with traditions and myths retold and a discussion of legal problems presented.

Other material includes a chapter on the "Cultivation of Psychoactive Tobacco." The author evidently believes that tobacco used in commercial products is inferior to "true herbal tobacco." Throughout the book, interspersed with practical advice, the author looks at what might be called the spiritual and psychic aspects of the subject. He calls marijuana a great force in the evolution of human consciousness, central to the liberation of feelings and ideas.

220. Elbert, Virginia F., and George A. Elbert. **Fun with Growing Herbs Indoors.** New York: Crown Publishers, Inc., 1974. 192p. illus. (part col.). bibliog. index. $7.95; $4.95pa. LC 74-80320. ISBN 0-517-5161-4; 0-517-51615-2pa.

Indoor herb gardening is becoming increasingly popular, especially with those who live in crowded suburbs or apartments. It is possible to grow a great many herbal plants indoors, and even those that normally grow only in tropical areas can be cultivated indoors in northern climates.

This beautifully illustrated book contains the following chapters: 1) All about Herbs; 2) A Ridiculously Short History of Herbals and Herb Gardens; 3) Annual, Biennial, and Perennial Plants; 4) Where to Grow Your Herbs Indoors; 5) Selecting the Right Plants; 6) General Culture of Herbs Indoors; 7) Herb Gardens in Terrariums; 8) Fluorescent Light Culture; 9) Step-by-Step Care of a Herb Indoors; 10) Growing Herbs from Seed; 11) Training Herbs Indoors; and 12) The Cultural Herb List. In addition, there is a list of commercial sources for herb plants and seeds.

Chapter 12 makes up about half the book and lists alphabetically by scientific name approximately 80 herbs which the authors feel are adaptable to growing indoors. Information on each plant includes common names, uses, usual habitat, description, and instructions for culture indoors. Photographs are usually provided for the plants.

This is a good how-to-do-it book.

221.   Fleming, Dave. **The Complete Guide to Growing Marijuana**. San Diego, CA: Sundance Press, 1969, 45p. illus. $1.00pa.

This booklet contains instruction on how to grow your own marijuana plants. In addition to a small amount of background information, there are discussions about the following: selecting a site (indoor and outdoor), intercropping, obtaining seeds, building a germinating box, preparing the soil, germinating, planting the seeds, transplanting, artificial light, care, and harvesting, curing, and preserving the crop.

Marijuana could probably be grown by following instructions given, but certain suggestions seem impractical. For instance, the following passage appears on indoor cultivation: "If you have a large house, take an empty room and line the floor with tar paper or similar substance....bring in the soil (each plant needs about a cubic foot of soil for root development), and you'll be in business."

222.   Fox, Helen Morgenthau. **Gardening with Herbs for Flavor and Fragrance**. New York: Macmillan, 1933; repr. New York: Dover Publications, 1971. 334p. illus. bibliog. index. $3.00pa. LC 71-99762. ISBN 486-22450-2.

The first quarter of this reprinted work is made up of historical information concerning medicinal and food uses of herbs. A chapter entitled "The Written Word" is an interesting essay on references made to herbs throughout recorded history. All of the introductory essays are delightfully written in a style that is unusual for most currently published herbals.

The main part of the book is a section called "Dramatis Personae" which is an alphabetical listing by Latin name of over 65 herbs. A common name index precedes this arrangement. Each entry includes a fairly extensive description of the plant, historical information, medicinal and food uses, and specific information on culture and harvesting. Each entry is from two to three pages, and some include drawings of the plant. All of the descriptions are well written. The final section of the book concerns cooking with herbs and includes specific recipes, which, for the most part, sound reasonably appetizing, except perhaps those for nasturtium sauce, marigold custard, and tansy pudding. The author's personal experience in growing and using herbs makes this a very practical book for herb culture and uses, especially for food uses.

223.   Frank, Mel, and Ed Rosenthal. **The Indoor/Outdoor Highest Quality Marijuana Grower's Guide**.   San Francisco, CA: And/Or Press, 1974. 94p. illus. $3.50pa.

This small book provides detailed instructions on how to grow your own marijuana plants, particularly indoors, although a shorter section on outdoor cultivation is also included. In addition, there is a section on an available commercial growing unit, and one on artificial lighting for plants. The authors claim that high quality, very potent plants can easily be grown using fluorescent lights, flower pots, and a good soil mixture.

224.   Frank, Mel, and Ed Rosenthal. **Marijuana Grower's Guide**. Deluxe edition. Berkeley, CA: And/Or Press, 1978. 330p. illus. (part col.). bibliog. index. $8.95pa. LC 77-82452. ISBN 0-915904-8.

This book begins with a foreword which makes a plea for legalization of marijuana use, or at least a reform of the laws. A section follows on "General Information about *Cannabis*," including history, chemical composition, and information about the plant. The second section is on indoor growing of the plant; the third on outdoor cultivation; the fourth on flowering, breeding, and propagation; and the last on harvesting, curing, and drying. A comprehensive treatment of the subject is presented, with many photographs of apparatus and equipment, colored micrographs of the plant, and lengthy bibliographic notes.

225.   Genders, Roy. **Growing Herbs As Aromatics.** Illustrated by Linda Diggins. New Canaan, CT: Keats Publishing, Inc., 1977. 95p. illus. (part col.). index. (Keats Living with Herbs Series: v.3). $2.50pa. LC 77-86544. ISBN 0-87983-155-3.

In earlier times, growing and using aromatic herbs (plants with fragrant properties) was a popular art. This is a charming but practical book that presents the history of pomanders, potpourris, scented waters, aromatic hanging baskets, rose perfumes, and other uses of aromatics and spices. Suggestions for use today are included.

The presentation is in three parts: history of aromatics, the aromatic herb garden, and further practical information. Chapter headings are: 1) Aromatics in Earlier Times; 2) The Middle Ages: Aromatics in the House; 3) The Distillation of Aromatics in the Middle Ages; 4) Aromatics about the Person; 5) The Medicinal Properties of Aromatics; 6) Other Health-Giving Properties; 7) Layout of the Garden; 8) The Aromatic Herb Border; 9) Aromatics in the Smaller Garden; 10) Less Hardy Aromatics; 11) The Propagation of Aromatics; and 12) Harvesting, Drying and Storing.

226.   Gilbertie, Sal, with Larry Sheehan. **Herb Gardening at Its Best: Everything You Need to Know about Growing Your Favorite Herbs.** New York: Atheneum/SMI, 1978. 245p. illus. index. $12.95. LC 77-23678. ISBN 0-689-10863-X.

The author of this practical, readable guide has operated with his family a popular garden center and herb nursery in Connecticut for many years. He frequently lectures on herb and vegetable gardening. In the book, he takes into account individual tastes, needs, and space available for gardening. Information on growing and cooking herbs is presented first; then 15 herbs are described in detail, and over 30 plans are provided for various kinds of herb gardens.

227.   Grubber, Hudson. **Growing the Hallucinogens: How to Cultivate and Harvest Legal Psychoactive Plants.** New York/Hermosa Beach, CA: High Times/Golden State Publishing, 1976. 32p. bibliog. $2.00pa.

This booklet presents general information on cultivation and propagation of plants, then gives specific instructions on growing and harvesting a variety of psychoactive plants, all of them legal, according to the author.

The following plants are discussed: belladonna, the brooms, betel nut, cabeza de angel, calamus, California poppy, catnip, chicalote (prickly poppy), coleus, colorines, damiana, daturas, doñana, fennel, Hawaiian baby woodrose, Hawaiian woodrose, heliotrope, henbane, hops, hydrangea, iochroma, kava kava, khat, lion's tail, lobelia, Madagascar periwinkle, mandragore (mandrake), maraba, maté, mescal beans, Mormon tea, morning glory, nutmeg, ololuique, passionflower, pipiltzintzintli, psilocybe mushrooms, rhynchosia, San Pedro, sassafras, shansi, silvervine, sinicuichi, so'ksi, Syrian rue, tobacco, wild lettuce, and wormwood. In addition, a short list of suppliers of seeds, cuttings, and dried herbs is included as well as a glossary and list of botanical names used, with pronunciation indicated.

228.   Harris, Bob. **Growing Wild Mushrooms: A Complete Guide to Cultivated Edible and Hallucinogenic Mushrooms.** Berkeley, CA: Wingbow Press, 1976. 82p. illus. (part col.). bibliog. $3.50pa. LC 76-6613. ISBN 0-914278-17-2.

The emphasis of this work is on cultivation of mushrooms, although there are some descriptions of species. There is a separate section on North American psilocybin mushrooms, a type which contains hallucinogenic agents. Some of the species discussed are currently restricted by law because of their chemical content.

Chapter titles are: 1) An Introduction to the Mushroom; 2) A Note on Cultivation; 3) Equipment for Sterile Culture Work; 4) Media; 5) Starting Cultures; 6) Incubation; 7) Sources of Materials; and 8) North American Psilocybin Mushrooms. The "Sources of Materials" chapter tells where supplies and equipment necessary for mushroom cultivation can be obtained. The last chapter contains descriptions and cautions that will help one distinguish lethal mushrooms from those sought.

229.   Hazlitt, W. Carew. **Gleanings in Old Garden Literature.** London: Elliot Stock, 1887; repr. Detroit, MI: Gale Research Co., 1968. 263p. bibliog. index. LC 68-21773.

This reprinted work reviews the early literature on gardening and herbs. Following are some of the topics considered: literary antiquities; the first English work on gardening; Elizabethan gardening; gardens in France, Holland, and Scotland; herbals, physic-gardens, and bees; the kitchen garden; the Kew Gardens about 1691; window-gardening; cottage gardens in 1677; influence of astrology; Bacon as a gardener; herbs and vegetables; fruit trees; flora; market gardens; Walpole and gardeners of the eighteenth century; bibliography of gardening literature and herbals. Included are many suitable discussions and quotations from classical literature and less well-known works.

230.   Hewer, D. G. **Practical Herb Growing.** Revised and continued by Kay N. Sanecki. London: G. Bell and Sons, 1969. 87p. illus. SBN 7135-1560-0.

The late author of this work was manager of a commercial herb farm. Her book is not intended for those who are already expert at growing herbs, but rather for those who wish to start cultivating them on a modest scale. The book does not deal with extremely poisonous plants. Three classes of plants are dealt with: medicinal herbs, fragrant and essential oil plants, and culinary and salad herbs.

Chapter titles are: 1) Introductory; 2) The Cultivation of Herbs; 3) The Harvesting of Herbs; 4) The Drying of Herbs; 5) Uses of Herbs; 6) Dyeing with Herbs; 7) Herb Gardens and Farms; and 8) A Catalogue of Herbs. The last chapter takes up about half the book, and lists plants alphabetically by common names, although scientific names are also given. Brief notes on the plants, a paragraph or so, are provided. Most of the information is on propagation, but uses are indicated.

The book is small, but it contains good basic information.

231.   Hyams, Edward. **Great Botanical Gardens of the World.** Photography by William MacQuitty; Foreword by Sir George Taylor. Camden, NJ: Thomas Nelson and Sons, 1969. 288p. illus. (part col.). index. ISBN 17-143004-2.

The beauties and rarities of about 50 of the world's greatest botanical gardens are described in this book. The first botanic gardens are presumed to have been physic (drug) gardens, but the idea of scientific collections of plants took hold in Europe by the mid-sixteenth century and, by the mid-twentieth century, over 500 such gardens were found in Europe, according to the book. These botanical gardens serve three major purposes: 1) They make possible the comparative study of the plants in them, making possible the development of modern taxonomy and experimental botany; 2) They have served as acclimatization stations where economic plants such as rubber, coffee, tea, chocolate, cotton, hemp, vanilla, and many other plants native to only one part of the world have been introduced in other areas; and they have provided a horticultural service.

Historical background on the gardens is included. Gardens of the U.S. featured include the Arnold Arboretum (Boston), Brooklyn Botanic Garden, Longwood (Pennsylvania), Missouri Botanic Garden, Strybing Arboretum (San Francisco), Huntington Garden (Los Angeles), and the Fairchild Tropical Garden (Miami).

232.   Jacobs, Betty E. M. **Growing and Using Herbs Successfully.** Charlotte, VT: Garden Way Publishing, 1981. 223p. illus. index. $6.95pa. LC 80-28802. ISBN 0-88266-249-X.

This is a comprehensive book about growing herbs for fun and profit. Thirty-two common herbs are discussed as well as 32 additional ones that are useful but more unusual. The book is made up of 10 chapters and six appendices, discussing just about everything about growing, selling, and using herbs. Specific cultivation, marketing, harvesting, and utilization information is given. Considerable directory type "source" information is also included. Historical and medical information is not emphasized in this work.

This is a good up-to-date book.

233.   Law, Donald. **Herb Growing for Health.** London: John Gifford Ltd. (125 Charing Cross Road, London, WC2), 1969. 223p. illus. bibliog. SBN 707-10341-X.

The author of this work encourages growing herbs at home. Plants discussed grow in England, but most are common in the United States also. Contents of the book is as follows: 1) Why grow herbs?; 2) Botanic medicine is safe; 3) Plants and their uses; 4) Correct scientific Latin names of herbs given to facilitate identification; 5) How to grow the herbs listed in chapter 3; 6) Woodman spare that tree!; 7) How to prepare medicines from herbs; and 8) Herbs you can grow indoors.

Chapter 3 is nearly half the book; it discusses herbs individually in short monographs. Chapter 4 gives correct scientific names of plants listed in chapter 3 and includes a few notes. Chapter 6 is about the valuable medicinal properties of trees and bushes. Although the author is said to be a lecturer and noted authority on botanic medicine, he makes some misleading statements. For example, Chapter 2 contains the following headings: "Why Botanic Medicine Is Safe," "Jungle Cure for Cancer Reported," and "No Toxic Elements in Herbs." The work is interspersed with examples of how commercial medicines have harmed users while herbal remedies have proved beneficial. Pesticides are denounced. The section on how to grow the plants may be useful; the material on medicinal uses of herbs should be considered carefully.

234.   Leighton, Ann. **Early American Gardens: "For Meate or Medicine."** Boston: Houghton Mifflin Co., 1970. 441p. illus. bibliog. index. $10.00. LC 68-26957. ISBN 0-395-07907-1.

When the Puritans emigrated to the New World in the seventeenth century, they were aware that they faced a wilderness where they would have to grow most of their own food. Housewives grew more than food in their gardens. The garden also provided other household aids such as flavorings, drinks, medicines, narcotics, cosmetics, insect repellants, and dyes.

In this book, the author describes the early American gardens, what they grew, and how the plants were used. The first chapter presents background material on gardening; the second discusses what was found already growing in the wilderness. Chapter 3 reports the findings of two men, William Wood and John Josselyn, who chronicled the growing of plants and gardens in New England. The fourth chapter shows the stature of early gardeners and the fifth is an account of what the early settlers thought and believed. Chapter 6 deals with food, chapter 7 with medicine; chapter 8 reports on the works of three leading authorities of the period on gardening. Chapter 9 deals with the form and shapes of early gardens. The tenth chapter discusses various plants grown in the area, based on material collected from books, letters, and recipes written by people of the early times.

The second half of the book, "An Appendix of Plants Described Individually by Their Own Authorities," lists about 200 plants alphabetically with botanical names and the names of sponsors or growers in seventeenth century New England. Also provided is a description of each plant and its uses, taken from three contemporary seventeenth century authorities, Johnson-upon-Gerard, Parkinson, and Culpeper. Illustrations included in the work are, for the most part, from the 1633 edition of Gerard's *Herball* (see entry 150).

This is an exceptional book with considerable detail about the lives of early Americans.

235.   Loewenfeld, Claire. **Herb Gardening: Why and How to Grow Herbs.** London: Faber and Faber, 1964. 256p. illus. index. $5.50pa. ISBN 0-571-09475-9.

Information on more than 50 herbs is provided in this book, which lists plants alphabetically by common name. Each entry includes historical data, a description of the plant, information on habitat, growing, and harvesting, and important uses. Most of the uses given are culinary, but some medicinal, cosmetic, and household virtues are mentioned. These discussions make up about three-fourths of the book. Introductory chapters include general discussions on history, harvesting, preserving, organic methods, uses, and hints on protecting and maintaining the winter garden. A "growing" chart and a "use" chart are two useful devices found at the end of the book. Both charts include concise practical information for quick reference.

236.   MacDonald, Christina. **Garden Herbs for Australia and New Zealand: Their History and Cultivation, Their Use in Cookery, Perfumery and Medicine.** Wellington, New Zealand: A. H., & A. W. Reed, 1969. 96p. illus. bibliog. index. $8.25. ISBN 0-589-00066-7.

This work was written because the author saw a need for a "small book on herb cultivation for southern-hemisphere gardeners" since the seasons and planting directions differ from those of Great Britain. The author also thinks "countrywomen should know more about the curative properties of these plants." Although the author had grown herbs for 30 years at the time of publication of this work, she claims it is by an amateur for amateurs. It contains "the simple and most easily cultivated herbs, and those that contain the most essential oils and food values."

The book begins with a short history on herbs and garden designs. The main body of the work is a listing of herbs. Included with each entry are common and scientific names of the plant, history, descritpion, uses, recipes, and a simple line drawing. The last chapters are on drying and storage, pot pourris, herb teas or tisanes, culinary recipes, and perfumes and cosmetics.

237.   McLean, Teresa. **Medieval English Gardens.** London: Collins, 1981. 298p. illus. bibliog. index. £12.50. ISBN 0-00-211535-2.

Using mostly manuscript sources, account rolls, charters, surveys, and registers, the author of this work has put together good descriptions of English gardens of the Middle Ages. In addition, chapters are devoted to detailed consideration of flowers, herbs, vegetables, fruit trees, and bushes that were cultivated for the needs of the medieval people.

The author describes monastic gardens that provided food and herbal medicines for monks and helped the general economy of the monastery. Plants also provided pigments for inks and illuminating aids. When church establishments were dissolved by King Henry VIII, such gardens came to an end; however, gardening was continued by town inhabitants, and small church gardens provided strewing herbs. In the days of castle building, gardens were placed outside the walls and often were not safe places for strolling. In more settled times, palaces, manors, and vicarages had ground for cultivating. Town inhabitants grew their own leeks, onions, garlic, and beans.

This is a unique and interesting book.

238.   Meltzer, Sol. **Herb Gardening in the South.** Houston, TX: Pacesetter Press, a division of Gulf Publishing Co., 1977. 77p. illus. index. $3.95. LC 77-0106. ISBN 0-88415-366-5.

Since growing conditions in the southern region of the United States are different from those in other parts of the country, Meltzer takes up the cultivation of herbs that are especially appropriate for that area. Many of the herbs that are grown as annuals in the North are perennials in the South. Also, there are a few herbs that are difficult to grow at all in the South.

The first chapter of this book is a general discussion of herb gardens; the next is on growing herbs, particularly preparing the soil. Propagation is then discussed, along with greenhouse growing; indoor herb growing; harvesting, drying, storing, and using the herbs. The latter section takes up herbal sprays to use as insecticides; herb oils, baths, rinses, and body lotions; a few reported medicinal uses; and herbal dyes. Some recipes for using herbs in foods are included. The last half of the book is a listing of more than 60 herbs alphabetically by common name. The following information about each is provided: scientific name, propagation, width and height, type of soil needed, exposure, water required, a descriptive paragraph, culture, uses, and miscellaneous remarks. Illustrations are provided. A few herbs are given brief treatment in an appended section. Also included are a chart "Herbs at a Glance," a short list of herb names in several languages, and a list of sources where herbs can be purchased.

It's a nice book, attractive and well-written with amusing and realistic comments scattered throughout. In one instance, a "priceless prescription, author unknown, for constipation" is given; Meltzer says he is afraid to try it. In another case a recipe for baldness is given; Meltzer says, "Did you see my picture? Didn't work on my head." In regard to herbs he advises: "Enjoy growing them, tasting the culinary ones; be careful when you use any medicine, herbal or otherwise."

239.   Owen, Millie. **A Cook's Guide to Growing Herbs, Greens, and Aromatics.** Illustrations by Karl Stuecklen. New York: Alfred A. Knopf, 1978. 263p. illus. index. $6.95pa. LC 77-20368. ISBN 0-394-73454-8.

In this book, Owen shares her experience in herb growing and also presents recipes for using the plants. The dishes sound appetizing; for instance, there is a recipe for ripe tomato and green oregano pizza. Little is said about folklore or medicinal uses of herbs.

The book is in two parts. The first part covers growing, preserving, and using fresh mixed herbs; the second lists about 50 common herbs and greens alphabetically by common name with several pages of information about each. Each plant is pictured with a line drawing, and the following information is usually provided: botanical and synonymous names, description, habitat and optimum growing conditions, cultivation, and preparation of the plants for use as food or seasoning. Several recipes are given using each plant. Appended is a list of sources (with addresses) for buying seeds and plants.

This is an attractive book, nicely done and practical.

240.   Pollock, Steven H. **Magic Mushroom Cultivation.** San Antonio, TX: Herbal Medicine Research Foundation, 1977. 64p. illus. (part col.). bibliog. (Psychomyco-logical Studies No.1). $5.00pa. LC 77-82244. ISBN 0-930074-01-7.

The author of this small book states that interest in growing magic mushrooms (types containing hallucinogenic psilocybin) at home has increased tremendously in recent times. A number of techniques for their cultivation are offered.

The following chapters are included: 1) The Magic Mushroom Life Cycle; 2) The Simplest Technique from Stratch; 3) Culture on Agar Media; 4) Growing Spawn on Seed; 5) Casing Spawn to Promote Mushroom Flushes; 6) The Rice-Cake Technique; 7) Cultivation on Compost; 8) Storing the Harvest; 9) The Magic Mushroom Agape.

It is noteworthy that psilocybin is a controlled substance in the United States, and unauthorized possession of the drug constitutes a violation of federal and most state regulations. However, there are evidently no laws in the United States prohibiting possession of the magic mushrooms per se.

241.   Prenis, John. **Herb Grower's Guide: Cooking, Spicing, and Lore.** Philadelphia, PA: Running Press, 1974. 96p. illus. $9.80; $2.50pa. ISBN 0-914294-37-7; 0-714294-07-5pa.

The paperback edition of this book is unique in that three packets of seeds are attached to the front cover. The reader is advised to plant the parsley, dill, and cress seeds for a harvest of healthgiving and tasty plants.

Brief general material on growing herbs outdoors, indoors, and from seeds is present first. There are also general hints on cooking with herbs. The main part of the work is a listing of 25 common, interesting, and useful herbs with line drawings of them included. About a page of information is given for each herb, including history, lore, description, best growing conditions, and uses in cooking. A set of symbols is used as a compact guide to characteristics and requirements of growing herbs. Plants best suited to available growing conditions can be determined at a glance. More detailed information is provided in the text. Appended are the following: a short section on drying herbs, a chart showing typical amounts of herbs to use for various dishes, a section on other uses for herbs (such as teas, vinegars, butters, and potpourris), and a list of sources for buying herb seeds, plants, and products.

This is a good, practical beginner's guide.

242.   **The Primo Plant: Growing Sinsemilla Marijuana.** By Mountain Girl. Berkeley, CA: Leaves of Grass/Wingbow Press, 1977. 96p. illus. bibliog. $4.50pa. ISBN 0-915070-04-9. (Distributed by Bookpeople, 2940 Seventh St., Berkeley, CA 94710).

The stated purpose of this small book is "to inform the public about growing marijuana, in all its diversity, to full perfection in America's different climate regions." Instructions are given especially for growing "sinsemilla" marijuana, the seedless variety, prized because it gives a superior "high." The reader is duly reminded that "growing marijuana is a natural act."

There are sections on: 1) Before planting; 2) Planting; 3) Growing; 4) Pruning and plant care; 5) Flowering; and 6) Harvest.

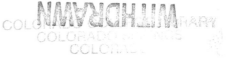
WITHDRAWN
COLORADO ... LIBRARY
COLORADO ...
COLORA...

The booklet should be of value (should one wish to get involved in this illegal activity) as it offers practical tips and inspiration. Note the following passages: "Five or six big, healthy, female plants will supply a heavy smoker for a year with pure, organically-grown harmoniously attuned grass," and also: "Don't forget that this stuff *is* a weed and will grow under difficult conditions, depending on the soil and the sun, but the perfect plant requires loving attention."

243.   Rea, C. B., and J. Rea. **Circa Instans.** Bryan, TX: The authors (810 E. 30th St., Bryan, TX 77801), 1973. 426p. bibliog. index. $10.00pa.

This work, published as a limited edition, is a history of drug plant gardens and a survey of those that presently exist. The authors feel that classical literature gives answers in medicine beyond the reach of science, and there are many references to the classics in the text. Other views developed are that Stonehenge was a drug plant garden or teaching hospital and that the pharmaceutical symbol "Rx" also stands for poetry. An appendix lists universities of the world that have drug plant gardens. Notes and an annotated index make up more than half the book.

The title of the book was suggested by a twelfth-century work that had no title and was known as *Circa instans* (about what is pressing and important). It's a curious book. The authors say "it presents the idea of medicine as co-existing with the critical spirit" and that "it is the critical spirit that is on call."

244.   Rohde, Eleanour Sinclair. **A Garden of Herbs.** Rev. and enl. ed. New York: Dover Publications, Inc., 1969. 300p. illus. bibliog. $3.00pa. LC 75-81736. ISBN 0-486-22308-6.   (An unabridged republication of the edition published by Hale, Cushman and Flint in 1936).

Plant an herb garden, the author of this book encourages. Only well-known English wild and garden herbs are dealt with. Medicinal uses of the plants are not emphasized; rather recipes are given for teas, syrups and conserves, drinks, wines, candied flowers and leaves, and sweet waters.

The following chapters are presented: 1) Of Herb Gardens; 2) Of Sundry Herbs; 3) Of Sallets; 4) Herb Pottages; 5) Herb Puddings; 6) Herb Drinks and Home-Made Wines; 7) Additional Recipes; 8) Of the Picking and Drying of Herbs; and 9) Of Sweet Scents. Chapter 2 makes up about half of the book; in it, plants are listed alphabetically by common name. Scientific names are usually not provided. The pattern of presentation usually followed is: first, a quotation from some classic work regarding the plant, then a general discussion of the herb, followed by several recipes. The bibliography is a list of classic works dating from 1440 to 1912. A few early manuscripts are also mentioned. The literature references contain only date, title, and author.

245.   Simmons, Adelma Grenier. **Herbs to Grow Indoors: For Flavor, Fragrance, for Fun.** New York: Hawthorn Books Inc., 1969. 146p. illus. index. $3.50pa. LC 73-85441. ISBN 0-8015-3416-X.

This is a practical little book for the person who wants to grow various herbs throughout the house for decoration and culinary purposes. It contains specific details about indoor culture and decorative growing arrangements, but illustrations are sparse.

There are three main sections in the book which list specific herbs and their uses, i.e., for flavor, fragrance, and fun. Almost all the plants are well known; the author doesn't stray into anything too exotic. Most good herb nurseries would carry these plants or have seeds. A short discussion on using herbs for entertainment purposes, such as pomander balls and centerpieces, is included. About 20 pages of the book provide culinary recipes. Uses of herbs as medicine are not mentioned except in passing. A good index completes the work. It is interesting to note that the book's introduction comments that growing plants indoors in the winter was once considered going against nature.

246.   Superweed, Mary Jane. **The Complete Cannabis Cultivator.** San Francisco, CA: Stone Kingdom Syndicate (Available from Flash Mail Order Post Express Co., Dept. S, P. O. Box 16098, San Francisco, CA 94116), 1969. 16p. illus.

The intent of this booklet is to inform the reader of various methods for growing marijuana depending on the circumstances. Brief instructions are given for raising plants out of doors, in a greenhouse, a living room, basement, or closet. The book addresses seed sprouting, harvesting, soil conditions, fertilizers, watering, lighting, concealing, plant diseases, and breeding methods to develop seeds which produce only female plants. The author of the pamphlet believed the time was near when marijuana could be grown legally.

247.   Superweed, Mary Jane. **Home Grown Highs: How to Grow Peyote, Psilocybe and Other Organics.** San Francisco, CA: Flash Mail Order (Dept. S, P.O. Box 16098, San Francisco, CA 94116), 1972. 16p. illus.

The author of this booklet remarks that "because of an increasing difficulty in procuring reliable organic psychedelics it has become necessary for people to grow their own." Instructions are provided on how to grow psilocybe mushrooms, peyote and other psychedelic cacti, pipizintzintli, coleus, morning glories, and Hawaiian baby wood rose. Also included are the names and addresses of suppliers of seeds.

Although the activity suggested may be illegal, plants could probably be grown by following instructions. Some of the information was evidently gleaned from scientific papers.

248.   Superweed, Mary Jane. **The Super Grass Grower's Guide: A Handbook for High Power Pot Farming.** San Rafael, CA: Stone Kingdom Syndicate (Available from Flash Mail Order, Dept. S, P. O. Box 240, San Rafael, CA 94902), 1970. 16p. illus.

Information on how to grow high quality marijuana is presented in this booklet. There are sections on hydroponic growing, lighting, special nutrients, and producing mostly female plants (which have the most resins). In addition, a section on how to graft hops to marijuana and produce plants that do not look like marijuana is included. It is claimed that these plants contain as much cannabinol resins as the original marijuana plants would have produced. Other methods of producing high quality marijuana are outlined, such as stimulating growth with hormones and mixing marijuana with dry ice. Even prayer is mentioned as being beneficial to the plants' growth; as is sitar music.

249.   Webster, Helen Noyes. **Herbs: How to Grow Them and How to Use Them.** New ed., rev. and enl. Boston, MA: Ralph T. Hale and Co., 1942. 198p. illus. bibliog. index.

Interest was being revived in the old herb gardens of the past about the time this book was written. The author has collected scattered bits of information on herb culture; herb use in cooking and medicine; and folklore, superstitions, and legends connected with herbs.

Contents of the book is as follows: 1) Early periods and designs of the herb garden (discusses bee gardens, medieval gardens, renaissance gardens; also includes a list of herbs known in medieval England and a list for a Shakespeare garden); 2) Colonial gardens (includes lists of plants known to have been grown in colonial gardens);

3) A garden of wild herbs (includes suggestions for native plants of herb interest);
4) A few important herb families and their genera; 5) Doctrine of signatures; 6) Medicinal herbs; 7) General horticultural directions for herb gardens; 8) Commercial growing of herbs; 9) Drying and curing herbs; 10) Uses of an herb garden (includes recipes for an old cough remedy, aromatic vinegar, and snuffs); 11) Herbs as a cottage industry; 12) Cooking with herbs (gives recipes); 13) Check list of herbs for modern gardens (herb genera and species which might be represented in a modern herb garden.

This is a nice book that has been popular. The photographs of gardens are especially noteworthy.

250.   White, Katharine S. **Onward and Upward in the Garden.** Edited and with an Introduction by E. B. White. New York: Farrar, Straus, Giroux, 1979. 326p. illus. bibliog. $10.00. LC 79-4522. ISBN 0-374-22654-7.

The text of this charming book originally appeared in *The New Yorker* in a series of pieces published from 1958 to 1970. The late Mrs. White was an amateur gardener and a professional editor. The work covers many aspects of gardening and includes reviews of many books on the subject. In addition, seed and nursery catalogues are discussed at some length.

Chapter titles are as follows: 1) A Romp in the Catalogues; 2) Floricordially Yours; 3) Before the Frost; 4) The Changing Rose, the Enduring Cabbage; 4) War in the Borders, Peace in the Shrubbery; 6) Green Thoughts in a Green Shade; 7) For the Recreation and Delight of the Inhabitants; 8) An Idea Which We Have Called Nature; 9) The Million-Dollar Book; 10) The Flower Arrangers; 11) More about the Arrangers; 12) Winter Reading, Winter Dreams; 13) Winterthur and Winter Book Fare; 14) Knots and Arbours—and Books. Appended is a list of seed and nursery dealers with addresses, a few in the United Kingdom. Also included is a list of gardening and plant books in print.

This is an unusual and interesting book by a person who obviously loved plants, books, and other publications about them.

7
HERB COOKERY

Books in this section deal specifically with the cookery of herbs, spices, and wild plants; virtually all provide recipes. Many of the general works on herbs listed in chapter 5 also include sections on culinary uses of herbs and some recipes. In addition, related materials on the use of wild plants for food can be found listed in chapter 17, and chapter 15 contains materials on the use of plants as "natural" foods.

Unusual subjects treated among the more mundane in this section are herbal teas, flower cookery, and the (illegal) use of marijuana in cooking.

* * * * *

251.   **The ABC of Herb and Spice Cookery.** With decorations by Ruth McCrea. Mount Vernon, NY: Peter Pauper Press, 1957. 61p. illus. $1.25.

Peter Pauper Press has published several other pretty little cookbooks similar to this one in format and style. Over 50 recipes are included, all of them interesting but not unusual. The book is arranged with one or two recipes under each letter of the alphabet. Each recipe uses at least one common spice or herb, all of which are available in most grocery stores.

252.   Adrian, Ann, and Judith Dennis. **The Herbal Tea Book.** Poorboy Press; distr. Simi Valley, CA: Benedict Lust Publications (P. O. Box 777, Simi Valley, CA 93065), n.d. 32p. $ .75pa.

This booklet lists plants from which herbal teas may be made. Arrangement is alphabetical by common name. The following is usually given about each herb: scientific name, synonyms, habitat, description, conditions for which the herbal tea is used, and a little history and/or folklore. Few instructions for making the teas have been provided.

253.   Albright, Nancy. **The Rodale Cookbook.** Emmaus, PA: Rodale Press Book Division, 1973. 486p. illus. (part col.). index. $12.95. LC 73-5161. ISBN 0-87857-071-3.

The author of this compilation is the chef-manager of Fitness House, the Rodale Press dining room which serves "organic" food as much as possible. The recipes provided in the book make use of the so-called "organic" and "natural" foods. Foods containing preservatives and processed foods are avoided as are foods grown with the use of chemical fertilizers, pesticides, herbicides, and insecticides. Honey is substituted for sugar in the recipes; flour other than wheat flour is usually used; unsaturated oils are used instead of animal or hydrogenated fats. In addition, brown rice, peanut flour, wheat germ, sunflower seeds, dried peas, beans, boybeans, nuts, and carob are used in cooking.

A variety of recipes are included. There are sections on: 1) Appetizers, snacks, nuts, seeds, relishes, and beverages; 2) Soups; 3) Salads and salad dressings; 4) Meats, poultry, fish and sauces; 5) Soybeans, eggs and cheese; 6) Vegetables; 7) Grains; 8) Breads; and 9) Desserts. The last section is a list of growers, distributors, and shops that market "natural" foods, arranged by state.

Some of the comments and cooking hints are good, some questionable. For instance, most would agree that natural cheeses are superior to processed cheeses; but it's difficult to accept the implication that our grandmothers used only food grown without the use of insecticides. Chemicals used may have been different in the past, but arsenate of lead and Paris green were used in the reviewer's grandmother's garden, and both chemicals are rated very poisonous.

254. Claiborne, Craig. **Cooking with Herbs and Spices.** New York: Harper and Row, 1970. 355p. illus. index. $12.95. ISBN 0-06-010784-7.

This is an updated and revised edition of an earlier book entitled *An Herb and Spice Cook Book.* Like other cookbooks, recipes are listed with ingredients firsts followed by directions on preparation and cooking. Notes on yield are also included. Arrangement of the book is by name of herb, and 54 different herbs are included. Each group of recipes is preceded by an illustration of the herb and a few notes about history and uses. Most herbs are well known and can be found in fresh or dried form in most grocery stores. Woodruff, sorrel, savory, rocket, and cassia are probably the most uncommon ones included.

The usefulness of the book is enhanced by a listing of all the recipes arranged by category of food, and by a good general index. The combination of more than one herb or spice in many of the recipes makes possible some interesting dishes.

255. **Cooking with Herbs and Spices.** Des Moines, IA: Better Homes and Gardens Magazine (Meredith Corp.), 1967. 24p. illus. $ .50pa.

This pamphlet is included as an example of the kind of publication available from many of the home, garden, and farm magazine publishers. They are usually updated from time to time and advertised in the magazine itself. This particular one has more than 50 recipes that use common herbs available on the dried herb and spice racks at most grocery stores. The pages contain a table which lists various herbs and spices and the typical foods they may enhance.

256. Crowhurst, Adrienne. **The Flower Cookbook.** New York: Lancer Books, 1973. 198p. illus. (part col.). index. $2.25.

Over 80 different flowers are used in the recipes in this most unusual cookbook. Like most cookbooks, specific ingredients are listed, followed by directions for preparation; it's the flower ingredients that make the work unique.

Recipes for the following indicate how unusual this book is: lilac fritters, candied jonquils, iced burnet soup, chardoons (thistles) with cheese sauce, stuffed tulips, yucca flower salad, tansy sauce, pansy wine, orange blossom souffle, mimosa cream, and motherwort tea. Many of the 164 recipes in the book are for teas. A brief discussion of habitat, history and a description of the flower plant precede each group of recipes that make use of a particular flower. The recipe section of the book includes color plates of each plant (and flower) and makes up about three-fourths of the book. Another section discusses flower drying and suggests the best method to use for various plants. Also included is a section that discusses in some detail uses of herbs for cosmetic purposes; specific formulations and applications are given. A final section discusses potpourris, sachets, and strewing herbs (those that may be strewn about for deodorizing and pleasant effects).

For those interested this is a good presentation for a reasonable price.

257.   Gottlieb, Adam. **The Art and Science of Cooking with Cannabis.** The Most Effective Methods of Preparing Food and Drink with Marijuana, Hashish and Hash Oil. New York/San Francisco, CA: High Times/Level Press, 1974. 79p. $2.50pa.

The author says this publication is not merely another cookbook; it serves as a guide to teach about the nature of cannabis, how it combines with different foods, how it is best assimilated in the human digestive tract, and how to get the most highs for the least expense.

The first section compares the results of ingesting cannabis to those from smoking it. (There is slower action from ingestion, but there are stronger, longer-lasting effects.) The second section explains the physical and chemical nature of cannabis, while the third describes such basic materials as canna-butter (the Sacred Ghee of India) and cannabis tar, both which are called for in some of the recipes included in the booklet. The recipe section contains directions for about 30 different dishes and/or beverages, including concoctions such as hash oil honey, cannabis chocolate icing, curried hash, creme de gras, and cannabis milk shake.

258.   Grieve, M. **Culinary Herbs and Condiments.** New York: Dover Publications, Inc., 1971. 209p. index. LC 70-153058. ISBN 0-486-21513-X.

The amateur gardener and the housewife will find in this manual useful information about herbs used for flavoring foods. Although originally intended for use in Great Britain, plants discussed grow equally well in North America.

More than half the book is a section on "sweet or culinary herbs—their cultivation and propagation—plant list." Herbs are first discussed in general, including information on cultivation and propagation and how to harvest and prepare them for market or home consumption. Each one is then dealt with separately, with plants arranged alphabetically by common name. Also given are the scientific name, local names, uses, description, cultivation, and instruction on preparing foods using the herb. The second section contains recipes for home-made wines, herbal beers, teas, and other herbal beverages. The last section deals with the condiments mustard, pepper, vinegar, salt, and oils.

The material included in this work has been well selected from older works or comes from the author's own experience. The book is nicely done.

259.   Hall, Walter, and Nancy Hall. **The Wild Palate: A Serious Wild Foods Cookbook.** Illustrations by David Frampton; designed by Joan Peckolick. Emmaus, PA: Rodale Press, 1980. 374p. illus. index. $7.95pa. LC 80-12530. ISBN 0-87857-303-8; 0-87857-302-Xpa.

The authors of this compilation live in the Rocky Mountain area where they hunt, fish, and gather wild foods. The book contains many practical tips for the hunter, fisherman, and forager, but it is mainly a collection of about 250 recipes using the wild foods.

An introductory chapter discusses gathering, preparing, and preserving the foods; wild seasonings are also listed and discussed. The 14 chapters listing the recipes are headed as follows: 1) Wild Appetizers; 2) Wild Beverages; 3) Raw Wild Vegetables, Salads, and Dressings; 4) Stocks and Soups; 5) Sauces, Gravies and Stuffings; 6) Seafood; 7) Freshwater Food; 8) North American Wildfowl; 9) North American Small Game; 10) North American Big Game; 11) Cooked Wild Vegetables and Greens; 12)

Wild Grains, Breads, and Cereals; 13) Wild Fruit and Nuts; and 14) Wild Desserts. Instructions are included on how to clean and field-dress game. Many recipes are exotic, indeed, (for instance, bear paw stew, braised woodchuck, arrowhead soup, violet tea, and pond lily tubers and greens). The authors advise against covering a "nutritious wild leafy vegetable with a manufactured dressing loaded with preservatives."

260. Harris, Ben Charles. **Better Health with Culinary Herbs.** Barre, MA: Barre Publishing, 1971. 163p. bibliog. index. $3.95pa. LC 74-163881. ISBN 0-8271-7124-2.

The book is divided into two sections: Culinary Herbs and Culinary Herbal. Most herbs in both sections are fairly well known and common. The first section provides general discussions of health and diet, problems with sugar and salt, and how to grow an herb garden. The major part of this section (about half the book) is given to specific culinary recipes. Integrated with these recipes are discussions of culinary uses of herbs. The second section of the book is an alphabetical listing of culinary herbs, divided into three groups and designated as major, minor, and wild herbs. Each entry in these groups includes the Latin and other names; historical information; description of the plant; information on cultivation, harvesting and preservation; and general remarks about medicinal and culinary uses. Specific medicinal applications and treatments are not given.

This is a good book with considerable detail. It should serve as a basic reference source on the subject.

261. Kavasc, Barrie. **Native Harvests: Recipes and Botanicals of the American Indian.** Illustrated by the author. New York: Vintage Books, 1979. 202p. illus. bibliog. index. $10.00; $5.95pa. LC 78-21792. ISBN 0-394-72811-4.

The first edition of this work was sponsored by the American Indian Archaeological Institute and covered New England only. This edition extends coverage to the whole continental United States. A large number of wild and cultivated plants are included with information about uses. There are chapters on herbs as food and seasoning, along with their uses in cosmetics and beverages and as poisons. Also, wild game and foods from fresh and salt water are considered. Recipes have been provided that sound quite good; each includes at least one wild, native ingredient. Botanical information is included in the recipe chapters, and a glossary and botanical charts are appended.

262. Loewenfeld, Claire, and Philippa Back. **Herbs, Health, and Cookery.** New York: Gramercy Publishing Co., 1967. 320p. index. $6.95. LC 66-22312. ISBN 0-517-105659.

More than half of this book is devoted to culinary recipes in typical cookbook format. Recipes are arranged under broad categories such as salads, soups, sweets, vegetables, and meat. Some unusual recipes are given, such as wild herb salads, but most do not use any exotic ingredients or herbs. Some British terminology is used. Other useful and interesting sections include discussions of the health properties of specific herbs, how to make various herbal teas, uses of herbs for cosmetic purposes, recipes of "healthy" eating, and herbs in invalid cooking. Another section entitled "Herbs for Cookery: Twenty-four Herbs in a Chest," includes all kinds of information about these fairly common herbs and their popular uses in cooking. This section lists the page numbers of specific recipes containing these herbs. There is also a general index for the entire book.

This work is fairly comprehensive and a good basic herbal cookbook.

263. Menzies, Rob. **The Herbal Dinner: A Renaissance of Cooking.** Millbrae, CA: Celestial Arts (231 Adrian Rd., Millbrae, CA 94030), 1977. 216p. illus. bibliog. index. $5.95pa. LC 76-53334. ISBN 0-89087-136-1.

This work is mainly a recipe book, but it also includes much other material about herbs and useful wild plants. Medicinal uses and nutritional value of the plants are frequently mentioned. Details are provided on planting, picking, gathering, drying, and storing roots, barks, berries, flowers, leaves and fruits. Plants mentioned in the recipes are mainly West Coast plants and may not be available wild elsewhere. However, a great many are available commercially.

Chapters are headed as follows: 1) It's All Spirit; 2) The Planting, Picking, Gathering; Drying and Storing of Roots, Barks, Berries, Flowers, Leaves and Fruit; 3) Simples; 4) Teas; 5) Soups; 6) Salads and Their Dressings; 7) Grains, Beans, and Nuts; 8) Breads, Their Heads, and the Pleasures of Kneading; 9) Mushrooms or Soma; 10) Meats, Fish, and Poultry; 11) Brews; and 12) Other Extracts. In addition, the following sections have been appended: Explanation of medicinal properties and abbreviations; Botanical list of plants; Utensils and measurements; Seed procurement stores, retail and wholesale.

Menzies, like many authors of books on herbs, has a philosophy about using "natural" foods and herbs. He seems to believe that some spiritual as well as physical good comes from the use of such substances.

264. Michael, Pamela. **All Good Things Around Us: A Cookbook and Guide to Wild Plants and Herbs.** Illustrated by Christabel King. New York: Holt, Rinehart and Winston, 1980. 240p. illus. (col.). bibliog. $19.95. LC 79-27956. ISBN 0-03-057296-7.

The author says this book is not meant to be about survival or how to live off the land; it is instead intended as a guide for using herbs and wild plants in the same way that our ancestors used them before we lost the old knowledge and came to rely on commercial products for our food and cosmetic preparations.

The book lists nearly 100 plants alphabetically by Latin name, and includes fine full-page color illustrations that show the edible parts at the best time for picking. Common names are supplied, a description given, history discussed, and a number of recipes listed. The book was written in Great Britain, but the plants are generally native in the United States also.

This quarto-sized book is very attractive. All recipes may not be entirely appealing, but they recapture the way of life of our ancestors. No index as such is provided, but the contents arrange the plants alphabetically by common name and list recipes for each plant.

265. Muenscher, Minnie Worthen. **Minnie Muenscher's Herb Cookbook.** With illustrations by Elfriede Abbe. Ithaca, NY: Comstock Publishing Associates, a division of Cornell University Press, 1978. 241p. illus. bibliog. index. $9.95. LC 77-90908. ISBN 0-8014-1166-1.

Unlike most other herb cookbooks, this one includes more unusual herbs; more than 40 are considered. In addition, over 250 recipes are presented, ranging from familiar favorites such as cookies, desserts, main dishes, and soups, to more unusual items such as herb jellies and butters, candied leaves, herb salts, sugars, and teas. Recipes are grouped under the predominant herb used and then cross-referenced to the other recipes that call for the herb as a secondary seasoning. There is a short section on preserving herbs and also one on their use in a salt-free diet. The author provides a description of the herbs and tells what they taste like.

266.   **Prize-Winning Recipes from the Golden Harvest Kitchens.** With an Introduction and valuable household and cooking hints by Beatrice Trum Hunter. New Canaan, CT: Keats Publishing, Inc., 1974. 96p. (Pivot Original Health Book). $1.26pa. LC 74-75105. ISBN 0-87983-087-5.

This collection of prize-winning recipes show how "natural" foods can be used in making dishes claimed to be superior in taste and nutritional quality. Emphasis is given to cooking "from scratch," that is, avoiding the use of convenience foods or processed foods as ingredients. Household and cooking hints, such as how to store herbs, are interspersed throughout the book. Included are discussions on the following: breakfast dishes; soup and salad; vegetables; beverages; breads; cookies; bars and squares; and desserts, cake and confections. There is also a special section on "natural" food preparation hints.

Some of the dishes seem appetizing; others are a bit too unusual, for instance, peanut butter soup, alfalfa leaf tea, and soybean aspic.

267.   Rohde, Eleanour Sinclair. **Culinary and Salad Herbs: Their Cultivation and Food Values, with Recipes.** New York: Dover, 1972. 106p. illus. index. $2.00pa. LC 72-84768. ISBN 0-486-22865-7. (Reprinted edition of a work first published in 1940).

The following chapters are presented in this little book: 1) Planning a Herb Garden; 2) Culinary Herbs; 3) Drying Herbs; 4) Use of Herbs; and 5) Salads. The chapters on planning the garden and drying herbs include only one or two pages of general remarks, giving almost no detailed information. The longest chapter (culinary herbs) is an alphabetical arrangement by common name of some of the most common herbs plus a few that are a little more unusual. Each entry includes historical information, a description of the plant, remarks about cultivation and nutrition, and some specific uses and recipes. Culinary uses only are mentioned. The chapter on uses includes a few recipes under general topics such as butters, vinegars, cheeses, salts, teas, and candies. The chapter on salads gives recipes for salads and salad dressings.

The book does not include a large collection of recipes, but it is a good basic introduction to culinary uses of herbs.

268.   Smith, Leona Woodring. **The Forgotten Art of Flower Cookery.** Drawings by Liz Thompson. New York: Harper and Row, 1973. 180p. illus. $6.96. LC 73-4124. ISBN 0-06-013934-X.

This is an unusual book about the use of common flowers in cooking. Recipes and menus are provided. Also included are legends, lore, and anecdotes about the plants. Each flower is presented in a separate chapter with recipes and ideas for use. If recipes are old, they have been updated in modern terms.

269.   Sounin, Leonie de. **Magic in Herbs.** New York: Pyramid Books, 1972. 159p. index. $0.95pa. ISBN 0-515-02855-X.

This is a reissue of a book originally published in 1941. Although it doesn't look like a typical cookbook, it is indeed a cookbook which places emphasis on the use of herbs and spices. Only common ones are dealt with.

One chapter is a listing of herbs and spices, with brief historical remarks and general culinary uses of each given. Most of the book is devoted to recipes (in non-tabular form) under the usual categories of sauces, vegetables, meats, fish, soups, and salads. Several complete meal demonstrations are included in one chapter. A final section describes how to start a herb garden. Medical uses of herbs are not discussed.

270.   **Supermother's Cooking with Grass.** San Rafael, CA: Sunshine Manufacturing and Import Co. (Available from Flash Mail Order, Dept. S, P. O. Box 240, San Rafael, CA 94902), 1971. 15p. illus.

This booklet contains nothing but 15 recipes, each using marijuana. Among other concoctions are recipes for banana coffee cake, brownies, pot tea, shrimp creole, spaghetti sauce, and wacky cake.

8

INDIVIDUAL
HERBS/SUBSTANCES

Materials grouped in this section consider individual herbal plants (or groups of plants) and a few substances of recent popular interest, such as honey, pollen, propolis, and ordinary sugar. The latter, incidentally, is not considered "natural" by "natural" food buffs, and honey is frequently suggested for use in its place as a sweetening agent.

The largest number of titles (about 10) deal with ginseng, a plant that is receiving a great deal of attention. It grows wild in the United States as well as in the Orient, and it is currently being gathered in the United States and sold, chiefly to an Oriental market. The Orientals believe it has great healing powers and is a kind of cure-all. There are also several works on garlic, another plant that is believed by some to have miraculous powers. Several works discuss hallucinogenic mushrooms that are believed to have mystical power and are legitimately used in religious ritual among Indians of North America, as is the peyote cactus. Other plants considered include kelp and other algae, comfrey, basil, cinchona tree, devil's claw, nightshades, holly, creosote bush, Japanese plum, Japanese mushrooms, coca, hawthorne berry, cannabis, arnica, kava-kava, laetrile, and goldenseal.

Claims made for the medicinal value of herbs are often exaggerated, but many of the plants provide valuable medicines. Some of them, of course, contain substances that are abused or have the potential for such, e.g., peyote, psilocybin mushrooms, coca, kava-kava, and cannabis.

* * * * *

271.   Airola, Paavo. **The Miracle of Garlic.** Phoenix, AZ: Health Plus Publishers (P. O. Box 22001, Phoenix, AZ 85028), 1978. 47p. bibliog. $2.00pa.

"Eat onions in March and garlic in May—then the rest of the year, your doctor can play." This is an old folk saying that the author quotes, and it fairly well sums up the approach of this little book. Garlic is a "wonder food."

Several scientific studies are cited that show such diseases as high blood pressure, atherosclerosis and heart disease, anemia, rheumatic diseases, diabetes, and hypoglycemia responding to garlic therapy. It is also claimed that more common medical problems such as upset stomach, pimples, constipation, and colds are prevented or cured by the substance. These latter claims are not necessarily backed up by scientific studies. Several other brief discussions of various properties of garlic are included along with four pages of commonly asked question about the plant. The 42-item bibliography completes the book.

272.   Anderson, Edward F. **Peyote: The Divine Cactus.** Tucson, AZ: University of Arizona Press, 1980. 248p. illus. bibliog. index. $7.95pa. LC 79-20173. ISBN 0-8165-0613-2.

The author of this work is a professor of biology who has examined, in an encyclopedic volume, most aspects of the peyote cactus and its use.

Indians have long used peyote as a medicament and in religious rituals. It gained notoriety, however, in the 1960s as a cult hallucinogenic plant. Contents of the book is as follows: 1) Peyote in Mexico, 2) Peyote in the United States; 3) Ceremonies; 4) The peyote user's experience; 5) Medical use; 6) Pharmacology; 7) Chemistry; 8) Botany; and 9) Legal aspects. There are several appendices: A) Peyote systematics; B) Peyote alkaloids; and C) Public law and regulations. A bibliography of over 600 entries is provided.

The author concludes that this insignificant-looking cactus has had a remarkable effect on Native American culture. The Indians of Mexico and some parts of the U.S. believe they can, through its use, reach out of physical life, communicate with spirits, and "become complete." The governments of Mexico and the U.S. have discouraged its religious and medicinal use. Anderson, however, is hopeful that his book will help eliminate some of the "prejudices and untruths that have presisted about this plant which these people so respect and honor."   .

273.   Binding, G. J. **About Comfrey, the Forgotten Herb.** Wellingborough, Northamptonshire, England: Thorsons Publishers Ltd., 1974. 63p. (The About Series). $1.75pa. ISBN 0-7225-0235-4.

At the time this booklet was written, the author felt that comfrey, an ancient wayside herbal plant, had all but disappeared from gardens and growers' catalogues. The aim of the book was to make the versatile plant's medicinal and culinary properties known. It has been used for composting and as a forage crop for livestock. The book also discusses borage, another herb in the same family of plants as comfrey.

Chapter headings are as follows: 1) History of Borage and Comfrey; 2) Some Therapeutic Applications; 3) A Forgotten Wonder Herb; 4) Cultural Instructions; 5) Farm and Garden Uses; 6) Organic Farming with Comfrey; and 7) Cooking with Comfrey. The last chapter includes recipes.

The plant enjoyed a comeback until recent research, reported after the book was published, provided evidence that comfrey contains a toxic substance and should not be used internally, at least not until more studies are carried out.

274.   Binding, G. J. **About Garlic: The Supreme Herbal Remedy.** Wellingborough, Northamptonshire, England: Thorsons Publishers, Ltd., 1970. 64p. bibliog. (The About Series). $1.75pa. ISBN 0-7225-0148-X.

This is a small book which is one of a series about various herbs and foodstuffs. It is written in simple terms and is easy to read. About half the book is given to a history of the uses of garlic, especially in England, France, and Egypt. A short discussion about all members of the onion family is also included. Other sections include a listing of illnesses supposedly cured by garlic, and a selection of kitchen recipes in which garlic is used. The author believes there is no "secret" ingredient in garlic that cures diseases, but that it is the substance which causes the odor that is the "germ killer."

275.   Binding, G. J., and Alan Moyle. **About Kelp: Seaweed for Health and Vitality.** Wellingborough, Northamptonshire: Thorsons Publishers Ltd., 1974. 63p. (The About Series). $1.75pa. LC 74-595056. ISBN 0-7225-0256-7.

Certain seaweeds can be useful to mankind, according to this small book. Kelp consists mainly of larger algae of many species, but the one most commonly used for processing kelp tablets is the *fucus vesiculosus*. Kelp has, in the past, been used as a source of algenic acid, agar-agar, carrageenin, and manure.

The book describes cultivation and harvesting of this "crop" and its agricultural, gardening, and food uses. Kelp is said to have therapeutic properties. There are sections on its use for respiratory diseases, indigestion and ulcers, gastric catarrh and mucous colitis, gall bladder disease and obesity, constipation, intestinal disorders, genito-urinary and reproductive system disorders, and musculo-skeletal and neuromuscular disorders. The authors conclude with the comment that seaweed is very versatile; the supply is virtually untapped; and it has high nutritive value.

276.   Binding, G. J. **About Pollen.** London: Thorsons Publishing Limited (37/38 Margaret St., London, W.1), 1971. 63p. (The About Series, No. 42). $1.75pa. ISBN 0-7225-0182-X.

The introduction to this work says that pollen is now accepted as a health food and medicine. The booklet attempts to answer some of the questions concerning it. Testimonials regarding its curative powers are included.

Chapter headings are as follows: 1) What Is Pollen; 2) Pollen throughout the Ages; 3) Sweden: Home of the Fabulous Pollen Industry; 4) Pollen in England; 5) The World of the Bee; 6) Pollen as a Food; 7) Pollen in Europe; 8) Pollen in the United States of America; 9) Medical Uses of Pollen and Royal Jelly; and 10) The Future of Pollen.

277.   Chapman, V. J. **Seaweeds and Their Uses.** 2d ed. London: Methuen and Co., 1970. 304p. illus. bibliog. index. £4.00.

The first edition of this work was directed primarily to the general public; this one is more for the professional worker in the field and the industrialists. It provides a good description of commercial uses of seaweeds, which include iodine production, potash, animal fodder, agricultural manure, food, agar-agar, algin, and alginates. A chapter on "Minor Uses of Algae and Their Products" contains information on uses in folk medicine in various parts of the world. The last chapter covers the geographic distribution of the world's supply of seaweeds.

278.   Cooper, Richard. **A Guide to British Psilocybin Mushrooms.** Rev. ed. London: Hassle Free Press (BCM Box 311, London WCIV 6XX, U. K.), 1979. 32p. illus. (part col.). bibliog. £1.25pa. ISBN 0-86166-004-8.

The purpose of this booklet is to assist in finding and identifying psychoactive (hallucinogenic) mushrooms of the British Isles. About a dozen are said to fall in this category when taken in the correct dosage. Other mushroom species that may be confused with the hallucinogenic ones, but which are poisonous, are pointed out, for instance, two members of the amanita family. There are sections on history and identification; then a short descriptive monograph on each species is presented with a line drawing of the plant. Sections follow on chemistry and dosage, collecting and preserving, effects, spore printing, spore details, legal position, and a glossary.

Information presented in the booklet seems to be reasonably correct, although it is dangerous to experiment in using these plants, as the author admits.

279.   Crane, Eva. **A Book of Honey.** New York: Charles Scribner's Sons, 1980. 193p. illus. bibliog. index. $15.95. LC 80-50475. ISBN 0-684-16651-8.

The author of this work is director of the International Bee Research Association and is a world authority on bees. Her book will remove many popular misunderstandings about bees and honey.

The book begins with a general account of the collection and nature of honey. Bees do not collect honey but nectar that they later convert to honey. Nectar collection is a laborious process, but it is important economically because bees pollinate flowers while gathering nectar.

Chapter headings are: 1) Bees. The Honey Producers; 2) Plants: The Honey Resources; 3) Constituents and Characteristics of Honey; 4) Honey in the Home; 5) Honey in the Past and Present; and 6) Bees and Honey in the Minds of Men. In addition, there is an appendix on producing your own honey. Tables of facts and figures are provided, such as a list of plants that are important sources of honey and where they grow, information on the life of the bee, and a list of sugars whose presence has been established in honey. (About 70% of the total is glucose and fructose.)

The scope of the book is wide. The chapter on "Honey in the Home" contains a number of recipes for foods and cosmetics using honey. The fifth chapter is a history of honey, and chapter 6 presents legends, beliefs, and customs.

The book has wide appeal; parts of it will interest the expert, and other parts are for the beginner.

280.   Darrah, Helen H. **The Cultivated Basils.** Illustrated by Dorothy S. Wilbur. Independence, MO: Buckeye Printing Co., 1980. 40p. illus. bibliog. LC 80-123301.

The author of this concise, authoritative work is a recognized expert on cultivated basils and their uses. She discusses 12 species or varieties of *Ocimum*. Included is information on morphology; descriptions of the species; basil oils; horticultural notes; sources for seeds; medicinal, culinary, and industrial uses; folklore; and history. The book contains an extensive bibliography and 12 leaves of plates. It is suitable for both popular and technical audiences.

281.   Dufty, William. **Sugar Blues.** Radnor, PA: Chilton Book Co., 1975. 194p. bibliog. index. $7.95. LC 75-28175. ISBN 0-8019-5954-3.

White table sugar is poisonous and addictive, according to the author of this work, a New York newspaperman. He tells the story of how actress Gloria Swanson convinced him of this "fact." Written in a somewhat sensational journalistic style, the book explores the history and extent of the use of sugar, including its use in soft drinks and packaged and canned foods. A plea is made for a diet free of sugar and for the use of "natural" foods. Instructions for preparing a few sugar-free dishes are included. Few scientific publications are listed in the bibliography or cited in the notes.

Incidentally, Dufty married Gloria Swanson.

282.   Duran-Reynals, M. L. **The Fever-Bark Tree: The Pageant of Quinine.** Garden City, NY: Doubleday and Co., Inc., 1946. 275p. bibliog. index.

This book is a historical account of the fight against malaria, how it has affected history (including military history), and the discovery of quinine from the cinchona tree to control the malady.

The story begins with the ancient Greeks and covers the World War II era when malaria accounted for more than half of total casualties. Quinine until recently was the only effective agent against malaria, and it is still useful in the treatment of acute attacks, although other drugs are now available. The book recounts many stories; for instance, how the cinchona tree was sacred to the natives of the high Andes where it grew, and white men at first were punished by death for exploiting its magic.

In the time of King Charles II, an English quack physician kept his use of quinine a secret to avoid being involved in a religious-political plot, although he cured the aristocracy of two countries.

The book covers a significant phase of medical history in an interesting, readable fashion.

283.   Fulder, Stephen. **About Ginseng: The Magical Herb of the East.** Wellingborough, Northamptonshire, England: Thorsons Publishers, Ltd., 1976. 64p. $1.75pa. (The About Series). ISBN 0-7225-0327-X.

This small book, intended for the lay public, covers a number of aspects of ginseng, long claimed in the East to be a universal remedy. Information is provided on the natural habitat, cultivation, evidence of properties, effects (particularly on the aging process), forms available, where to purchase, dosage, and the herb's future in the field of medicine.

284.   Hanssen, Maurice. **About Devil's Claw: The Natural and Safe Treatment of Rheumatism and Arthritis.** Wellingborough, England: Thorsons Publishers Ltd., 1978. 64p. illus. bibliog. index. $1.75pa. ISBN 0-7225-0450-0.

This is another booklet in the "About Series" from Thorsons Publishers. It discusses the origin of this African herb (*Harpagophytum procumbens*) and medical evidence of its value in treating rheumatism and arthritis. Underground tubers are the useful part of this plant. It is called devil's claw because it protects its seed with a vicious barbed claw. A complete program of managing arthritis is included as one section of the book. Testimonials (British case histories) praising the value of devil's claw take up about 15 pages. The bibliography adds considerably to the value of this book. References are to German language works of some importance. Most of the original papers on the plant are written in that language.

285.   Harding, A. R. **Ginseng and Other Medicinal Plants: A Book of Valuable Information for Growers as Well as Collectors of Medicinal Roots, Barks, Leaves, etc.** Columbus, OH: A. R. Harding, 1908; repr. Charlestown, MA: Emporium Pubns. (28 Sackville St., Charlestown, MA 02129), 1973. 367p. $7.50; $4.00pa. LC 72-87757. ISBN 0-88278-009-3; 0-88278-007-7pa.

This work covers mainly the growing or gathering of ginseng to sell. Other medicinal plants, considered valuable and marketable, are also covered. Golden seal is discussed in some detail. The author claims that roots are usually the most valuable part of a plant, although the bark and leaves of some are useful.

The book begins with a discussion of "plants as a source of revenue" and, in addition, lists medicinal plants with information on the cultivation of them. The main body of the work is on ginseng, covering its history, habits, cultivation, shading, diseases, marketing, and letters from growers. The sections on golden seal provide similar information. Other plants discussed individually are cohosh, snakeroot, pokeweed, mayapple, seneca snakeroot, and lady's slipper. The rest of the book is divided into sections on forest roots, forest plants, thicket plants, swamp plants, field plants, dry soil plants, rich soil plants, medicinal herbs, and medicinal shrubs. Plants in each section are discussed briefly, giving scientific name, other common names, habitat and range, description of plant, description of root stock, collection, prices, and uses. Both line drawings and photographs are scattered throughout the work.

286.   Harriman, Sarah. **The Book of Ginseng.** New York: Pyramid Books, 1973. 157p. illus. bibliog. index. $1.25pa. ISBN 0-515-02988-2.

Dissatisfaction with the quality of life conventionally offered has caused many to seek alternatives, according to this book, which focuses on the neglected folk medicine of Asian peoples.

Long used in the Orient, ginseng has been considered a cure for such diseases as diabetes and heart disease and to be of value in restoring youth, increasing fertility, prolonging life, and acting as an aphrodisiac and a tranquilizer. The book begins with the history of the plant, gives recipes or formulas for its use, provides evidence of its efficacy, and gives information on growing, gathering, and marketing it. A list of places where Asiatic and American ginseng may be purchased is appended.

287.   Harris, Ben Charles. **Ben Charles Harris's New Fact Book on Ginseng: What It Is ... What It Can Do for You.** New Canaan, CT: Keats Publishing, Inc. (36 Grove St., New Canaan, CT 06840), 1978. 126p. bibliog. $1.95pa. LC 78-59174.

This small book adequately presents the history and other information concerning ginseng. The author's aim, he says, is to dispel the mysterious panacea syndrome, myths, and superstitions associated with the plant. It is not a cure-all as many claim, although therapeutic properties and uses are presented in the book. Other chapter topics include cultivation, collection, preparation, marketing and pricing, home growing, and preparation of remedies. There is also a chapter on aphrodisiac herbs including ginseng. Each chapter has a list of references, and a good bibliography is included at the end of the book. This work presents a balanced view of this almost universally known herb.

288.   Harris, Lloyd J. **The Book of Garlic.** 3rd rev. ed. Los Angeles, CA: Panjandrum/Aris Books (11321 Iowa no.1, Los Angeles, CA 90025), 1979. 286p. illus. bibliog. $8.95pa. LC 79-20972. ISBN 0-915572-29-X.

It is difficult to describe this book because it covers so many aspects of garlic. The style is whimsical (occasionally even silly), and one wonders whether to take the material seriously. However, much information is included, literature references are provided, and the book has evidently been well received, at least in some circles.

The work is divided into four main sections: 1) A serious history in which the use of garlic as food, medicine, and magic throughout the world is discussed; 2) Garlic, the super herb, a survey of clinical and experimental studies indicating its effectiveness as a medicinal agent; 3) Garlic in literature and art; and 4) Culinary uses of garlic, including a number of recipes. The book has only a recipe index; however, it is not intended as a quick reference work but is to be read.

For additional information on garlic, the author offers membership in an organization called "The Lovers of the Stinking Rose (or LSR)," which puts out a newsletter on the subject. (Harris is also publisher of Aris Books.) Despite some outrageous suggestions (such as garlic ice cream), the book may serve as a basic work on the subject.

289.   Heffern, Richard. **The Complete Book of Ginseng.** Millbrae, CA: Celestial Arts (231 Adrian Road, Millbrae, CA 94030), 1976. 127p. illus. bibliog. index. $3.95pa. LC 75-28757. ISBN 0-89087-151-5.

The ginseng plant is covered thoroughly in this book, including botanical variations, history and legends surrounding it, methods of cultivation, and recent research findings. A great deal of mystery and lore has surrounded the plant and in some cultures (Oriental), it has held a prominent place in medicine; in others (some American Indian Tribes), it has been considered a form of magic. The root of the plant often bears some resemblance to the human form, and fortunes have been paid for a near perfect root.

Ginseng has been used for many physical ailments; for instance, to increase endurance, as a tonic, for small pox eruptions, for fever, and for every kind of stomach ailment. It has served as a love charm, presumably as an aphrodisiac, and has been a kind of panacea in some cultures.

Contents of the book is as follows: 1) Botany of the plant; 2) History of ginseng; 3) Ginseng legends; 4) Grades of ginseng; 5) *Eleutherococcus senticosus* ("Siberian ginseng"); 6) The use of Asiatic ginseng; 7) The use of North American ginseng; 8) Early research; 9) Modern research findings; 10) Cultivation and marketing; and 11) Collection of the wild plant.

The author cites recent research that has isolated some of the chemical constituents of ginseng. The plant seems to act on the adrenal cortex so that when a body is subjected to stress the ginseng constituents replace the hormones of the adrenal cortex and do not allow the latter to become overworked. Ginseng is evidently a kind of stimulant. The author believes that pharmaceutical companies should market some of the constituents of the plant. Ginseng is now available only in crude form at a rather high price.

290.   Heiser, Charles B., Jr. **Nightshades: The Paradoxical Plants.** San Francisco, CA: W. H. Freeman and Co., 1969. 200p. illus. bibliog. index. $5.95. LC 70-85798. SBN 7167-0672-5.

The nightshade family of plants (*Solanaceae*) has figured conspicuously in human history, literature, and science. Some members of this family are useful and include important food plants; others are deadly because of the alkaloids they contain.

This book discusses a number of the nightshades, a family made up of more than 75 genera and 2,000 species. Most of the members of the family are herbs, although some are shrubs and a few small trees. Plants discussed include chili peppers, potatoes, eggplant, the wonderberry, tomatoes, lulo, pepinos, mandrake, Jimson weed, henbane, deadly nightshade, tobacco, petunias and a few other flower garden plants.

The author has collected a great deal of historical material, information on cultivation, anecdotes, and lore about the nightshades. Uses are discussed as well as preparation for eating edible species. The author of the book is a professor of botany. He has lived periodically in Latin America, and the book makes frequent references to the way nightshades are used in those countries.

291.   Hensley, David L., and others, eds. **Proceedings of the First National Ginseng Conference.** Lexington, KY: May 1-2, 1979. Frankfort, KY, Governor's Council on Agriculture (Capital Plaza Tower, Frankfort, KY 40601), 1979. 124p. illus. bibliog.

This publication contains about 20 papers on a broad range of subjects that were covered at a conference, such as "ginseng production techniques, cultural research, chemical analysis of the roots, monitoring of wild ginseng populations, regulation and control of ginseng harvest and marketing, and commercial use of ginseng." The conference was co-sponsored by the Kentucky Ginseng Association, the Governor's Council on Agriculture, and the University of Kentucky College of Agriculture in cooperation with the United States Endangered Species Scientific Authority, Washington, D.C. A list of participants and bibliographic references add to the value of the publication. It is hoped that this conference will be held on a continuing basis so people interested in ginseng can be kept up-to-date on the subject.

292.   Hills, Lawrence D. **Comfrey: Fodder, Food, and Remedy.** New York: Universe Books, 1976. 253p. illus. bibliog. index. $4.95pa. LC 75-33485. ISBN 0-87663-932-5.

This is a comprehensive work about a well-known but somewhat controversial herb, comfrey. Various aspects of the plant are discussed, history, growth, cultivation, analysis, and use as food and medicine for man and animals. The emphasis is on comfrey as a feed for animals.

There is much data throughout the work showing nutritional values, feed ratios for animals, and comparison yields in test plots. The plant is an inexpensive source of high quality protein. The author has obviously studied the plant thoroughly over many years and has supplied a tremendous amount of information. Sections on the use of comfrey as a medicine, and on the chemical analysis of alkaloids found in it, complete the book and add to its value as a reference work. The book has been criticized because the section on medicinal uses is dated, and much of the evidence is testimonial. However, some scientific observations have been included, and they should stiumulate an interest in further research on the subject.

The plant has attracted attention recently in health food stores, and an herbal tea made of it has enjoyed some popularity. However, it is noteworthy that the copy of the book reviewed had a warning label, prepared by the author, attached to it, stating that comfrey has recently been found to contain a dangerous factor, and further investigations should be completed before it is used for food.

293.   Hou, Joseph P. **The Myth and Truth about Ginseng.** South Brunswick, NJ: A. S. Barnes & Co., 1978. 245p. illus. bibliog. index. $9.95. LC 77-74114. ISBN 0-498-02083-5.

This is a clearly written, up-to-date book concerning all aspects of the famous herb, ginseng. The author is a pharmaceutical chemist and Senior Research Scientist at the Squibb Institute for Medical Research and is therefore well prepared to present a book that is well researched and documented.

The first part of the work discusses the history and medical uses of ginseng in China, Korea, Japan, the Himalayas, and North America. Several specific medicinal preparations and their uses are described in this section. The second part of the book concerns the economics of the ginseng business and how to go about growing the plant commercially. Much of this information on cultivation has been taken from the U.S. Department of Agriculture, Farmer's Bulletin series. Nearly half of the book discusses recent scientific studies from around the world concerning the chemical basis and uses of the plant. Comprehensive lists of references and additional bibliography make this a good reference work.

A list of ginseng dealers in the United States and a good index and glossary add to the value of the book. This is one of the most complete and well-documented works on this subject published in recent times. The author admits that the "age-old panacea tonic" is not popular in the Western countries, particularly the U.S. It was deleted from the official U.S. drug compendia in 1950. However, the American public is now searching for new evidence about the plant even if the scientific sector is not very interested.

294.   Hudson, Charles M., ed. **Black Drink: A Native American Tea.** Athens: University of Georgia Press, 1979. 175p. illus. bibliog. index. LC 78-18751. ISBN 0-8203-0462-X.

According to the editor, the purpose of this book is "to clear away the extraordinary confusion about an important ethnobotanical and ritual complex among the

Indians of the Southeast and to describe the true nature of a caffeinated beverage...,"
i.e., yaupon, cassina, or Ilex vomitoria—various names for a species of holly found in
North America. The drink is evidently used mostly as a ritual emetic.

In addition to introductory material, five studies by various scholars are included in this work: 1) The botany of yaupon; 2) Ilex vomitoria among the Indians of the
Southeast and adjacent regions; 3) Origins and prehistoric distributions of Black Drink
and the ceremonial shell drinking cup; 4) The function of Black Drink among the
Creeks; and 5) Black Drink and other caffeine-containing beverages among non-Indians.

This is a readable work on an interesting subject essentially unknown to most
people in the United States. Good bibliographies with each article and an overall general bibliography for the book make this a particularly valuable study.

295.   Illinois Department of Conservation. Division of Forestry. **Conserving Wild
Ginseng in Illinois.** Springfield, IL: Illinois Department of Conservation, Division of
Forestry (R. R. No. 5, Conservation Area, Springfield, IL 62707), 1979. 12p. folder.
illus. (part col.).

This attractively illustrated leaflet contains succinct information about native
wild ginseng and how it should be conserved and handled. Information is given under
these headings: some common names, varieties, history, today, botany of the plant,
collection, be a good collector, digging and drying roots, selling the root, uses and
products, and cultivating ginseng. In addition, there are good illustrations of ginseng,
a map of Illinois showing the range of the plant, another showing district foresters, a
list with addresses of the district foresters, and location of regional offices where
more information may be obtained.

Due to the high prices paid for ginseng, many people have been gathering the
wild type, and some have begun cultivating it. Cultivation is somewhat difficult, according to the publication. It is pointed out that most ginseng is used in the Orient. About
95% of it is exported to Hong Kong for processing. Although certain components of
the root may have practical medicinal applications, it has not yet gained any real acceptance in the United States. Its value still needs to be established.

296.   Kimmens, Andrew C., ed. **Tales of the Ginseng.** New York: Wm. Morrow
and Co., 1975. 208p. illus. bibliog. index. $3.95pa. LC 75-9888. ISBN 0-688-
02942-6.

This is an interesting and well-documented book containing all kinds of tales,
narratives, lore, and historical information about ginseng. Most of the folk tales are
from China and Korea and contain Taoist and Confucian ginseng lore. There are discussions of Chinese ginseng laws, scientific studies, European discoveries of ginseng, and
American ginseng history and stories. Practical advice about the use of the plant is
scattered throughout. The bibliography is extensive and includes actual excerpts from
the references cited.

297.   Lyngheim, Linda, and Jack Scagnetti. **Bee Pollen: Nature's Miracle Health
Food.** North Hollywood, CA: Wilshire Book Co., 1979. 90p. illus. bibliog. index.
$3.00. LC 79-56633. ISBN 0-87980-371-1.

Both authors of this work are said to be health enthusiasts, and this is probably the main qualification they have for writing such a book. Lyngheim was formerly an airline stewardess, more recently a school librarian, and Scagnetti, is a journalist
and free-lance writer. The book is all about how wonderful bee pollen is, "an excellent
source of proteins, vitamins, minerals, amino acids, hormones, trace elements, and
enzymes to help build and maintain a healthy body." It is claimed that it helps

arthritis and allergy sufferers, prevents prostate disorders, helps cancer victims, and aids athletic performance and digestion. In addition, it is said to be a beauty aid and to increase life. The book contains ancient history of bee pollen and comments about bee products and their uses. A short glossary is provided.

References are made throughout the text to scientific studies on bee pollen. However, the only bibliography is at the end of the work, and it lists only popular books and articles, mainly from magazines such as *Track and Field Notes* and *Prevention Magazine* (see entry 118).

298. Mabry, T. J., J. H. Hunziker, and D. R. DiFeo, Jr., eds. **Creosote Bush: Biology and Chemistry of Larrea in New World Deserts**. Stroudsburg, PA: Dowden, Hutchinson and Ross, Inc., 1977. 284p. illus. bibliog. index. (U.S./IBP Synthesis Series: 6). $24.00. LC 76-58381. ISBN 0-87933-282-4.

This book is one of a series of volumes that report results of research by U.S scientists participating in the International Biological Program. Cresote bush is the dominant shrub in certain arid areas of Argentina and in the southwestern U.S. and Mexico. The basic aim of the work is to answer the larger questions concerning origin, structure, and function of the desert ecosystems.

The book contains contributions by 27 authors. Topics covered include: adaptive strategies, geographical distribution, morphology, hybridization, cytogenetics, evolution, growth and development, reproductive biology, animal associations, natural products and chemistry, community structure, and practical uses.

The plant is best known for the presence of Nordihydroguaiaretic Acid in the resins deposited on the surface of leaves, a substance that is a strong antioxident and has been used to preserve food and pharmaceuticals and as a stabilizer in Vitamin A, lubricants, and rubbers. In addition, it evidently has anti-mold and anti-tumor properties. Indian tribes use the plant for a variety of ailments.

Only a small portion of the volume is devoted to practical uses and products of *Larrea*. Most of the chapters are well–written scholarly papers on other aspects of the subject. It is a good example of a highly scientific work on a plant of potential medicinal value.

299. Matsumoto, Kosai. **The Mysterious Reishi Mushroom: Its Powers for Health and Longevity and in the Treatment of Cancer and Other Incurable Diseases**. Santa Barbara, CA: Woodbridge Press Pub. Co., 1979. 63p. illus. bibliog. index. (Lifeline Book). $2.95. LC 78-71030. ISBN 0-912800-52-6.

This is a translation of a Japanese work. Its purpose is to present information about the reishi mushroom (sarunokoshikake) which grows on old plum trees in Japan, China, and other northern areas of the temperate zone. It is rare; out of 100,000 old Japanese plum trees only a few have reishi on them. However, a successful method for artificial cultivation has been developed. The book presents the history of the mushroom, purported uses (for longevity, for cancer and other incurable diseases), cultivation, testimonials to the plant's efficacy, explanation of the action of the substance, preparation, and dosage.

300. Matsumoto, Kosai II. **The Mysterious Japanese Plum: Its Uses for Healing, Vigor, and Long Life**. Santa Barbara, CA: Woodbridge Press (P. O. Box 6189, Santa Barbara, CA 93111), 1978. 90p. illus. $2.95. LC 78-71029. ISBN 0-912800-51-8. (Translated from the Japanese).

The author of this book is known in Japan for his study of Ume, or Japanese plums, a "health food" known for more than a thousand years in the Orient. Traditional foods are undergoing an awakening in Japan, and Matsumoto's books on the subject have sold well. The plum is said to prevent disease, and it was used in ancient time to cure a wide variety of diseases and conditions.

The book begins with a history of the use of the Japanese plum from early times until today. Following are some of the many virtues attributed to the fruit: for cough, an antifebrile, an expectorant, to stop nausea, for headaches, dysentery, food poisoning, restoration of acid-alkaline balance, to metabolize sugar, as an antibacterial, to combat radioactivity (useful after the Hiroshima bombing), to balance the spirit, for problems of pregnancy, for skin troubles, a source of stamina, to slow the process of aging, to prevent anemia, prevent colds, for liver troubles, stomach ulcers, high blood pressure, athlete's foot, snake bites, and as a contraceptive. In addition, it was even believed at one time to improve one's luck at gambling.

The plums are used in everyday cooking. The final third of the book is a presentation of recipes for Japanese traditional health foods using the plums, which are usually marketed as salted plums, preserved by pickling in salt brine. The best salted plums, according to the author, are picked from the tree by hand and processed with roasted natural salt (whatever that is). The plums are then sun dried for several days and later exposed to night air.

301.   Mori, Kisaku. **Mushrooms as Health Foods.** Tokyo: Japan Publications, Inc.; distr. Japan Publications Trading Co. (1255 Howard St., San Francisco, CA 94103), 1974. 88p. illus. $3.25pa. ISBN 0-87040-332-X.

Mori, who is Director of the Japan Institute of Mushroom Research, offers this work in support of the view that the shiitake mushrooms of Japan are good for the health and have a therapeutic effect on a wide range of diseases. He says he has divided their effects into four major categories: 1) Prevention of sickness; 2) Recovery from fatigue; 3) Increase of stamina and sexual powers; and 4) Improvement of personal appearance. The claim is made that influenza and cancer are affected by the mushroom spores, and that the fungi contain a substance which will lower the amount of cholesterol in the blood and be effective in treating such diseases as artherosclerosis, high blood pressure, diabetes, gallstones, and other conditions.

The work of several scientists is mentioned to support these claims, although there are no direct literature references to publications reporting research results. The work is presented in three parts: 1) Mushrooms as food; 2) Effects of mushroom foods; and 3) Appetizing shiitake dishes. The mushrooms can be obtained fresh, dried, and in extract form, and the recipes in the last section seem appetizing. Illustrations are cartoons that somewhat humorously depict the power of the mushrooms.

302.   Mortimer, W. Golden. **Peru History of Coca: "The Divine Plant" of the Incas.** With an introductory account of the Incas, and of the Andean Indians of today. New York, J. H. Vail and Co., 1901; repr. Berkeley, CA: And/Or Press, 1978. 576p. illus. bibliog. index. $8.50. ISBN 0-915904-01-2.

This classic work undertakes to trace associations and uses of coca (the plant from which cocaine comes) from the earliest accounts to the time the book was written. The story begins with the Empire of the Incas and shows a connection between these people and the history of the use of the plant. Industries, science, arts, poetry, drama, laws, social system, and religious rites of the Incas are all interwoven with the uses and applications of coca. Mortimer's work includes accounts of contemporary travelers and scientists, as well as the scientific material about the plant that was known at the time. The following chapters are presented: 1) An Introduction to the History of Coca; 2) The Story of the Incans; 3) The Rites and Acts of the Incans; 4) The Conquest of the Incans; 5) The Physical Aspect of Peru; 6) The History of Coca; 7) The Present Indians of Peru; 8) The Botany of Coca; 9) In the Coca Region of Peru; 10) The Products of the Coca Leaf; 11) The Production of Alkaloids in Plants; 12) Influence of Coca upon Muscular Energy; 13) Action of Coca upon the Nervous System; 14) The Physiological Action of Coca; 15) Adaptation of Coca to Voice Production; and 16) The Dietetic Influence of Coca.

There are some additional appended materials, such as results of a collective investigation among several hundred physicians on the physiological action and the therapeutic application of coca. This monumental book, which includes 178 illustrations, is quite interesting.

303.   Myerhoff, Barbara G. **Peyote Hunt: The Sacred Journey of the Huichol Indians.** Ithaca and London: Cornell University Press, 1974. 285p. illus. bibliog. index. LC 73-16923. ISBN 0-8014-0817-2.

This book is one of a series on symbol, myth, and ritual, the aim of which is to bring to public attention works by anthropologists on these subjects. This work describes an annual pilgrimage made by members of the Huichol Indian tribe of Mexico to their sacred land of Wirikuta where they hunt the peyote cactus. The plant's "button" contains a powerful hallucinogenic agent which is used in religious ceremonies. The myth, rituals, religious symbols, and culture of the people are all painstakingly treated by the author who accompanied the Indians on their trip.

The interesting account does not focus entirely on the effects of the hallucinogen in the peyote. It treats peyote as only one constituent of the Huichols' ritual complex. This complex is made up of the deer, maize, and peyote as symbols in a sacred unity.

304.   Ott, Jonathan, and Jeremy Bigwood, eds. **Teonanacatl: Hallucinogenic Mushrooms of North America.** Seattle, WA: Madrona Publishers, Inc., 1978. 175p. illus. (part col.). bibliog. index. (Psycho-Mycological Studies, No.2). $14.50; $8.95pa. LC 78-14794. ISBN 0-914842-32-3; 0-914842-29-3pa.

This book is based on the proceedings of the Second International Conference on Hallucinogenic Mushrooms, held in Port Townsend, Washington, in October 1977. Leading authorities in the field, such as R. Gordon Wasson, Albert Hofmann, Andrew Weil, and Richard Evans Schultes (some of them respected scientists), presented papers. The history of the use of hallucinogenic mushrooms is traced; their use in religious ritual is discussed; and their botanical identification and cultivation outlined. In addition, an appeal for responsible use in modern society is made, doubtlessly a controversial matter.

The editors and contributors take the subject seriously. At lease some of them believe that these mushrooms have had mystical power, although it may have been lost in modern times because of their use by a "profane and puerile, largely hedonistic cult which has succeeded its venerable ancestor." Wasson has observed that the superficial use by ignorant thrill-seekers is a desecration. It is hoped that there might be a resurgence in their use as sacraments.

305.   Rivier, L., ed. **Coca and Cocaine, 1981.** Lausanne, Switzerland: Elsevier Sequoia, 1981. 106-379p. illus. bibliog. index. (**Journal of Ethnopharmacology,** v.3, nos.2-3, March/May, 1981).

Included here are updated articles based on papers presented at the Symposium on *Erythroxylon*—New Historical and Scientific Aspects, sponsored by the Botanical

Museum of Harvard University and Casa de la Cultura del Ecuador, Quito, Ecuador, December 3-5, 1979.

Coca has been a part of human affairs in South America for several thousand years, has remained an integral part of Andean culture, and plays a vital role in many Indian societies in the western Amazon. The custom of chewing coca leaves is poorly understood from many points of view. Some consider it a noxious habit while others think it is physiologically beneficial for Andean Indians in their adaptation to the harsh environment of hunger, cold, and fatigue at high altitudes. The use of cocaine in western societies, which is on the increase, has recently focused attention on the plant.

The papers in this special issue of a periodical focus on the history, aboriginal use, chemistry, and medical potentialities of the coca plant. Legal, social, or political aspects of the subject are not considered. The following papers are included: 1) Sundry episodes in the history of coca and cocaine; 2) Coca and cocaine as medicines; an historical review; 3) Social function of coca in pre-Columbian America; 4) Coca in northwest Amazon; 5) Amazonian coca; 6) Determination of varieties and cultivars in Peruvian coca; 7) Systematic anatomy of *Erythroxylum* P. Browne: practical and evolutionary implications for the cultivated cocas; 8) The comparative phytochemistry of the genus *Erythroxylon*; 9) Chemotaxonomy of Erythroxylaceae (including some ethnobotanical notes on old world species); 10) Constituents of *Erythroxylon coca*; 11) Mass-analyzed ion kinetic energy (MIKE) spectrometry and the direct analysis of coca; 12) Analysis of alkaloids in leaves of cultivated *Erythroxylum* and characterization of alkaline substances used during coca chewing; 13) Guide to the analysis of cocaine and its metabolites in biological material; 14) Cocaine pharmacokineics in humans; and 15) The therapeutic value of coca in contemporary medicine.

306.   Rodale, J. I. **The Hawthorn Berry for the Heart.** Emmaus, PA: Rodale Books, Inc., 1971. 125p. $ .95pa. SBN 87596-050-2.

The author says he has written this book about an obscure berry because, at one time, it was used extensively in heart disease, and there exists a good deal of clinical data about it (most of it done before 1910) that should be made known. He sets about the task of doing this, making references to many publications in the text. There is no formal bibliography.

Several case histories are provided. In addition, the book contains reprinted articles and quotations from diverse periodical publications such as the *Journal of the American Medical Association*, the *British Medical Journal*, *Homeopathic Recorder*, *Biochimica e Terpia Sperimentale* (translated), *Prevention*, *Journal of Clinical Nutrition*, *Acta Phytotherapeutica*, and *Nutrition Reviews*. Material from monograph publications is cited also, some as old as *Culpeper's Complete Herbal* (see entry 139).

The book possibly brings to light valuable buried information. It does provide a curious mixture of material from scientific, clinical, and popular sources.

307.   Rubin, Vera, ed. **Cannabis and Culture.** The Hague: Mouton Publishers; distr., Aldine, 1975. 598p. illus. bibliog. index. (World Anthropology). $24.92. ISBN 90-279-7669-4; 0-202-01152-6 (Aldine).

The papers in this volume were originally presented at a Conference on Cross-Cultural Perspective on Cannabis, held in Chicago in 1973, during the Ninth International Congress of the International Union of Anthropological and Ethnological Sciences.

The papers help provide an understanding of the sociocultural differences in reactions to the ancient and widespread substance, cannabis. Also, the volume introduces new botanical classifications and presents data on clinical studies of cannabis users.

Scientists from a number of disciplines participated—anthropologists, botanists, geneticists, pharmacologists, psychiatrists, and sociologists. The 35 papers are arranged under the following section headings: 1) Ethnobotany and diffusion; 2) Sociocultural aspects of the traditional complex; 3) Medical, pharmacological, and ethnometabolic studies; 4) Traditional usage of other psychoactive plants; and 5) The modern complex in North America. An abstract is included with each paper.

The work makes apparent the fact that psychoactive plants have been used for a variety of purposes in the world, secular as well as sacred, to serve a wide range of human needs, and that different emphases have been placed on the use of such substances in various cultures.

308. Sandford, Jeremy. **In Search of the Magic Mushroom: A Journey through Mexico.** New York: Clarkson N. Potter, Inc.; distr. Crown Publishers, 1973. 176p. illus. bibliog. index. $2.95pa. LC 72-80846. ISBN 0-517-501546.

This is an account of the author's travels through Mexico in search of the mysterious magic mushrooms of the mountains. Sandford first heard of the mushrooms while on assignment in Mexico for a London newspaper. These mushrooms, when eaten, induce hallucinations said to be frightening, but they produce splendid hallucinations of color, profound emotions, beautiful visions, and the like. The author, like others, believes these mushrooms (*Amanita miscaria* and *Psilocybe Mexicana*) are at the heart of many religions.

The book describes life in Mexico, the scenes, the poverty, and the beauty as well as the mushroom search. An appendix quotes information about the mushrooms, taken from several other works. Methods of preparation of the fungi for hallucinogenic doses is provided, along with cautions, as the plants are poisonous.

309. Speight, Phyllis. **Arnica, the Wonder Herb: The Remedy That Should Be in Every Home.** Holsworthy, England, Health Science Press, 1977. 45p. illus. (Health in the Home Series). $2.00pa. ISBN 0-85032-138-7.

The author of this small book has written several other titles in the Health in the Home Series. After a short introduction, a verse, and some historical material about the herbal plant *Arnica Montana*, its medicinal uses are taken up individually. Arnica is one of the best-known old homoeopathic remedies. Its uses include treatment for bruises and shock, sleeplessness, healing of dental surgery, tired feed, over-tiredness, playground injuries, sprains, rheumatism, surgical trauma, and athletic injuries.

The book suggests that arnica should be purchased in the proper strength from a pharmacy specializing in homoeopathic pharmacy. In some instances, the proper strength is specified in the text in homoeopathic standards. Homoeopathic products are ordinarily extremely dilute. Also included in the work are a few case histories on the value of arnica and some extracts from works of "old homoeopathic masters" in which references are made to the medicinal plant.

310. Stamets, Paul. **Psilocybe Mushrooms and Their Allies.** Seattle, WA: Homestead Book Co. (Distributed nationally by And/Or Press, Box 2246, Berkeley, CA 94702). 1978. 160p. illus. (part col.). bibliog. $9.95pa. LC 77-26546. ISBN 0-930180-03-8.

The primary purpose of this work is to identify the hallucinogenic and poisonous mushrooms of the U.S. and to separate them from those which are not. It can serve as a field guide. In addition, information is included on how to cultivate mushrooms. There are five chapters as follows: 1) Mushrooms: Habits and Habitats; 2) Taxonomy; 3) The Keys; 4) Species Descriptions; and 5) Mushroom Cultivation. Also included are two appendices, "The Mushroom Life Cycle" and "The Microscopic Dimension," and a glossary. The book is well illustrated with many color photographs, drawings, and diagrams. It is an accurate presentation.

311.   Steinmetz, E. F. **Piper Methysticum, Kava - Kava - Yaqona; Famous Drug Plant of the South Sea Islands.** Amsterdam, the Netherlands; E. F. Steinmetz, 1960. 46p. illus. bibliog. (A 1973 reprinted edition entitled **Kava-Kava, Famous Drug Plant of the South Sea Islands** is available from High Times/Level Press, Box 386, Cooper Station, New York, NY 10003 for $2.00).

This booklet contains information about the kava plant and the beverage made from it that is used primarily as a ceremonial drink in the South Pacific islands. The drink is habit-forming and occasionally abused, although it may have medicinal properties. There are short chapters on the habitat of the plant, cultivation, description and varieties, structure of the root, harvesting the rootstock, history, preparing the beverage, effects, chemical composition, and use in therapy.

312.   Taylor, Norman: **Cinchona in Java: The Story of Quinine.** With an introduction by Pieter Honing. New York: Greenberg, 1945. 87p. illus. bibliog. index.

This work is about the production of cinchona in Java for making quinine to be used for treating malaria. It covers the development of agriculture in Java, the history and cause of malaria, the discovery of cinchona, British and Dutch attempts to introduce cinchona into the old world, and the development of cinchona production in Java. The bibliography is a selected list of cinchona literature. There are black and white photographs and some line drawings throughout the text. The book is by a noted botanist and is still of historical interest.

313.   Veninga, Louise. **The Ginseng Book.** Santa Cruz, CA: Ruka Publishing (P. O. Box 1072, Santa Cruz, CA 95061), 1973. 152p. illus. bibliog. $4.95pa. LC 74-151211.

This book has 13 chapters covering most everything about ginseng. The information comes from the author's first-hand experience, Chinese herbalists, cultivators, collectors, pharmacologists, and doctors. A discussion of medical research concerning ginseng is included.

A large amount of historical and geographical information is provided as well as extensive discussions about cultivation, harvesting, identification, and foraging for the plant. The chapter entitled "Root Buyer's Guide" is a detailed discussion of the varieties of ginseng found in different parts of the world and the quality of the plants. The book contains a good deal of practical information. The author's aim in writing this book is to promote the herbal alternative in medical practice.

314.   Veninga, Louise, and Benjamin R. Zaricor. **Goldenseal/Etc.: A Pharmacognosy of Wild Herbs.** Santa Cruz, CA: Ruka Publications (P. O. Box 1072, Santa Cruz, CA 95060), 1976. 193p. illus. bibliog. $3.95pa. LC 75-41630. ISBN 0-915178-03-7.

This book is a comprehensive discussion of the herb, goldenseal, which the authors consider the "Universal Herb." After an introduction which includes historical material and a short discussion of early American medical publications, the first half of the book is taken up with specific information about goldenseal.

Description, habitat, pioneer and commercial history, cultivation, and preparation of goldenseal are discussed in detail in the first part of the book. Several formulas using the herb are given, along with the illnesses which they may treat. Several notes of warning are given throughout the text about overuse of the plant. The second half of the book contains discussions on other American herbs. Each discussion includes the scientific name, several common names, the chemical compounds found in the usable part of the plant, the therapeutic uses of the herb, the preparation and dosage, historical notes, habitat (including a map of the U.S.), proper times to harvest, and how the herb is cultivated. Ink drawings or black and white photographs are shown for each herb.

315.   Vosnjak, Mitja. **The Miracle of Propolis: The Story of the Rediscovery of the Remarkable Healing Properties of This Product of the Beehives.** Wellingborough, England: Thorsons, 1978. 93p. $3.95pa. LC 78-317500. ISBN 0-7225-0408-X.

Propolis, a brownish resinous material of waxy consistency, collected by bees from the buds of trees and used as a cement, has caught the interest of those seeking "natural" remedies. It is presumed, by the author of this book at least, to be a powerful antibiotic. Vosnjak reports on his personal experiences with the substance and provides case histories of others who are reported to have benefited from internal or external use of propolis.

316.   Watanabe, Tadashi. **Garlic Therapy.** Tokyo: Japan Publications, Inc.; distr. Japan Publications Trading Co. (200 Clearbrook Road, Elmsford, NY 10523), 1974. 66p. illus. $3.95pa. LC 74-79313. ISBN 0-87040-272-2.

The author of this monograph is a Japanese known for his numerous writings on the wholesome effects of garlic on health. His view is that people generally have a vague notion that garlic is good for the health but do not know why. He attempts to show scientifically that garlic is indeed a health food because it improves general physical condition. Also included are a section on specific effects of the plant (which are rather general) and recipes for garlic dishes. Watanabe has included suggestions on how to eliminate garlic odor. The book is illustrated with cartoons.

The author does not make a good case for garlic as a medicine or "health food" (if such exists). He points out that it has long been part of general Oriental folk medicine, much of which originated in China where medicines are often used to promote general good health rather than for specific symptoms. Any food can probably be considered a health food if all it has to do is promote general good health.

317.   Weniger, Del. **Cacti of the Southwest: Texas, New Mexico, Oklahoma, Arkansas and Louisiana.** Austin and London: University of Texas Press, 1970. 249p. illus. (col.). index. (The Elma Dill Russell Spencer Foundation Series. No.4). $25.00. LC 78-104326. ISBN 0-292-70000-8.

The author's introduction to this work points out that cacti grow naturally only in the Western Hemisphere. They had not been seen by the so-called civilized world until Columbus discovered America. Accounts of them, however, evidently spread rapidly because Gerard described four species in his *Herball* of 1597 (see entry 150). The introduction further describes how cultivation of cacti became popular in many parts of the world and tells about botanists who have been interested in them.

The book lists all forms of cacti known to be growing in the five states mentioned in the title. The 119 species and 171 varieties are listed by scientific name with common names following, including Spanish and Indian names in some cases. A long description is given, range, and miscellaneous remarks. The remarks include unusual and interesting information. The book is large in page size, and 64 full-color plates are included. Most of the plants are in bloom. A glossary and indexes of scientific and common names are provided. References are made throughout to literature, but no formal bibliography is included.

It is noteworthy that the peyote cactus (discussed at some length in the book) is famous out of all proportion to its size and appearance. It is the sacred hallucinogenic plant of the Indians.

Folk medicine of peoples of early times and of various cultures of more recent times is discussed in the books listed in this section. Virtually all the groups have relied heavily on herbal plants for their medicines, although some animal and mineral products also have been utilized. Magic and witchcraft have played a role, but books covering these areas more exclusively are listed in chapter 13. A few books on Biblical medicine are included with the miscellaneous materials in chapter 21. Works listed in the field of ethnobotany cover more than medicines made from plants, but medicines are an important segment of such studies.

An unusually large percent of the works listed in the following section are reports of scholarly research studies, and most seem to be well done and valuable as well as interesting.

Many of the books deal with folk medicine of China, perhaps a reflection of the current interest in that country among Americans. Other geographic areas and cultures studied include the following: early American, Californian, Texan, Zulu, Welch, American Indian, black American, Hawaiian, African, Pennsylvania German, Vermont, Russian, Shaker, Sea Island, Low Country of South Carolina, Ancient Egyptian, Gypsy, Sicilian, Mayan, Indian, Mexican, Southwestern U.S., British of the seventeenth and eighteenth centuries, southern U.S., rural U.S., Oriental, Australian, and the British.

* * * * *

318.   Aikman, Lonnelle. **Nature's Healing Arts: From Folk Medicine to Modern Drugs.** Washington, DC: National Geographic Society, 1977. 199p. illus. (col.). bibliog. index. LC 76-56997. ISBN 0-87044-232-5.

This book is in keeping with publications put out by the National Geographic Society. It is profusely illustrated with excellent color photographs and a few paintings, a great many showing people using or gathering various medicinal herbs and remedies.

Most of the book is devoted to discussions of the experiences of individuals from various parts of the world who use folk remedies. Many actual quotes from these people are reported. Discussion of nineteenth-century patent medicines and Chinese herbal medicine are included in the book. The latter part of the work tells how modern medicine has drawn upon many "old time" herbs in discovering cures for various diseases and in synthetically reproducing these or similar compounds. Also discussed is the renewed interest in "natural" medicinal cures both by the lay public and scientists.

The work makes no attempt to help the reader to identify a particular plant for recognition in the field, but it does specifically mention many herbs and plants commonly found throughout the U.S. Specific preparation and use of the various plants for medicinal purposes is not given. The book is written simply for the lay public. An alphabetical listing of common names for various plants and animals mentioned in the book is given at the end of the text, and scientific designations are also included.

319.   American Herbal Pharmacology Delegation. **Herbal Pharmacology in the People's Republic of China: A Trip Report.** Submitted to the Committee on Scholarly Communication with the People's Republic of China. Washington, DC: National Academy of Sciences, 1975. 269p. bibliog. $8.00. LC 75-39772. ISBN 0-309-02438-2.

Twelve U.S. scientists in the fields of chemistry, medicine, pharmacology, pharmacognosy, pharmacy, and Chinese culture visited in 1974 some major Chinese cities to assess the current status of herbal pharmacology in the country. It was hoped that something would be learned about current Chinese uses of herbal medicines and that plant materials could be identified that might be utilized by Western scientists in developing new drug products. Visits were made to medical schools (both traditional and Western type), research institutes, hospitals, pharmacies, pharmaceutical plants, and plantations.

The report begins with an introductory essay that emphasizes the inseparability of politics and medicine in China. Traditional medicine (which is mainly herbal-based) is especially encouraged in China. The Western scientists are critical of many of the practices of the Chinese; for instance, if a drug (or herb) appears to be beneficial, time and effort are not devoted to chemical experiments to isolate its active principles and little attempt is made to determine what specific herb is responsible for a patient's improvement (a number are often used simultaneously). Westerners are skeptical of traditional remedies, but the Chinese believe that medicines used for centuries *must* be effective and safe. In the U.S. it is mandated by law that proof of efficacy and safety be established before a remedy can be marketed, the scientists point out. Despite criticisms, the essay concludes that botanicals and botanically derived drugs are a major source of some of the most useful drugs known.

Other sections of the book are: 1) The wedding of Western and traditional medicine; 2) The clinical use of herbal medicines; 3) Chinese pharmacology; 4) Laboratory researches emanating from herbal medicine; 5) Medicinal plant gardens in China; 6) Pharmacy and pharmaceutical manufacturing in China; 7) Drug control in China; 8) The validation of claims for traditional medicines; 9) Biomedical education in China; 10) General medical care in China; and 11) Concluding remarks.

There is an appended table (about one-half of the book) that is an evaluation of 248 plant and animal drugs used in the People's Republic of China. They are listed alphabetically by scientific name, and for each is given uses and an analysis of the value. The latter includes a review of available literature and comparison with reports from other countries. There is no index by common name, which limits the usefulness of the book for non-scientists.

This is one of the few objective, scholarly, and scientific works on the subject.

320.   Anderson, John Q. **Texas Folk Medicine: 1,333 Cures, Remedies, Preventives, and Health Practices.** Woodcuts by Barbara Mathews Whitehead. Austin, TX: Encino Press, 1970. 91p. illus. bibliog. (Texas Folklore Society, Paisano Book, No.5). $5.95. ISBN 0-88426-013-5.

Material that makes up this compilation was selected from data collected by students in the author's folklore class at Texas A and M University. Anderson begins by stating that the general reader of the book will probably be convinced that his ancestors were a hardy race or they could not have survived their own medical practices.

He also notes that some of the beliefs implied in the cures seem incredible, although some remedies will be familiar. Such attitudes are part of the lore of folk medicine, Anderson believes.

There is an introductory chapter on folk medicine. Then ailments are listed alphabetically with various remedies given. The geographical source of the information is indicated, most from Texas, but some material comes from other states and a few foreign countries as well.

321.   Balls, Edward K. **Early Uses of California Plants.** Berkeley, CA: University of California Press, 1962. 103p. illus. bibliog. index. (California Natural History Guides, No.10). $12.95. LC 62-17531. ISBN 0-520-02989-5.

The seven chapters of this book cover food plants; drink plants; fiber and basketry plants; medicinal plants; soap and fish poison plants; dye, gum and tobacco plants; and present-day uses of a few California plants. Certain plants could be placed in more than one category of use, but each is included only once.

The food plant section is almost one-third of the book and covers only 18 plants. The medicinal plant section includes only seven entries. Each entry includes some historical information, a disucssion of Indian and early settler uses of the plant, the Latin name, a brief description, and remarks about habitat. Many entires include ink drawings. Most discussions are fairly comprehensive, but specific recipes are not given. The bibliography lists mainly references to California plants and history.

322.   **A Barefoot Doctor's Manual: The American Translation of the Official Chinese Paramedical Manual.**   Philadelphia, PA: Running Press (38 S. Nineteenth St., Phila-delphia, PA 19103), 1977. 948p. illus. index. $6.95pa. ISBN 0-914294-92-X. (Translation of Ch'ih chiao i sheng shou ts'e. Reprint of 1974 edition published by U.S. Dept. of Health, Education, and Welfare, Public Health Service, National Institutes of Health, Bethesda, MD, in series DHEW publication no. [NIH 75-695]).

This manual was published in China in 1970 to supply the "barefoot doctors" with a guide to help them in their work in rural areas of the People's Republic of China. The "barefoot doctors" are defined by the government as being "peasants" who have had basic medical training and can handle medical emergencies, prescribe for simple injuries and illnesses, and apply treatments prescribed by a qualified doctor.

About two-thirds of the book is taken up with material on rudimentary anato-my, physiology, hygiene, diagnostic techniques, and treatment of common diseases. A listing of more than 500 common Chinese herbs, including about 390 line-drawing illustrations, makes up about one-third of the book. Also included is an introductory section of general facts about medicinal plants. For each plant listed is given: Chinese common name (transliterated), botanical name, synonyms, morphology, properties and action, conditions used for, and preparation. There is no index by plant name, and the listing seems to be in somewhat random order.

The publisher warns that some Chinese herbs may bear a close resemblance to varieties found in North America, but they cannot be assumed to act in the same way. The book should not be used as a blueprint for self-treatment. It has some appeal as a view of a distant and largely unknown culture.

323.   Bauer, W. W. **Potions, Remedies and Old Wives Tales.** Garden City, NY: Doubleday and Co., Inc., 1969. bibliog. index. $5.95. LC 69-10977.

The late author of this work was a noted physician-author who was interested in medical folklore. In the book, he has examined hundreds of common folk beliefs and practices and has pointed out facts and fallacies regarding them. Many he found to be superstition only, although some are based on sound scientific principles. A good deal of history is presented where myth, magic folklore, and religion are intermingled.

Chapter titles are: 1) How Did Folklore Begin?; 2) Folklore, Religion, Medicine; 3) Witches, Witchcraft and Witch Doctoring; 4) Man's Emerging Image of Himself; 5) Medicinal Plants and Herbs; 6) Medicinal Properties in Foods; 7) Animals in Folk Medicine; 8) The Quest for Beauty; 9) Grandma Is Not Always Wrong; 10) New Therapy from Old Remedies; 11) Our Debt to Medical Folklore; 12) Poisons in Your Plantings?; 13) Is Folk Medicine Coming Back?; and 14) Popular Beliefs that Are Not So.

The last chapter points out that history is repeating itself; there is a renewed interest in folk medicine, especially in plants and herbs. Some of this is good, the author thinks, because part of the interest is scientific and may lead to development of more valuable drugs. Unfortunately, though, there is "exploitation of old, outmoded discredited or purely fictitious properties attributed to substances which have been found to have little or no value under the scrutiny of modern scientific evaluation." These claims may lead to false hopes that are cruel and misleading, the author believes.

The book is interesting and authoritative.

324.   Black, William George. **Folk-Medicine: A Chapter in the History of Culture.** New York: Burt Franklin, 1970. 226p. bibliog. index. (Burt Franklin: Research and Source Works Series 486; Selected Essays in History, Economics, and Social Science 136). $11.00. LC 74-124308. ISBN 0-8337-0298-X. (Originally published in 1883).

This 1883 publication has been reprinted with no new preface or introductory material. It is a thoughtful scholarly account; the author has attempted to "classify the explanations of the causes of disease which come to light in folk-lore." He presents a philosophical and analytical view of the subject with ample reference to works of other authors.

Chapter titles are: 1) Introduction: Origin of Disease; 2) Transference of Disease; 3) Sympathy and Association of Ideas; 4) New Birth and Sacrifice; 5) Our Lord and the Saints in Folk-Medicine; 6) Charms Connected with Death or the Grave; 7) Colour; 8) Number—Influence of the Sun and Moon; 9) Personal Cures; 10) Animal Cures; 11) Specific Charms: Magic Writings—Rings; 12) Domestic Folk-Medicine; and 13) The Place of Folk-Medicine in the Study of Civilization.

The last paragraph of the book asks: "What place can Folk-Medicine claim in the great book of culture?" The author hopes that "illustrations of man's intellectual history will be found by study of collections of classified facts, and that the investigation of spells and amulets, of superstitions and witcheries, may not be unworthy of systematic analysis."

325.   Bryant, A. T. **Zulu Medicine and Medicine-Men.** Cape Town, South Africa: C. Struik, 1966. 115p. illus.

When the author of this work undertook his study he assumed that the Zulu had advanced little in 6,000 years and that his knowledge of disease, although considerable, had changed little.

Following are the chapter titles: 1) Introduction; 2) The General Status and Initiation of the Medicine-Man; 3) Origin of the Zulu Name *I-nyanga* (medicine-man); 4) The Medicine-Man and Witch-Doctor Compared; 5) The Nature of Native Medical Practice; 6) The Native Medicines; 7) The Preparation of Medicines and General Treatment; 8) Physical and Constitutional Traits of the Native; and 9) Treatment of Diseases.

The longest chapter, Treatment of Disease, lists ailments and tells what remedies are used to treat them. The last section of the book is a list of about 240 Zulu medicinal plants, giving what the natives believe to be their properties and how to use them. The author thinks many more are known to the natives, perhaps 700 in all. The list also serves as an index to the contents of the book, as page references are given that refer to sections where remedies are discussed.

326.   Conway, David. **The Magic of Herbs.** New York: E. P. Dutton and Co., 1973. 158p. illus. index. $4.50. LC 73-79539. ISBN 0-525-47417-X.

The author of this work grew up in a rural part of Wales and learned most of what he reports about the use of herbs from a descendant of the great Welsh herbal doctors known as *Meddygion Myddfai.* These doctors, Conway says, are not known widely outside of Wales.

The following chapters are presented: 1) Botanical Medicine; 2) Herbalism and Astrology; 3) The Doctrine of Signatures; 4) The Preparation of Herbs; 5) Tonics and Physics; 6) Cosmetics and Narcotics; 7) Wines from Herbs and Flowers; 8) The Language of Flowers; and 9) Herbal *Materia Medica.* The last chapter, which makes up about half the book, is an alphabetical list of herbs (by common name), most of them common to temperate regions. Brief descriptions of the plants are given, as are scientific names, uses, and lore. The index lists ailments and herbs for their treatment.

The book is of interest for the folklore it contains, but suggested medicinal uses of the plants seem unusually primitive.

327.   Curtin, L. S. M. **Healing Herbs of the Upper Rio Grande.** Los Angeles, CA: Southwest Museum (P. O. Box 128, Highland Park Station, Los Angeles, CA 90042), 1965. 281p. illus. bibliog. index. $7.50.

This book is a reprint of the original work published by the Laboratory of Anthropology in Santa Fe, New Mexico, in 1947.

The main part of the work is an alphabetical arrangement (by popular Spanish name) of plant names and miscellaneous other folk medicine cures. More than 400 entries are included. Some examples of non-plant cures listed are: rattlesnake oil, mineral lime, alum stone, skunk lard, rabbit milk, tierra de rata (earth drug up by gophers), blood of various animals, red ants, and remolino (roasted hive cells of the Mason bee).

Each entry includes the Latin name and several popular English and Spanish common names. Most descriptions are written in a folksy style and include some historical information, miscellaneous quotes from books and actual users of the cure, a general description of the plant or cure, and how the cure is applied. Specific formulations and applications are usually not given.

A separate section includes about 30 black and white photographs of selected plants with their Spanish names. A general index and a remedy index add considerably to the value of this work. The bibliography contains only old and presumably out of print items, but some interesting citations are included. The book is interesting, but its value as a practical home medical guide or as a field identification guide is limited. Its greatest value probably lies in the anthropological and ethnobotanical contribution it makes, and it has been well received for that reason.

328.   Densmore, Frances. **How Indians Use Wild Plants for Food, Medicine, and Crafts.** (Formerly titled **Uses of Plants by the Chippewa Indians**). New York: Dover Publications, Inc., 1974. 279-397p. illus. bibliog. $3.00pa. LC 73-92500. ISBN 0-486-23019-8.

This work is an unabridged republication of an article originally appearing in the *Forty-fourth Annual Report of the Bureau of American Ethnology, 1926-27.* The author, who was an ethnologist with the Smithsonian Institution, reports on nearly 200 plants used by the Chippewa Indians of Minnesota and Wisconsin. She captured many of the traditions of these groups, showing how they used plants for food, medicine, arts, crafts, and dyeing. Emphasis is on wild plants and lesser-known uses.

The publication begins with lists of plants arranged according to botanical name, common name, and native name, respectively. Then a list of medicinal properties of plants and a list of principal active medicinal constituents of plants follow. There are sections on plants as food, plants as medicine, plants used in dyes, plants used as charms, and plants used in useful and decorative arts. The publication ends with sections on the legend of Winabojo and the birch tree, legend of Winabojo and the cedar tree, gathering birch and cedar bark, and articles made of birch bark. Many plants discussed are native to the Great Lakes region only; others are found throughout a wide area. Special attention is given to making maple sugar and gathering wild rice. Over 30 plates are included.

329.   Dimond, E. Grey. **More than Herbs and Acupuncture.** New York: W. W. Norton and Co., 1975. 223p. $7.95. LC 74-11166. ISBN 0-393-06400-X.

The author of this book is a cardiologist who played a key role in developing medical exchanges between the U.S. and China. The book is an account of his experiences and observations in China while studying their medical system. The Chinese typically use a combination of traditional and modern Western treatments. A modern drug and an herbal medicine may be used together. The viewpoint expressed in the work is that the world, particularly the underdeveloped nations, can learn much from the Chinese, and research efforts into all aspects of Chinese medicine should be carried out.

330.   Elmore, Francis H. **Ethnobotany of the Navajo.** A Monograph of the University of New Mexico and the School of American Research. New York: AMS Press, 1978. 136p. bibliog. index. $22.50. LC 76-43698. ISBN 0-404-15530-8. (Reprinted from the edition of 1943, which was issued as v.1, no.7 [whole no. 392] of the Monograph series of the University of New Mexico).

The author of this work spent three summers working first-hand with Navajo informants who assisted in identifying plants in the field that are used by their tribe. Only a portion of the plants used by the Navajo are included in the book, but the author hoped it would serve as a preliminary study to stimulate more research among the Indians. Unfortunately, not a great deal of medicinal data has been included in the book, largely because other workers were making such studies, and it was not felt necessary to duplicate efforts.

Arrangement of the plants is alphabetical under family headings. Information given includes synonymous names, other names (including the Navajo), authors, references to the bibliography, and text material which includes folklore, uses, and descriptions. There are tables of plants arranged by uses, such as medicinal, for witchcraft, ceremonial, food, wood, dye, basketry, and beverage. The bibliography lists 87 references. There are three indexes: Navajo names, scientific names, and a general index. This is an interesting scholarly effort.

331.   Fiedler, Mildred. **Plant Medicine and Folklore.** New York: Winchester Press, 1975. 268p. illus. bibliog. index. $12.95. LC 75-9262. ISBN 0-87691-205-6.

The author of this attractive book says belief in medicinal virtues of wild plants is deeply entrenched in American folklore, a belief that was born of necessity. There were few, if any, doctors available on the frontier, and people sought remedies in the woods and wilds. Old ways are not entirely gone, the author points out. Modern medical research has proved some folk remedies really worked; others have been found to be worthless, even harmful. The book presents folklore and facts, information about healing properties, real or imagined, and historical anecdotes connected with plant medicines.

Plants are grouped according to ailment treated as follows: bites, wounds, and parasites; burns, abrasions, rashes, and skin infections; disorders of head and throat; disorders of stomach and bowels; disorders of other internal organs; childbirth and child care; colds, neuralgia, and rheumatism; and general tonics. There is also a chapter on poisonous plants. Illustrations are nice photographs and line drawings. Many common plants are covered.

The book is of high quality. No claims are made for the value of the plant medicines discussed, and the reader is warned to be cautious about trying any of them as many of the plants are now considered poisonous.

332.   Gilmore, Melvin R. **Uses of Plants by the Indians of the Missouri River Region.** Foreword by Hugh Cutler. Lincoln, NE: University of Nebraska Press, 1977. 109p. illus. bibliog. index. $11.95; $3.50pa. LC 77-89833. ISBN 0-8032-0935-1; 0-8032-5872-0pa. (Originally presented as the author's thesis, University of Nebraska, 1914; a reprint of the 1919 ed. which appeared in the 23rd Annual Report of the Bureau of American Ethnology).

In this classical work in the field of ethnobotany, the author attempts to show that primitive peoples and their culture were tied together with plants and the environment, an idea that is still held by many. Gilmore also hopes to show that plants used by American Indians might be used by others to good advantage, also a popular idea today. Information in the book was obtained first-hand from older persons in the Indian tribes and was checked with other members of the same or different tribes of the region.

Section headings are as follows: 1) Introduction; 2) Neglected opportunities; 3) Ethnic botany; 4) Influence of flora on human activities and culture; 5) Influence of human population on flora; 6) Taxonomic list of plants used by Indians of the Missouri River region; 7) Ancient and modern phytoculture by the tribes; 8) Conclusion; and 9) Glossary of plant names mentioned in this monograph.

The taxonomic list makes up most of the book. Each plant is identified with scientific, common English, and Indian names. The various Indian tribes used different names for the same plant. Habitat is described briefly, and uses are discussed at some length. The plants were used for medicine, food, dyes, charms, weapons, and in religious ceremonies.

333.   Gordon, Lesley. **Green Magic: Flowers, Plants, and Herbs in Lore and Legend.** New York: Viking Press, 1977. 200p. illus. (part col.). bibliog. index. $14.95. LC 77-6338. ISBN 0-670-35427-9.

This book is not a typical herbal but a comprehensive, documented study of the role that plants, flowers, and herbs have played in the varied aspects of human experience. These roles are discussed as they apply to literature, art, crafts, religion, communication, medicine, ceremony, witchcraft, cosmetics, and miscellaneous areas. The book is heavily illustrated and includes several color plates.

A selection from the 24 chapter headings will give an idea of the subjects covered: 1) Christian Flower Legends; 2) Plants and Planets; 3) A Few Flowers from

Shakespeare; 4) Poison Gardens; 5) Political and Historical Flowers; and 6) Flowers and the Craftsman. Each chapter is intended to be read as a whole rather than used as a reference source for facts and figures. An appendix provides information on telling the time of day by the opening and closing of various flowers. There is a table that gives specific opening and closing times for 20 flowers. Another appendix lists hundreds of herbs and the "sentiments" they represent.

This is an entertaining, well-researched, and well-written book, one of the best available on this fascinating subject.

334. Grimé, William E. **Ethno-Botany of the Black Americans.** Algonac, MI: Reference Publications, Inc. (218 St. Clair River Drive, Algonac, MI 48001), 1979. 237p. illus. bibliog. index. $29.95. LC 78-20356. ISBN 0-917256-10-7. (Published in 1976 under the title: **Botany of the Black Americans**).

This work is primarily a compendium of about 245 species of plants that have been utilized by Negroes for food, medicine, or other purposes during their enslavement in North and South America and the Caribbean. Plants are divided into two main categories, those introduced by the slaves from Africa and those indigenous to the New World. Most are in the latter category, although it is noteworthy that peanuts, marijuana, and black-eyed peas are in the former category.

The plants are listed alphabetically by Latin names. With each listing is given: common names, use, literature references, and quotations from source literature. Additional features of the book include a chapter of historical perspectives, a summary tabulation of currently accepted botanical names, indexes of scientific and common names, and a key to genera and families.

The book has been well received as making a contribution to a little-explored area.

335. Gutmanis, June. **Kahuna La'au Lapa'au: The Practice of Hawaiian Herbal Medicine.** Translations by Theodore Kelsey, illustrations by Susan G. Monden. Honolulu, HI: Island Heritage Limited (828 Fort Street Mall, Suite 400, Honolulu, HI 96813), 1979. 144p. illus. (part col.). bibliog. index. $12.50. LC 76-1510. ISBN 0-89610-027-8.

The kahuna la'au lapa'au mentioned in the title of this book were Hawaiian priest doctors who were herbal practitioners. Material presented is based on interviews with Hawaiians and on a variety of written sources including legal medical records that were required of native medical practitioners. The book is not a typical herbal but rather a history and discussion of Hawaiian herbal medicine.

The book includes 13 chapters and eight appendices. Chapter headings give an idea of subjects covered: 1) Prologue; 2) The Beginnings of Medical Practices; 3) The Kahuna: Choice and Training; 4) The Diagnosis; 5) The Treatment; 6) First Aid; 7) The Illnesses and Medicines of Women; 8) The Herbal Medicines of Children; 9) The Medical Plants; 10) The Herbal Prescriptions; 11) Ancient Medical Prescriptions; 12) A Kahuna Notebook; and 13) The Herbal Medicines of Hawaii Now. Chapters 11 and 13 include listings of illnesses and complaints with suggestions for using various herbal remedies.

Hawaiian vocabulary is used heavily throughout the book, which makes reading somewhat difficult, but a Hawaiian language glossary is included along with a list of Hawaiian plant names and a good general index. Thirty full-page color plates illustrate many plants mentioned, giving an idea of their appearance. To make identification easier, scientific names as well as Hawaiian common names are indicated.

This is an interesting, attractive, and informative work that provides a rather comprehensive treatment of the subject. It includes many references to literature and to personal informants.

336.   Hamel, Paul B., and Mary U. Chiltoskey. **Cherokee Plants and Their Uses—a 400 Year History.** Sylva, NC: Herald Publishing Co., 1975. 72p. illus. bibliog. index. $1.50pa. LC 75-27776.
This booklet deals with plants and uses made of them by Cherokee Indians during the past 400 years. Much of the material was gathered from conversations with older people at Cherokee, North Carolina, and from reference works.
The presentation is in two parts. The first provides general information on how and why plants are used. There are sections on plants in religion and medicine, plants in social activities, and plants in daily living. The second section is made up of lists of plants from the sixteenth through the twentieth century. Brief information given about each plant includes: common names, scientific name, translation of Cherokee names, uses, and occasionally something about method of preparation and dosage. If the plant is not native, it is so indicated.

337.   Hand, Wayland, ed. **American Folk Medicine: A Symposium.** Berkeley, CA: University of California Press, 1976. 347p. bibliog. index. $12.95. LC 74-30522. ISBN 0-520-02941-0.
This work presents the papers of a meeting, the UCLA Conference on American Folk Medicine, held December 13-15, 1973, and sponsored by the Center for the Study of Comparative Folklore and Mythology in cooperation with the Medical History Division of the UCLA School of Medicine and the Society for the History of Medical Science, Los Angeles. The papers were presented by 25 scholars representing many fields, including the biological sciences, biochemistry, ethnobotany, ethnopsychology, ethnology, cultural history, anthropology, and folklore.
Following are some of the topics covered: 1) Folk medicine and history; 2) The use of madstones in healing; 3) The role of animals in infant feeding; 4) The mole in folk medicine; 5) Restoration of lost body parts; 6) The nightmare tradition; 7) Interrelationship of scientific and folk medicine; 8) Shamanism; 9) American Indian folk medicine; 10) Plant hypnotics; 11) Medical folklore in Spanish America; 12) Folk medicine in French Canada and Louisiana; 13) Amish and other Pennsylvania German folk medicine; 14) Black American folk medicine; 15) The relationship of case history accounts to curing; and 16) Southwest medical lore.
The editor writes that the appeal of folk medicine is pervasive in all cultures, including the most advanced.

338.   **Herbal Medicine Revisited.** Special feature in **American Pharmacy.** Washington, DC: American Pharmaceutical Association, 1979. p.16-33. illus. (part col.). bibliog. (**American Pharmacy,** vol.NS19, No.10, September, 1979).
This issue of a periodical has a special feature on naturally occurring folk remedies that have long been ignored by modern medical sciences. New studies of herbal medicines in China and Western countries are revealing some of the mysteries of ancient cures. In addition, increasing use of marijuana and some other natural products is providing information about their possible therapeutic value.
The following articles review the subject: 1) Herbal medicine revisited: science looks anew at ancient Chinese pharmacology; 2) Chinese traditional medicine; 3) The herbal pharmacy; 4) Fertility control sought from plants in worldwide effort;

5) Marijuana by prescription; 6) Marijuana's health effects probed by Congress; and 7) Legal grass farm supplies government pot.

339.   Hume, Edward H. **The Chinese Way in Medicine.** Baltimore, MD: Johns Hopkins Press, 1940. 189p. illus. bibliog. index.

This historical work focuses on three aspects of Chinese medicine: 1) the universe and man in Chinese medicine; 2) the founders and chief exemplars of Chinese medicine; and 3) distinctive contributions of Chinese medicine. There is a section on each topic.

The author provides an account of how the Chinese have contributed to medicine by establishing medical libraries and writing significant monographs. They have also stressed treatment using herbs, animal products, and minerals. Physical therapy (including acupuncture, massage, special exercises, and counter-irritation) and diagnosis have been important.

Plant remedies are discussed throughout the book.

340.   Hyatt, Richard. **Chinese Herbal Medicine: Ancient Art and Modern Science.** With Therapeutic Repertory by Robert Feldman. New York: Schocken Books, 1978. 160p. bibliog. index. $12.95. LC 77-87891.

Herbal medicine is evidently held in high esteem in China, although Western medicine is often used concurrently with it. This book is designed as an introductory work on Chinese herbal medicine, and it is not a complete catalogue of the subject.

The first chapter is historical background. Chapter 2 takes up the theory and fundamental principles of Chinese herbal medicine. Chapter 3, on symptomatic medicine and therapeutic repertory, divides illnesses by symptoms and enumerates specific conditions. Chapter 4 is on diagnosis and discharge. Four methods of diagnosis are employed: looking, listening and smelling, questioning, and touching. The next section presents teas and other herbal preparations, including teas most commonly used in the Chinese Pharmacopeia. Entries are in Romanized alphabetical order with annotated Chinese characters. Another section presents a list of commonly used Chinese herbs, also in Romanized alphabetical order with annotated Chinese characters. The appendices are indexes. A list of places to buy Chinese herbs has been provided.

The author remarks that to a person unacquainted with Oriental culture, the principles of Oriental medicine may seem vague, archaic, and superstitious. Indeed they do.

341.   Imperato, Pascal James. **African Folk Medicine: Practices and Beliefs of the Bambara and Other Peoples.** Baltimore, MD: York Press, Inc., 1977. 249p. illus. bibliog. index. $16.00. LC 77-5465. ISBN 0-912752-08-4.

The author of this scholarly work is a physician who has had much experience in tropical medicine. His book is an introduction to traditional medical beliefs and practices of various African peoples, particularly the Bambara people of Mali. It is a compilation of the knowledge of Bambara healers, herbalists, Koranic teachers, diviners, patients, and old sages.

The author's preface cites earlier work of authorities on West-African herbal medicines. Titles of the 18 chapters are as follows: 1) Introduction to Mali and the Bambara; 2) The Therapeutic Process; 3) Disease Causation and the Spirit World; 4) Bambara Social Organization and Religious Beliefs; 5) Folk Medicine among Rural Bambara; 6) Folk Medicine and Modern Health Care among Urban Bambara; 7) Folk Medicine in Timbuctoo; 8) Mental Illness; 9) Fertility and Reproduction; 10) Childhood

Diseases; 11) Measles; 12) Communicable Diseases of Adults; 13) Chronic Diseases; 14) Smallpox and Variolation; 15) Traditional Surgery; 16) Traditional Dentistry; 17) Snakebites and Other Bites and Stings; and 18) The Traditional African Pharmacopeia. Appended are a snyopsis of major disease problems in Africa and a glossary of Bambara terms.

The author points out in chapter 18 that, while most authorities agree that the African pharmacopeia possesses some valuable and useful products, there is a need to elucidate the pharmacology of these preparations to the satisfaction of modern science. National pride and revalorizing traditional medicine do not create an atmosphere in which critical and objective evaluations can be made.

342.　**The Inglenook Doctor Book.** Choice Recipes contributed by Sisters of the Brethren Church, Subscribers and Friends of the Inglenook Magazine. Elgin, IL: Brethren Publishing House, 1903. Reprinted 1975 with an introduction by Walter C. Alvarez. 157p. index. $1.50pa.

Presented in this book are 916 remedies that were passed from generation to generation from farms, homes, and kitchens of the nineteenth-century members of the Brethren Church, a conservative branch of the Dunkards, German Baptist Brethren, who settled originally in Pennsylvania and whose members were usually farmers.

This reprinted edition is an honest presentation. The late respected Dr. Walter Alvarez, noted medical columnist and Mayo Clinic consultant, has provided the introduction. He makes no exaggerated claims for the "recipes." Rather, he calls the book a "charming and delightful look at the not-too-distant American past." He says the remedies reflect the innocence of a young people and a struggling medical profession largely unavailable to them. Alvarez cautions that the "cures" may not work today; the twentieth-century reader should not try them. He does allow, however, that drug houses are constantly looking for new drugs in the pouches of witch doctors, and that there may be some good drugs hidden away in the book.

Chapters of the book are presented by type of ailment, such as infantile diseases, eruptive diseases, and each suggested remedy is numbered. There are several suggestions given for some conditions. Each suggested remedy is followed by the name and address of the person making the contribution, most of them women. Many of the surnames are familiar to the reviewer, a Midwestern descendant of members of the Church of the Brethren. The book indeed is a charming nostalgic look at our frontier heritage when life was simpler but harsher, and home remedies were born of necessity.

343.　Jarvis, D. C. **Folk Medicine: A Vermont Doctor's Guide to Good Health.** New York: Holt, Rinehart and Winston, 1958. 182p. $5.95. LC 58-6454. ISBN 0-03-027410-9.

This was one of the first books written in the recent revival of interest in unconventional and folk medicine. Jarvis, a Vermont physician, explains folk medicine as practiced by the people of rural Vermont and recommends the system for healthy living.

The emphasis of the book is on the use of a dietary supplement of apple-cider vinegar and honey to ensure good health. The preparation is especially recommended for chronic fatigue, headache, insomnia, high blood pressure, dizziness, sore throat, and obesity. The use of a few other substances is advocated in the book, including kelp, iodine, castor oil, and corn oil.

Jarvis marketed a product of honey and vinegar called Honegar, a step which brought him some trouble with the Food and Drug Administration as it is necessary to prove the efficacy and safety of commercial drug products.

The book has been widely criticized by the scientific community, but it has been a best seller, has been through many reprintings, and is still in print.

344.   Kordel, Lelord. **Lelord Kordel's Natural Folk Remedies.** New York: G. P. Putnam's Sons, 1974. 284p. index. $7.95. LC 73-78591. ISBN 0-399-11205-7.

Throw out the pills and get back to nature to preserve health, the author of this book suggests. His book contains remedies and herbal recipes drawn from sources in a number of countries and cultures.

Chapter headings are: 1) The Healing Power of Nature's Remedies; 2) The Real Flower Power; 3) Hints on Preparing Nature's Remedies; 4) Kitchen Cures for Whatever Ails You; 5) Remedies, Old and Updated, for Aches and Pains; 6) You Can't *Cure* a Cold, but. . .; 7) Fruits: The Remedies That Revitalize; 8) Natural Tranquilizers and Aids to Sleep; 9) Remedies the Gypsies Taught Me; 10) Garlic: The Natural Antibiotic; 11) Some Rediscovered Germ Killers; 12) Medical Magic from the Beehive; 13) Lactic Acid: The Fountain of Friendly Bacteria; 14) Water: The Medicine *Everyone* Can Afford; 15) Fenugreek: An Ancient Solution for Modern Pollution; 16) All the Comforts of Comfrey and Chamomile; 17) Medicine from the Sea around Us; 18) Sex Stimulants and Hormone Boosters; 19) Russian Secrets of Health and Super Energy; 20) Fifty Centuries of Chinese Folk Medicine; and 21) The Secret of Prolonging Youth.

Each chapter contains a general discussion and a selection of recipes. The author stresses "preventive remedies" and the use of "safe, natural home medication."

345.   Kourennoff, Paul M. **Russian Folk Medicine.** Translated, edited and arranged by George St. George. London and New York: W. H. Allen, 1970. 213p. ISBN 0-491-00484-2.

This work describes some of the medications and methods used by folk medicine practitioners in Eastern Europe and Asia, particularly Russia and Siberia. The book emphasizes throughout that qualified medical advice should always be sought; the book is merely a glance into a fascinating world of ancient wisdom of historical interest.

The introductory chapter contains historical notes on Russian-Siberian folk medicine. A plea is made for a scientific study of folk remedies. The next section lists disorders and afflictions and presents folk remedies. The following section covers emergencies, accidents, injuries, and personal body care, while the last part is a selection of popular herbal remedies in formula format. An appendix contains a list of medicinal herbs and plants of the British Isles and Ireland and their uses in the preparation of herbal remedies.

346.   Landy, David, ed. **Culture, Disease, and Healing: Studies in Medical Anthropology.** New York: Macmillan Publishing Co., 1977. 559p. bibliog. LC 76-2013. ISBN 0-02-367390-7.

This collection of scholarly essays came into being as a result of courses taught by the editor at the University of Pittsburgh and the University of Massachusetts. These courses had various titles, for instance, "Primitive and Folk Medicine," "Social and Cultural Factors in Health and Disease," "Medical Systems in Cultural Perspective," and "Medical Anthropology." Landry believes there is a close relationship among disease, medicine, and human culture. This book presents a representative selection of studies in medical anthropology. The writings deal mainly with accounts of those peoples who traditionally have caught the attention of anthropologists: the prehistoric, historic, and contemporary non-Western, largely preindustrial societies of the world.

The writings, most by noted historians and anthropologists, are presented under these headings: 1) The Field of Medical Anthropology; 2) Paleopathology; 3) Ecology and Epidemiology of Disease; 4) Medical Systems and Theories of Disease and Healing; 5) Divination and Diagnosis; 6) Sorcery and Witchcraft in Sickness and Health; 7) Public Health and Preventive Medicine; 8) Anatomy, Surgery, and the Medical Knowledge of Preindustrial Peoples; 9) Obstetrics and Population Control; 10) Pain, Stress, and Death; 11) Emotional States and Cultural Constraints; 12) The Patient: Status and Role; 13) The Healers: Statuses and Roles; and 14) Healers and Medical Systems in Social and Cultural Change. A bibliography of about 40 pages is included.

347.   Li, C. P. **Chinese Herbal Medicine.** A publication of the John E. Fogarty International Center for Advanced Study in the Health Sciences. Washington, DC: GPO, 1974. 120p. illus. bibliog. index. (DHEW Publication No. [NIH] 75-732).

The author of this work, a distinguished Chinese-born scientist, was invited by the Fogarty International Center to study and document ancient, and apparently successful, practices of the Chinese in utilizing medicinal herbs. This book is the result.

About half the book is taken up by discussions on "Traditional herbal medicine—an overview" and "Recent experimental studies and clinical applications." The other half of the work is an appendix "Pharmacognosy of individual herbs discussed in the monograph," which is a list of 44 plants arranged alphabetically according to scientific name. Each plant is illustrated. Most entries include Chinese name, a description, location, chemical action, and traditional use. Seventy-six literature references are provided.

The author concludes that in China today diseases are treated with a combination of Western and traditional Chinese methods, including herbal drugs. (Traditional Chinese medicine, however, is not precisely folk medicine.) Some success has been achieved. This blending could have great influence on future development of Western medicine, according to Li.

348.   Lucas, Richard. **Secrets of the Chinese Herbalists.** Plant drawings by Steven Talbott. West Nyack, NY: Parker Publishing Co., 1977. 244p. illus. index. $9.95. LC 76-25955. ISBN 0 13-797639-9.

This is a timely book because there has been a recent upsurge of interest in traditional medicines of China. The author's view is that the relief of human suffering should be of prime concern and that less emphasis should be placed on whether or not a remedy is conventional. Lucas reports on Oriental herb remedies, and he believes they are "natural, sensible, and beneficial."

The following chapters are included: 1) The Wisdom of Chinese Herbalists; 2) Chinese Herb Remedies for Stomach Disorders; 3) Chinese Herb Remedies for Respiratory Ailments; 4) Ginseng—Chinese Health Herb; 5) Oriental Herb Tonics and Blends; 6) The Chinese "Elixir of Life" Plant; 7) Chinese Herb Remedies for Rheumatism; 8) Chinese Herb Remedies for Urinary Disorders; 9) Chinese Herb Remedies for Men's Ailments; 10) Building Female Health with Chinese Herbs; 11) Chinese Herb Remedies for Bowel Complaints; 12) Chinese Herbs for Coping with Headaches, Nervousness, Stress, and Insomnia; and 13) Plant Remedies for Circulatory Disorders. Also included is a list of herb dealers.

Chapters usually begin with a general discussion of the medical problem, then various herbal remedies are listed under Chinese names with English names, botanical name, use, formula for a remedy, evidence of efficacy, and testimonials given. A chapter summary is also presented. Drawings of plants may be included. Many are familiar in the United States.

The book is of interest as a curiosity; some of the advice is sound, but the material should not be read uncritically. There is an aura of the medicine show about the book.

349.   Meyer, Clarence. **American Folk Medicine.** New York: Thomas Y. Crowell Co., 1973. 296p. bibliog. $8.95. LC 73-4300. ISBN 0-690-06693-7.

The author of this work believes it is important to collect and catalog herbal-medical folklore because it is rapidly disappearing. Even apparently ridiculous recipes should be scrutinized, the author recommends. He has gathered the recipes presented here for more than two generations, limiting entries to the most commonly used and restricting ingredients to those found in old-time households or available at general stores or from itinerant peddlers.

The first section is a discussion of early American practitioners, while the second lists common conditions treated in American folk practice and includes a description or recipe for remedies. Arrangement is alphabetical by ailment. A wide range is covered, including colds, croup, choking, fevers, hives, intoxication, mumps, poison ivy, warts, wounds, and many more. Frequently, a number of remedies are listed and, in most cases, the source of the recipe is given. Complete references to sources are listed in the bibliography. Appended is a list of common plant names with Latin names provided.

350.   Miller, Amy Bess. **Shaker Herbs: A History and a Compendium.** New York: Clarkson N. Potter, Inc.; distr. Crown Publishers, 1976. 272p. illus. (part col.). bibliog. index. $12.95. LC 76-40485. ISBN 0-517-52494-5.

The early Shakers believed that no study contributes more to the length, utility, and pleasure of existence than botany—it "adds to health, cheerfulness and enlarged views of creative wisdom and power and improves the morals, tastes and judgment."

The first part of this book (nearly half) is a history of the Shakers, covering the various societies in the United States from approximately the late 1700s until the early 1900s when most groups were dissolved. The Shakers were religious and were dedicated to making a society free of crime, poverty, and misery. They wished to be as self-sufficient as possible and spoke of "consecrated industry." None of their industries was more consecrated than the medicinal herb business. The Shakers published catalogs, advertising flyers, and broadsides of medicinal plants and vegetable medicines, and also provided herb and garden seeds. They sold herbs in bulk and, in addition, offered medicinal preparations of the patent medicine type. The historical chapters are headed by the names of the societies or communities and their geographical location. These chapters provide details about production of Shaker medicines.

The second section of the work lists herbs the Shakers collected, grew, or purchased for their own use or for sale, together with the names of communities participating and dates of participation. About 300 plants are included. Herbs are arranged alphabetically under common names. Information given includes Latin name, synonymous names, uses, properties, habitat, and names of the participating communities and dates. Delicate illustrations are provided for many plants.

The book is interesting, well researched, and attractive.

351.   Mitchell, Faith. **Hoodoo Medicine: Sea Islands Herbal Remedies.** Illustrated by Naomi Steinfeld. Berkeley, CA: Reed, Cannon and Johnson Co., 1978. 108p. illus. bibliog. index. $4.95pa. ISBN 0-918408-06-7.

Isolation has caused the Sea Islands (a chain of islands extending from the coast of North Carolina, along South Carolina and Georgia to the northern edge of

Florida) to retain a strong African tradition in their medicines, of which herbal medicine is one component, the author of this book points out. He adds, though, that there has been considerable intermingling of medical systems in the Sea Island culture despite isolation, for instance, plantation medicine has influenced black folk medicine. In the traditional black medical system, according to the author, illness originated from three causes. Those originating from natural causes (such as malnourishment) were cured by an herbalist. A hoodoo illness, resulting from occult or supernatural causes, could only be cured by a conjurer, while spiritual illness, caused by sin or the devil, was curable only by religious healers.

The first of the two sections of the book traces the history of the Sea Islands and describes the black traditional medical system; the second section presents plants and cures. The second section is sub-divided into two parts: "A Directory of Sea Island Medicinal Roots and Herbs" (more than half the book) and "Plant Cures Used in the Sea Islands." In the directory section, plants are arranged alphabetically by common name with the following information given: scientific name, description, part of plant used on Sea Islands, medicinal use on Sea Islands, officially recognized properties (those given in the *United States Pharmacopeia* and the *National Formulary*), use by other Afro-Americans, use by Native Americans, and use by Euro-Americans. Literature references are usually provided as are line drawings of plants.

Mitchell reports that old patterns that have held for hundreds of years on the Sea Islands are beginning to fade, and traditional herbal medicine is one of them. Conventional medicine has made herbal medicines seem old-fashioned and "country" to young urban people; yet older adults still use herbal remedies, especially when medication prescribed by a physician does not seem to be working, Mitchell notes.

This is a very well-researched, well-written, and interesting book.

352.   Morley, Peter, and Roy Wallis, eds. **Culture and Curing: Anthropological Perspectives on Traditional Medical Beliefs and Practics.** Pittsburgh, PA: University of Pittsburgh Press, 1979. 190p. bibliog. $14.95. LC 78-62194. ISBN 0-8229-1136-1.

Different societies have different systems of medicine and approaches to healing. This volume contains nine papers, all published for the first time, each covering medical beliefs of some societal group.

The chapter titles are: 1) Culture and the Cognitive World of Traditional Medical Beliefs: Some Preliminary Considerations; 2) Spiritualist Healing in Mexico; 3) *Bajanje*: Healing Magic in Rural Serbia; 4) Disease Etiologies of Samaran Filipino Peasants; 5) Sex Differences and Cultural Dimensions of Medical Phenomena in a Philippine Setting; 6) Melanesian Medicine: Beyond Culture to Method; 7) Magic and 'Medicine' in Ufipa; 8) Choices of Treatment among the Yoruba; and 9) From Honey to Vinegar: Lévi-Strauss in Vermont. The last paper analyzes D. C. Jarvis' book *Folk Medicine* (see entry 343).

The book lacks a general introduction to the subject, and there is no summary or integration of the papers. Some of the chapters are well done, however, and the material interesting. Most of the contributors are anthropologists or sociologists in academic institutions.

353.   Morton, Julia F. **Folk Remedies of the Low Country.** Miami, FL: E. A. Seeman Publishing, Inc., (P. O. Box K, Miami, FL 33156), 1974. 176p. illus. (col.). bibliog. index. $12.95. LC 74-81529. ISBN 0-912458-46-1.

This work is the result of research on the use of folk remedies by people of the Low Country of South Carolina. It is a compilation of herbs, their properties and uses by these people. The author hopes that plant lovers "will find this book an aid to better acquaintance with the economic plants of the Low Country and that the scientist may find herein inspiration for fruitful investigation of active plant constituents."

The plants are listed alphabetically by scientific name. Included for each is its family name, common names, description, season, habitat, range, current use in South Carolina, properties and historical medical uses, other uses, bibliographic sources, and a color photograph. The main section is called "Principal Plant Remedies"; in addition there are two short sections, "Sundry Plant Remedies" and "Other Remedies."

354.   **The Old Herb Doctor: His Secrets and Treatments.** Hammond Book Co., 1941; repr. Mokelumne Hill, CA: Health Research (P. O. Box 70, Mokelumne Hill, CA 95245), 1974. 200p. illus. $6.00pa.

This reprinted (facsimile) edition of a work published originally in 1941 is not of very good quality, but it is readable.

After six brief introductory articles (e.g., "How to keep young" and "Vitamin E–The sex vitamin"), the book is arranged alphabetically by disease or medical problem. Diseases run from Anemia to Yellow Jaundice, and information about them covers an average of three pages. One unusual section is "Habit breakers" in which several techniques for breaking the tobacco habit are included.

Under each disease is listed the "Herb Doctor's" choices of botanicals, often referring to a specific package number from the Calumet Herb Company's stock. (This book was evidently somewhat of an advertisement for this company.) Several home recipes and testimonials are given under each disease. The "Herb Doctor" often suggests other products (from his company) in addition to home remedies. Among other home remedies is the suggestion that one carry a buckeye for hemorrhoids.

The book ends with four pages of dietary advice for specific diseases. Health Research Publishers has also appended its own advertisement at the end of the book, listing other available titles mostly about diet and herbal medicine.

355.   **The Papyrus Ebers.** Translated from the German version by Cyril P. Bryan, with an Introduction by G. Elliot Smith. New York: D. Appleton and Co., 1931. 167p. illus. (Based upon a translation by Dr. H. Joachim).

The Papyrus Ebers is the longest and most famous document available relating to the ancient practice of medicine in Egypt. It was written about 1500 B.C., but the bits and pieces of folklore in it are probably of much earlier times, perhaps from five to 20 centuries older. Much of the terminology used is impossible to translate, although an attempt was made by a German, Dr. H. Joachim, many years ago. This book is based on his imperfect, but available, work. The Papyrus consists mainly of a large collection of prescriptions for various ailments, specifying names of the drugs, quantities of each, and method of administration. Some other materials are also included, such as spells and incantations.

This book contains material on the age, description, and contents of the Papyrus. It lists mineral, plant, and animal (called "organic") remedies. There is a chapter on the gods and the healing art. Diseases of various systems of the body are listed with representative remedies from the Papyrus. There are also chapters on diagnosis, the hair, cosmetics, and domestic hints. Remedies are given to stop the crying of a child (contains opium), to keep mice away (cat's fat), and to make hair grow on a bald head (a concoction made from the fat of a lion, hippopotamus, crocodile, cat, serpent, and goat). Ingredients of some vile concoctions cannot be deciphered, perhaps fortunately.

356.   Petulengro, Gipsy. **Romany Remedies and Recipes.** With a new Introduction by Walter F. Starkie. Hollywood, CA: Newcastle Publishing Co., 1972. 47p. illus. (A Newcastle Self-Enrichment Book). $2.25pa. ISBN 0-87877-016-X.

This reprinted work was first published in 1935. The new introduction provides historical background material about the Gypsies who for the past five centuries have wandered about the world. It was from his Romany (Roumanian Gypsy) mother, the author says, that he acquired knowledge of herbs and remedies that had been handed down for centuries. He has designed this small book to give the Romany remedies a more permanent form.

Contents of the book is as follows: 1) Remedies; 2) Ointments, embrocations, and liniments; 3) Recipes; 4) For the kiddies (suggestions for amusing children); 5) Dog hints (canine remedies); 6) Fishing, poaching, and other tricks and recipes; and 7) Fakes.

357.   Pitrè, Guiseppe. **Sicilian Folk Medicine.** Translated by Phyllis H. Williams. Lawrence, KS: Coronado Press (Box 3232, Lawrence, KS 66044), 1971. 314p. illus. bibliog. $48.50. ISBN 0-87291-013-X.

This is a handsome quarto-sized book printed in a limited edition. Pitrè wrote 25 volumes during his lifetime under the general title *Biblioteca della Tradizioni Popolari Siciliane.* This is number 19, *Medicina Popolare Siciliana*, published in 1896. The translation preserves, to a large extent, the dialect of the Sicilian people.

The introduction outlines the life of Pitrè, who died in 1916; then the author's preface discusses folk medicine in general. The main text presents five chapters as follows: 1) Popular Practitioners of the Medical Art; 2) Anatomy, Physiology, Physiognomy, Hygiene; 3) General Pathology; 4) Special External Pathology: Medical and Surgical; and 5) Special Internal Pathology. Also included is a list of Sicilian herbs mentioned in the book, an outline summary of the book's contents, and a section of plates picturing healing saints of Sicily.

As might be presumed in an early work of this kind, the medicine described is primitive and characterized by superstition.

358.   Roys, Ralph L. **The Ethno-Botany of the Maya.** New Orleans, LA: Department of Middle American Research, Tulane University of Louisiana, 1931; repr. Philadelphia: Institute for the Study of Human Issues, 1976. 359p. bibliog. (Tulane University of Louisiana, Middle American Research Series, Publication No.2; ISHI Reprints on Latin America and the Carribean). $29.95. LC 76-29024. ISBN 0-915980-22-3.

A considerable body of native Maya literature on the use of plants, especially medicinal plants, still exists in manuscript form. The library of the Tulane University of Louisiana, Department of Middle American Research, has a large valuable collection of such material along with a few published works. This study is based on that collection. It is of note that the Yucatan is unique in that it is the only part of America where there is found a considerable body of medical literature written by the Indians in their native language. None of the manuscripts are earlier than the eighteenth century, but they seem to have been compiled from earlier sources.

The book offers a survey of the botanical knowledge of the Maya Indians. The work is divided into chapters as follows: 1) Maya Medical Texts and Translations; 2) Aches and Pains; 3) Asthma, Colds and Diseases of the Lungs and Breathing Passages; 4) Birth, Obstetrics and Diseases Peculiar to Women; 5) Bites and Stings of Animals, Insects and Reptiles; 6) Bleeding; 7) Bowel Complaints; 8) Burns; 9) Charms, Magic; 10) Chills and Fever; 11) Convulsions; 12) Cupping; 13) Nervous Complaints, Irritability, Depression, Loss of Speech, Nightmare, Vertigo, etc.; 14) Dislocations and Complaints of the bones; 15) Ear Complaints; 16) Eye Complaints; 17) Fainting, Suspended

Animation, Unconsciousness; 18) Falling; 19) Hair, Diseases of the Scalp; 20) Complaints of the Head; 21) Hiccoughs; 22) Inflammation, Enlargement or Tumefaction of a Part; 23) Insanity; 24) Jaundice; 25) Complaints of the Knees; 26) Complaints of the Mouth and Tongue; 27) Complaints of the Nose; 28) Poisoning; 29) Skin Diseases, Ulcers, Abscesses, Cancer and Tumours, 30) Sunstroke; 31) Sweating; 32) Teeth and Gums; 33) Throat and Neck; 34) The Urine; 35) Wounds, Cuts, Bruises, and Ruptures; 36) Various Unidentified Diseases; 37) A Survey of the Ethno-Botany of Yucatan (includes vocabulary of Maya terms relating to the growth, parts and environment of plants; an annotated list of Maya plant names; and a table of nomenclature); 38) Annotated List of Maya Fauna Names; and 39) The Climate and Food Supply of Yucatan.

Diseases are listed in the main chapters with remedies given in the original language and in the English translation.

359.   Sanyal, P. K. **A Story of Medicine and Pharmacy in India: Pharmacy 2000 Years Ago and After.** Calcutta: Shri Amitava Sanyal (34/1G, Ballygunge Circular Road, Calcutta-19), 1964. 224p. illus. (part col.). bibliog. index.

This book gives a picture of the growth of medicine and pharmacy in India from ancient time to the present. Twenty centuries are covered.

Four "systems" of medicine are practiced in India: 1) the indigenous system called the Ayurveda (drugs from animal and mineral sources as well as plants are used); 2) the Unani (Greek medicine developed during Arab civilization and called Arab medicine by European historians); 3) modern European medicine; and 4) homeopathy (a system which uses drugs that produce a condition similar to the disease being treated).

A section is presented on each of the four system. The author concludes that the best of each system should be blended for the benefit of mankind. A special plea is made for more study of the Ayurvedic system. Illustrations in the work are noteworthy. There are some photographs, but many are reproductions of art on the history of medicine and pharmacy; some are in color.

360.   Schendel, Gordon. **Medicine from Mexico: From Aztec Herbs to Betatrons.** With the collaboration of Dr. José Alvarez Amézquita and Dr. Miguel E. Bustamante. Austin and London: University of Texas Press, 1968. 329p. illus. bibliog. index. (The Texas Pan American Series). $6.50. LC 68-24663.

Although written by a journalist in journalistic style, this is a scholarly work which presents a panoramic view of medical progress in Mexico from the Aztec days to the present. The history of medicine and public health is presented, with emphasis on the latter.

Since Mexico is a country of great cultural, socioeconomic, and geographic contrasts, old and new medical treatments are intermingled there. Some of the country's citizens are making the cultural leap to modern medicine rapidly, but the problem of quacks and "witches" still abounds. In many rural areas the only medical care available in the recent past was from the local witch doctor or quack. It is said that old women still sell medicinal herbs in open-air markets throughout Mexico. Some of these herbs are efficacious, some worthless, and some harmful. Vendors often "moonlight" as witches. The book provides limited information about the herbs and their uses.

361.   Scully, Virginia. **A Treasury of American Indian Herbs: Their Lore and Their Use for Foods, Drugs, and Medicine.** New York: Crown Publishers, 1970. 302p. illus. bibliog. index. $3.95. LC 75-108063.

Material in this book is divided into two nearly equal sections: "Food and Drink" and "Maladies and Medicine." Many of the same herbs and plants are mentioned in both sections. The author states that the hundreds of plants listed or discussed are limited to those used by the Indians in the Rocky Mountain area of the United States, but most grow in many areas of the country.

Both sections are arranged alphabetically by plant name, but the medicine section also includes diseases and ailments in the alphabetical arrangement. Each entry includes a brief description of the plant, remarks about its habitat in the Rocky Mountains, how the Indians used the herb or how the ailment was treated, and some historical information about pioneer use. Most entries are brief and do not give specific recipes or dosages, but the book provides a basic introduction to the usage of these herbs and plants. A good bibliography is included.

362.   Smith, Huron H. **Ethnobotany of the Menomini Indians** bound with **Ethnobotany of the Meskwaki Indians.** New York: AMS Press, 1978. (Repr. of two works published by order of the Board of Trustees of the Public Museum of the City of Milwaukee in 1923 and 1928, which were issues as vol.4, No.1-2 of its Bulletin). 326p. illus. index. LC 76-3836. ISBN 0-404-15690-8.

The author of these reprinted monographs attempts to identify plants or parts of plants used by two Indian tribes of Wisconsin. He felt this was an important task because at that time (the 1920s) the use of many plants was rapidly being abandoned by most tribes.

The largest number of plants were used as medicines, but also covered are plants used for food, fibers, dyes, and miscellaneous purposes. Plants are listed under their various broad uses and, under each of these captions, alphabetically by families. The literal translation of the Indian name is given when possible. Method of preparation for use is briefly described and specific use indicated.

Each of the two bulletins includes an introduction which is a general discussion of the ethnobotany and ancient lore of the Indians. Illustrations are photographs, most of plants, but a few are of individual Indians and the countryside. There are indexes, called "Finding Lists of Plants," for each bulletin, arranged by scientific names and by English names. In addition, the latter bulletin includes indexes of Meskwaki names and Prairie Potawatomi names.

363.   Spicer, Edward H., ed. **Ethnic Medicine in the Southwest.** Tucson, AZ: University of Arizona Press, 1977. 291p. bibliog. index. $16.50. LC 76-62553. ISBN 0-8165-0636-1; 0-8165-0490-3pa.

The editor, in his introduction to this work, points out that in complex societies like ours where many cultural traditions exist, a corresponding number of healing traditions can be found. Many groups do not believe that "Western" medicine is a universal cure-all, and they have carried along their own distinctive alternative beliefs and practices.

In this book, four anthropologists examine medical arts and practices of blacks, Mexican Americans, Yaqui Indians, and lower-income Anglo-Americans of the Southwestern United States. According to the book, these groups often believe that illness may be caused by overwork, exposure, witchcraft, or sin. Treatment often includes herbal food and medicine, prayer, massage, or some supernatural cure. Zodiac signs are important, as is finding the proper herbs.

The editor's view is that recognition of the characteristics of ethnic medicine is important because it provides a basis for the adaptation of the medical practitioner to the environment in which he works.

364.   Stevens-Cox, J., ed. **Dorset Folk Remedies of the 17th and 18th Centuries.**
2d ed., enl. With an introduction by K. J. T. Wilson. Mount Durand, St. Peter Port
Guernsey, C. I., via Britain: The Toucan Press, 1970. 22p. illus.

The author says in his preface that the term "folk remedies" used in this
pamphlet refers to those traditional cures and treatments, usually self-administered,
that were used by inhabitants of Dorset in the seventeenth and eighteenth centuries.
Although remedies usually were handed down verbally from generation to generation, some were written; these are reproduced in this work in the original spellings.
The manuscript sources are given. About 55 remedies are described.

As is usually the case with folk remedies, some concoctions probably were
effective, others useless (such as the blood of a hare to remove freckles), and some
harmful.

365.   Svensson, Jon-Erik. **Compendium of Early American Folk Remedies,
Receipts, and Advice.** New York: Berkley Publishing Corp., 1977. 166p. illus. (part
col.). $4.95pa. (A Berkley Windhover Book), $4.95 pa. ISBN 0-425-03367-8.

The author of this book of miscellaneous materials says it is his hobby to
recapture the good things of the past. In this work he says he has attempted to separate myth and religion from medical reality. A great deal of text is quoted from early
works.

The first section is on medicinal preparations. Discussed are herbs and herb
compounds, medicinal beverages, and patent medicines. Typical illustrations of patent
medicine advertisements are included. The next section is on beverages; both alcoholic
and "temperance drinks" are discussed. Directions for making various punches and
liquors are given. Presented next are sections on foods and desserts with recipes from
early books reproduced. The author believes in cooking from "scratch." Toilet and
beauty preparations are taken up in a separate section. Following the text are several
pages of early advertisements which include examples for foods and medicines as well
as toilet preparations. Remaining sections contain household tips and odds and ends.
Some of the advice gleaned from the old publications is quite good; however, "A View
of Women's Lib Circa 1855," reproduced from *The Mother's Book of Daily Duties*,
contains advice not entirely relevant today, as might be expected. A glossary of terms
and measures and a list of places to buy ingredients such as herbs and oils are appended.

This book creates nostalgia for the better good old days.

366.   Taylor, Lyda Averill. **Plants Used as Curatives by Certain Southeastern Tribes.**
Cambridge, MA: Botanical Museum of Harvard University, 1940; repr. New York: AMS
Press, 1977. 88p. bibliog. index. $14.50. LC 76-43866. ISBN 0-404-15725-4.

Little had been published at the time this work was written to show
whether Indian herbal remedies had any real medicinal value. The author undertook
this study with that in mind. She gathered material about Indian herbs from the Choc-
taw and Koasati tribes and took information from a few published works, comparing
those findings with medicinal data found in authoritative dispensatories and other
standard works in an effort to assess the value of the medicines.

The main part of the publication is a listing of about 185 plants by family,
genera, and species. Under each entry the common names are given, what tribe used
the plant, supposed medicinal properties, the part of the plant used, and the method
of preparing and applying it; then comments about the value of the remedy are given.
These comments include remarks such as, "This remedy is of no value," or "This
plant is beneficial as applied," as well as more detailed discussion. The book also contains a section that is a general analysis and discussion of the findings. The section

concludes with the statement that most tribes show a higher percentage of useful remedies than useless ones; for the area as a whole, 58% of the remedies were useful and effectively applied. As would be expected, it was found that some ailments were more effectively treated than others, and that no tribe had a useful remedy for such conditions as heart trouble, rheumatism, headache, and snakebite.

367.   Teaford, Ruth Romine. **Southern Homespun.** Huntsville, AL: Strode Publishers, Inc., 1980. 126p. $7.95. LC 79-91431. ISBN 87397-158-2.

This unique, earthy, and somewhat whimsical book is divided into three sections. The second section, which makes up almost half the book, is devoted to folk medicine. Four pages of this section contain some general hints and remarks about how to stay healthy, such as, "Don't go to bed with cold feet," and "Beets cleanse the blood." Another two pages contain a listing of chemical elements needed by the body and which plants contain them.

The major part of this section is an alphabetical listing of medical complaints and diseases. Under each entry various treatments are suggested, most of them herbal. In many cases, specific recipes and dosages are given. Entries also contain some "old wives' tale" remedies, such as cutting a notch in a peach tree limb for every wart you have and then burying the limb for a complete cure. Other sections of the book contain colloquialisms from Walker County, Alabama, and a fascinating discussion of superstitions and "spooks." This is a fun book, but, at the same time, it has true historical value.

368.   Thesen, Karen. **Country Remedies from Pantry, Field and Garden.** New York: Harper, 1979. 160p. illus. index. $4.95pa. LC 78-24701. ISBN 0-06-090687-1.

This heavily illuminated book is a bit showy but attractive. It is made up of seven chapters with about two-thirds of the text devoted to specific remedies and recipes under these chapter headings: 1) Homely Remedies; 2) Ancient Remedies; 3) Herbal Remedies; and 4) Herbal Teas. Entries in these chapters contain specific recipes, dosages, and treatments.

Another chapter is entitled "Spells" and includes information about how to prepare love potions, how to ward off evil spirits, and how to open a jammed lock (insert a sprig of wild chicory). A final chapter is a brief listing of nine herb suppliers in the United States and England. Addresses are included.

This is a nice little book with lots of useful information, but even the author admits that some remedies are more or less "old wives' tales," with doubtful efficacy.

369.   Toguchi, Masaru. **Oriental Herbal Wisdom.** New York: Pyramid, 1973. 141p. $1.50pa. ISBN 0-515-02906-8.

This concise work discusses in fairly general terms the Oriental approach to herbalism with some historical information included. Although there is mention of non-herbal remedies, the emphasis is on treatment of disease with herbal preparations.

Diseases, categories of sickness, or complaints are listed with detailed descriptions of the conditions and symptoms. Each entry contains suggestions for herbal treatment. Specific recipes and dosages are not given, and the suggested treatment is given in general terms only. A glossary of medical terms makes up the final section of the book.

It is difficult to use this book because Chinese terms are used throughout when referring to various herbs. There is a cross-referenced list to the English equivalent, but constant comparing makes reading tiresome. Many Chinese herbs mentioned do not have English equivalents, so they may not be available in the United States.

370.   Vogel, Virgil J. **American Indian Medicine.** Norman, OK: University of Oklahoma Press, 1970. 585p. illus. bibliog. index. (Civilization of the American Indian Series, vol.95). $17.50. LC 69-10626. ISBN 0-8061-0863-0.

The purpose of this scholarly book is to show the effect of American Indian medicinal practices on white civilization. Most books dealing with Indian medicine dwell upon the shamanistic and ritual aspects, but Indians also employed what can be called rational therapy, particularly in the use of botanical drugs. The book emphasizes the latter, although many aspects of Indian medicine are covered, such as sorcery, taboo violation, spirit intrusion, soul loss, unfulfilled dreams, and shamanistic practices used to combat them.

The author is a historian who based this book on his doctoral dissertation. He has made no judgment on the efficacy of the remedies discussed, but he does acknowledge help and advice of a number of experts in the field and has included excellent documentation.

Chapter titles are: 1) What the Red Men Gave Us; 2) Indian Theories of Disease, and Shamanistic Practices; 3) Early Observations of White Men on Indian Medicine; 4) Services of Indian Doctors to Whites; 5) The Influence of Indian Medicine on Folk Medicine, Irregular Practitioners, and Patent Medicines; 6) Indian Health and Disease; 7) American Indian Therapeutic Methods; and 8) Conclusions.

The influence of Indian medicine on pharmaceuticals used by the white man was great. Many have been accepted in the *Pharmacopeia of the United States* and the *National Formulary* (official drug compendia of the U.S.). About half of the book is an appendix listing and describing the "American Indian Contributions to Pharmacology" in separate sections as follows: 1) Official Botanical Drugs Used by North American Indians; 2) American Indian Nonbotanical Remedies; and 3) Official Drugs Used by Latin-American Indians. About 170 medicines were contributed by Indians north of the Rio Grande, and about 50 more came from Latin-American Indians.

371.   Vohora, S. B., and S. Y. Khan. **Animal Origin Drugs Used in Unani Medicine.** New Delhi: Vikas Publishing House PVT LTD (5 Ansari Road, New Delhi, 110002, India), Copyright Institute of Medicine and Medical Research, 1979. 137p. illus. bibliog. index. $9.60. ISBN 0-7069-0768-X.

The authors of this work have had considerable research experience in India in pharmacology and pharmaceutical chemistry. Extensive studies are being carried out in India and elsewhere on drugs from plant sources, but research on drugs of animal origin is not so common at this time. The authors have undertaken a thorough study of drugs of zoological origin used in the age-old system of Unani medicine. They have collected and classified available data with the hope that the work will assist in framing guidelines for future research workers in the field. Information on more than 200 drugs is presented.

The Unani system of medicine assumes that ingestion of animal organs invigorates the corresponding human organ. It is of note that Unani medicine ordinarily used whole organs while modern medicine extracts their active principle.

Material presented is classified in two ways. The first group discusses whole organisms, while the second deals with parts/organs/secretions and excretions of animals. More than half the book is a table, "Therapeutic Index of Animal Origin Drugs." Unani name, English name, parts used, and mode of administration are indicated.

372.   Wallnöfer, Heinrich, and Anna von Rottauscher. **Chinese Folk Medicine.** Translated by Marion Palmedo. New York: Bell Publishing Co.; repr. New York, New American Library, 1972. illus. index. $1.25pa. LC 65-24333.

Many treatments and alleged cures that have been used in China for many centuries are described in this book. Recipes and remedies are given exactly as they have been handed down from generation to generation. The intent of the work is to better acquaint the lay public and professionals with a complex system that is new and foreign to Western peoples.

Contents of the book is as follows: 1) The fundamentals of Chinese medicine; 2) The evolution of Chinese medicine; 3) Medicinal herbs, drugs, and love-medicines; 4) Chinese anatomy and physiology; 5) Chinese pathology; 6) Chinese treatment methods; 7) Aging and dying; 8) Tortures as "pillars of justice"; 9) The tortures of fashion—cosmetics; 10) Tales, dreams, and their interpretations; and 11) An end and a beginning. A glossary is appended.

The chapter on medicinal herbs is rather long and contains subheadings as follows: medicinal herbs in old China; recipes for the preparation of herb medicines, and their application; the main rules for preparing prescriptions; ginseng and other prescriptions; A B C of Chinese medicinal plants; the story of the poppy; human, animal, and mineral "medicines"; and Chinese love philters. Chapter 6 includes a discussion of acupuncture.

373.   Wannan, Bill. **Folk Medicine: A Miscellany of Old Cures and Remedies, Superstitions, and Old Wives Tales Having Particular Reference to Australia and the British Isles.** Melbourne, Australia: Hill of Content Publishing Co., 1970. 191p. illus. index. SBN 85572-035-2.

An authority on Australian folklore and tradition has collected the recipes, nostrums, and cures for this delightful book. Wannan does not treat the matter in a completely serious vein. He says he is merely seeking to throw light on a particular field of folk customs and practices as well as superstitions and fallacies surrounding them. This quotation from the introduction illustrates the tone and style of the book: "Should anyone, as a result of reading this book, have an overwhelmingly compulsive urge to swallow snail-water for his dropsy, or to feed a portion of cooked mouse to his bed-wetting offspring, I would suggest that he immediately consult his doctor instead. And in heaven's name, dear Reader, if you have a bad back don't go out and shoot a goanna and use its liver oil as liniment, or you'll probably have the Wildlife authorities and conservations on your back as well."

Wannan begins with the remark that the attitude of white settlers to the Aborigines in Australia was an ambivalent one, marked by fear of their supposed extra-human powers and contempt for their alleged mental inferiority. This view prevailed in other frontier areas and has had a direct bearing on folk medicine.

The main part of the book is a collection of remedies arranged alphabetically under such headings as "Abscesses," "Cuts and Wounds," "Garlic," "Camphor," "Gout," and "The Ears." No formal bibliography is included, but reference to early and more recent works follow descriptions of remedies. Sources include old English recipes imported with early immigrants, Aboriginal cures adopted by the bush settlers, medicaments of travelling quacks and pseudo physicians, letters in newspapers, cookbooks, household manuals, and folklore books.

374.   Weiner, Michael. **Earth Medicine - Earth Foods: Plant Remedies, Drugs, and Natural Foods of the North American Indians.** New York: Collier Books, a Division of Macmillan Publishing Co., 1972. 214p. illus. bibliog. index. $4.95pa. LC 73-167802. ISBN 0-02-082480-7.

Early settlers to the U.S. learned a great deal about herbal medicine from the Indians. Remedies described in this book came from records of the Indians' plant medicine and also from records of medicines used by our grandfathers' physicians. Several works are cited as having provided the material presented.

The author says he has followed the presentation of the various editions of the *Dispensatory of the United States* and has cited uses to which drugs have been put, but Weiner does not recommend their use. It is too difficult, he thinks, to make a decision about their value.

The work is in two sections. The first is called "Earth Medicine" and the second "Earth Foods." In the first section, plants are listed under the disease or condition for which the plants were used, such as asthma, burns, colds, or frostbite. Most plants are pictured. All are described with an account of their reported uses. The chemical constituents are usually named. The second section of the book is made up of 16 categories of American Indian foods. Some examples are squashes, the pine family, palms, grasses, acorns, and cacti. Under each plant mentioned, brief historical discussions and information on how the food was used are given. Specific recipes are not usually included.

Three indexes and a good bibliography enhance the value of this work. The indexes include both common English and Latin names of the various plants. This book is recommended as a well-written and interesting guide to the subject.

10

TREATMENT OF
SPECIFIC DISEASES/CONDITIONS

Books on herbal and other unproven remedies for diseases are often concerned with conditions for which there is no satisfactory treatment or cure known. Predictably, the largest number of titles in this section are on cancer treatment and prevention. Several books discuss nutritional treatment and laetrile, a relatively recent unproven remedy that has stirred controversy. Since the books in this section were written, the National Cancer Institute has published results of a well-conducted scientific study of the substance. That study concluded there was no evidence that laetrile either controls or reduces cancer in humans, and it was shown to be potentially dangerous. The conclusions seem fair, but it is questionable that the laetrile controversy will be quelled in view of the antiscience, antiestablishment bias of many of the proponents of the substance.

There are several books on aphrodisiacs, always a topic of interest, although it is unlikely that any such drugs exist. They have defied scientific detection and exist mainly in folklore.

Other conditions considered in books of this section are arthritis, skin problems, prostate and bladder disease, headache, and diabetes.

* * * * *

375.   American Cancer Society, Inc. **Unproven Methods of Cancer Management.**
New York: American Cancer Society, 1971. 226p. illus. bibliog. index.

Collected here are more than 50 articles, each describing an unproven or worthless method of cancer treatment. The introductory essay provides a historical account of various aspects of the subject; cancer remedies are as old as the disease itself. Also discussed are the roles of the proponents of unproven methods, patients, books, advertisements, magazines, radio, television, "health" organizations, prominent individuals, investigations, standards of investigation, associations, government, and education.

Methods described include some familiar and widely publicized ones such as the use of krebiozen and laetrile. Articles are arranged alphabetically by name of treatment method. An evaluation of the method heads each article; in all cases no evidence of value has been found. Summary information from the American Cancer Society files is included in the work. Information typically includes a description of the therapy, clinical reports, information about the proponents, legal actions, and literature references. Appended are three articles that describe proponent organization of unproven methods.

This is a valuable and authoritative book that will answer many questions about unconventional cancer treatment.

376.   Beckett, Sarah. **Herbs for Clearing the Skin.** Denington Estate, Wellingborough, Northamptonshire: Thorsons Publishers Limited, 1973. 64p. illus. (Everybody's Home Herbal No.4). ISBN 0-7225-0211-7.

This small book lists (alphabetically by common name) plants that are said to be of value in treating skin diseases and in soothing inflammation. Each herb is pictured by a line drawing. Information included is as follows: scientific name, common names, description, parts used, presumed therapeutic value, and directions for use. Although no bibliography or list of herbals referred to has been included, quotations from various classical works are found in the text, such as, "Culpeper says, 'It serves to purge the blood and body from all ill humours....' "

Most plants listed are familiar, such as bittersweet, burdock, chickweed, red clover, and sassafras. A short therapeutic index has been supplied.

It is probably true, as the introductory chapter states, that when all is well with the body internally, any eruptions of the skin are unlikely. Claims made for many of the herbs may leave one skeptical, however. Just as some of the supplementary advice is good; some is of doubtful value.

377.   Beckett, Sarah. **Herbs for Prostate and Bladder Troubles.** Drawings by Jill Fry. Wellingborough, Northamptonshire: Thorsons Publishers Limited, 1973. 63p. illus. ISBN 0-7225-0238-9.

This small book contains information on herbal remedies said to be valuable for treating enlargement of the prostate gland and for dealing with bladder troubles such as cystitis, stones, and renal colic. In addition, it includes introductory material on urinary tract problems and "supplementary advice" on fasting, diet, and the value of sitz baths to reduce problems in the pelvic area.

The main part of the book is an alphabetical (by common name) listing of plants, including a line drawing of each, scientific name, synonymous names, description, part of plant used, and directions for use. Historical material has been included in some instances. There is a brief Therapeutic Index.

378.   Berson, Dvera, with Sander Roy. **Pain-Free Arthritis.** New York: Simon and Schuster, 1978. 96p. illus. LC 78-520. ISBN 0-671-24042-0.

The author of this book says she suffered six years of debilitating pain and crippling from conditions diagnosed as rheumatoid arthritis, osteoarthritis, osteoporosis, and cervical spondylosis deformans. After extensive conventional treatment, medication, braces, and supports, she improved but little and only temporarily. Berson found by accident that exercising under water in a swimming pool alleviated the conditions. She developed an exercise program that is outlined in the book with diagrams, directions, and emphasis on beginning gradually and slowly lengthening time spent in the pool. Berson claims she is now free of disease and needs no braces or supports. She encourages others to try her plan.

379.   Cameron, Ewan, and Linus Pauling. **Cancer and Vitamin C: A Discussion of the Nature, Causes, Prevention, and Treatment of Cancer with Special Reference to the Value of Vitamin C.** Menlo Park, CA: Linus Pauling Institute of Science and Medicine; New York: distr. by Morton, 1979. 238p. illus. bibliog. index. $9.95. LC 79-91118. ISBN 0-393-50000-4.

Pauling is known as an advocate of the use of megadoses of vitamins, especially vitamin C, for prevention of certain diseases such as the common cold (see entry 590). He and Cameron make a case in this book for the use of the vitamin in large doses as protection against cancer. They also believe vitamin C has therapeutic value in certain advanced cases of cancer. Clinical trials are cited in which the vitamin has been effective. The treatment is controversial, and the work has been criticized because the number of patients tested is extremely small.

380.   Connell, Charles. **Aphrodisiacs in Your Garden.** New York: Taplinger Publishing Co., 1966. 143p. illus. $3.50. LC 66-17666. ISBN 0-8008-0275-6.

Connell says there is one personal attribute about which a man can never be sure—his virility. Countless numbers of pills and remedies have been sold because men naturally want "renewed vigor, increased potency, abundant energy, and extra stamina." The author points out that some supposed aphrodisiacs can be very dangerous, but that those recommended in this book are harmless, beneficial, and nourishing.

The book is about growing plants that are credited with having aphrodisiacal qualities. Some are common garden products. Literary history and medical lore are included as are recipes for dishes that use the plants. The contents of the book shows some of the plants discussed: 1) Come into the garden, Maud!; 2) Beans and crumpet; 3) Have your greens and eat them; 4) 'A box where sweets compacted lie' (a discussion of the window box); 5) Burdock on the balcony; 6) Radishes on the roof; 7) Fish, frogs and flags (about the water garden); 8) Mushrooms in the basement; 9) Don't knock the rock (rock gardens); 10) Yolks and honey; 11) Specialités de la maison; and 12) Bedding time.

The book is entertaining although hardly based on scientific fact, at least where the efficacy of the plants is concerned.

381.   Culbert, Michael L. **Freedom from Cancer: The Amazing Story of Vitamin B-17, or Laetrile.**   Seal Beach, CA: '76 Press (P. O. Box 2686, Seal Beach, CA 90740), 1976. 238p. illus. bibliog. index. $2.95pa. LC 76-43206. ISBN 0-89245007-X.

The author of this book is a journalist, and he has relied heavily on news media sources in his bibliographic references. He makes a case for the use of laetrile in prevention and treatment of cancer, primarily relying upon personal testimonials. Laetrile has remained controversial, and its use is illegal in most of the United States. It is no longer considered a vitamin and, since this book was written, it has become more evident that the substance is quite toxic; deaths from overdose have resulted. The main source of laetrile is apricot pits, also a source of cyanide.

In brief, the book accuses the medical/government "establishment" of suppressing the use of a substance that can save lives. Recent research has not found laetrile effective in cancer treatment, however, and the official viewpoint is that its use prevents cancer victims from receiving medical treatment of value. As the book indicates, laetrile treatment can be received in Mexico.

382.   Gosling, Nalda. **Herbs for Headaches and Migraine.** Drawings by A. R. Gosling. Wellingborough, Northamptonshire, England: Thorsons Publishers Ltd., 1978. 64p. illus. index. $1.75pa. ISBN 0-7225-0396-2.

This small book discusses the causes of headache, including the importance of correct diet in avoiding chronic headache and migraine.

Twenty-one herbs that may relieve headache and migraine are suggested. Each description includes an ink drawing, a historical note, the specific value of the herb, and the preparation and dosage. Some mention of how to locate these herbs is given, but the book is not intended as a field guide. Many of the plants are common. Two special features of the work are directions for making an herbal infusion and a therapeutic index giving the complaint and the herb to be used for a cure.

383.   Griffin, LaDean. **Insulin vs. Herbs and the Diabetic.** Salt Lake City, UT: Hawkes Publishing Inc. (3775 S. 500 W., P. O. Box 15711, Salt Lake City, UT 94115), 1977. 28p. $1.75.

Even though the author specifically states that getting a person to give up insulin treatment for diabetes is not the intention of this book, an herbal alternative is given that is claimed to be superior.

Over half the book is made up of discussions of diabetes and sugar. The "natural" treatment is then explained—adhering to a diet of mild food. The diet is said to rid the body of parasites. After a short testimony about this diet treatment, the conclusion of the book is that diet and the use of the herb golden seal is a superior treatment for diabetes.

384.   Jarvis, D. C. **Arthritis and Folk Medicine.** New York: Holt Rinehart and Winston, 1960; repr. New York, Fawcett, 1978. 179p. index. $1.95pa. LC 60-11318. ISBN 0-449-24160-2.

The author of this book is a Vermont physician, who has frequently been criticized for making unproven claims for certain remedies. He says that after his book *Folk Medicine* (see entry 343) was published he was flooded with letters, many asking questions about the treatment of arthritis by Vermont folk medicine. This folk medicine has been handed down from one generation to the next in Vermont for 2000 years, Jarvis says. His view is that arthritis, like other ailments, is due to the abandonment of childhood instinct by adults, "and so we have nothing to guide and direct us in observing nature's laws. As a result the laws are broken, and sickness and unhappiness begin to appear." The work is concerned with treatment of arthritis with various Vermont remedies which include "biologic food selection," and taking kelp tablets, apple cider vinegar, honey, and a drop of Lugol's solution of iodine. Remedies suggested in the book should be taken as folk medicine only, as most are not based on scientific fact.

385.   Kittler, Glenn D. **Laetrile: Nutritional Control for Cancer with Vitamin B-17.** Denver, CO: Royal Publications, Inc.; worldwide distr. Nutri-Books Corp., 1978. 325p. bibliog. $3.95pa. LC 78-111093. ISBN 0-918738-02-4. (First published in 1963 under the title: *Laetrile, the Anti-Cancer Drug*).

Details of the 25-year controversy over the value of the use of laetrile for cancer treatment are given in this book, written by a journalist. Kittler's view is that personality conflicts, power, and money have all been part of what should be only a scientific debate. He takes the stand (at the time this edition of the book came out) that laetrile is not a "cure" for cancer but rather a "control" or perhaps a preventive. (Notice the change in title from the first edition.) More than half the book is made up of an appendix, a bibliography, and a glossary. The appendix contains medical reports, case histories, and observations.

386.   Markle, Gerald E., and James C. Petersen, eds. **Politics, Science, and Cancer: The Laetrile Phenomenon.** Boulder, CO: Published by Westview Press for the American Association for the Advancement of Science, Washington, DC, 1980. 190p. bibliog. index. (AAAS Selected Symposium; No.46). $20.00; $9.75pa. LC 80-13466. ISBN 0-89158-854-X; 0-86531-046-7pa.

The papers presented in this publication are based on a symposium held at the 1979 AAAS National Annual Meeting in Houston, Texas, January 3-8. Contributors are an interdisciplinary group who give a scholarly analysis of the laetrile phenomenon. The efficacy of the substance, used for the treatment of cancer, has been debated for more than 25 years. Despite opposition from medical and scientific communities and recent federally sponsored research that shows the substance to be of no value for treating cancer, support for its use continues to grow and intensify. The matter has become highly politicized. The book attempts to answer the many questions surrounding this controversy and to analyze the behavior of organizations and individuals involved in it. The work has a sociological slant.

The papers discuss the following topics: an overview of the phenomenon; laetrile in historical perspective; laetrile at Sloan-Kettering; the political implications of laetrile; legal perspective; ethical aspects of the laetrile controversy; social context of the laetrile phenomenon; bias in analyses of the controversy; and science and technology in the pits.

387. Passwater, Richard A. **Dr. Richard A. Passwater's New Fact/Book on Cancer and Its Nutritional Therapies.** New Canaan, CT: Keats Publishing Co. (36 Grove St., New Canaan, CT 06840), 1978. 256p. bibliog. index. (A Pivot Original Health Book). $2.25pa. LC 78-57646.

Dr. Passwater is a biochemist who believes the body's immune response to cancer cells can be restored and strengthened by a program of nutrition. In addition, he feels that correct nutrition can cut chances of getting cancer.

The book gives basic facts of cancer, then presents and discusses evidence on the roles of vitamins, minerals, and the controversial substance laetrile in its treatment and prevention. (In regard to laetrile, the author concludes that there are such widely differing opinions about the substance that the government should take the responsibility for human testing.) The last section of the book outlines a personal program of nutritional therapy.

Passwater points out that his plan in no way conflicts with surgery, radiation, or chemotherapy used as cancer treatment. He advises combining nutrition with conventional treatment. While many may find some of Dr. Passwater's reasoning illogical and his suggestions of doubtful value, there is not much reason, perhaps, to think that his plan can do much harm, except possibly for the fact that large doses of certain vitamins have been found to have toxic effects on the body.

388. Superweed, Mary Jane. **Herbal Aphrodisiacs.** San Francisco, CA: Flash Mail Order (Dept. S, P. O. Box 16098, San Francisco, CA 94116), 1971. 16p.

The introduction to this booklet says it is "about the chemistry of sex and the natural substances which influence it." It covers more than substances that are supposed aphrodisiacs.

The statement is made that there are several undesirable aphrodisiacs known (such as cantharides, L-dopa, and amyl nitrite). Those disucssed in the booklet are all plant materials, "natural," and presumably desirable. There are short sections on the following: yohimbe, dita, night blooming cereus, sensitive plant, sarsaparilla, opium, ginseng, kola, saw palmetto, damiana, strychnine, burra gokerro, kelp, red capsicum, cotton root, fo-ti-tieng, and marijuana. Also provided are short sections on other aphrodisiac herbs, anaphrodisiacs, aphrodisiac foods, sex and nutrition, other sexual medicines from nature, where to procure materials described in this book, and a new approach to birth control (use of laetrile).

389. Timms, Moira, and Zachariah Zar. **Natural Sources: Vitamin B-17/Laetrile.** Millbrae, CA: Celestial Arts (231 Adrian Rd., Millbrae, CA 94030), 1978. 149p. bibliog. index. $4.95pa. LC 77-90009. ISBN 0-89087-217-1.

The authors of this work take the view that meat consumption is unhealthy (perhaps causes cancer) and that cancer is a deficiency disease, caused by a lack of vitamin B-17 (laetrile). The claim is not made that suggestions made in the book can *cure* cancer, but that they can *prevent* it.

The first section (over half the book) consists of 11 chapters on cancer and how to prevent it. Diet, environment, "organic" food, psychological factors, and propaganda are discussed. Section 2 discusses foods (do's and don'ts). The main message is to avoid processed and refined foods, additives and preservatives. Section 3 contains recipes containing vitamin B-17 foods that are meatless. Section 4 (an appendix) contains lists and charts, including foods containing vitamin B-17, food sources of vitamins and minerals, nutritional composition of some vitamin B-17 foods, and a protein guide for meatless meals. Also included is a list of organizations providing mostly unconventional help for cancer victims.

The book cannot be recommended. The authors do not seem to be authorities and, while some of the statements are based on scientific evidence, much material is of doubtful reliability, particularly in view of more recent findings. For instance, chapter 2 begins with the statement, "There is an increasing body of evidence indicating that cancer may well be the symptom of a modern deficience disease...—that deficient factor being vitamin nitriloside, a naturally occurring, nontoxic cyanide now known as vitamin B-17." Laetrile is a highly controversial substance, illegal in most states, and is no longer considered a vitamin. In addition, it *is* toxic. Cancer victims have died of overdoses.

390.   Walton, Alan Hull. **Aphrodisiacs: From Legend to Prescription.** A Study of Aphrodisiacs Throughout the Ages, with Sections on Suitable Food, Glandular Extracts, Hormone Stimulation and Rejuvenation. Introduction by Herman Goodman. Westport, CT: Associated Booksellers, 1958. 267p. illus. bibliog. index. $7.95. LC 58-13948.

Walton, an English scholar, has produced in this work a fascinating survey of the use of aphrodisiacs over the centuries. Much obscure literature was searched to provide a basis for the book.

Material is divided into three major sections. The first section, which makes up almost half the book, is a history of aphrodisiacs, covering the Jews, ancient Greeks and Romans, the Arabs, India, China, and the Middle Ages to 1800 in Europe. It is essentially a review of early literature on the subject. The second part is devoted to "The Cookery of Love." Proper nutrition is discussed, as are habits to avoid. Then a number of recipes are given, including meat, cheese, fish, poultry, and egg dishes. The last section, "Medicine and Secuality," shows how pharmaceutical preparations may affect virility.

The author does not make exaggerated claims for any particular program or treatment. He evidently believes in a healthy active life, nourishing food, and freedom from worry. He concludes that many historic aphrodisiacs have been fantastic and unreasonable, but that a good deal has been discovered about stimulative food.

391.   Whelan, Elizabeth. **Preventing Cancer.** Preface by Philip Cole. New York: W. W. Norton and Co., 1977. 285p. bibliog. index. $9.95. LC 77-26682. ISBN 0-393-06431-X.

The author of this work, an epidemiologist at the Harvard School of Public Health, takes the view that control of cancer will come from prevention more than from cure. Her book describes safeguards helpful in preventing the disease.

The book begins with a section on what causes human cancer and then presents statistics on cancer trends. The next section discusses factors known to increase odds on developing cancer, such as tobacco, diet, alcohol, radioactivity, sun, drugs, sex, and occupation. Dr. Whelan names some much-talked about factors that have *not* been shown to increase odds on developing cancer. These include chemicals in food, stress, and air pollution. The last chapter, called "Cancer: A Perspective," discusses ways to minimize risks by changing lifestyles. The reader is urged to influence cancer research policy through legislation and to promote education regarding the matter. The book includes three appendices as follows: A) Tips for kicking the cigarette habit; B) Prudent eating made elegant; and C) Cancer's seven warning signals.

This is an authoritative work that puts the matter of cancer prevention in proper perspective.

11

MEDICINAL PLANTS
AND THEIR CONSTITUENTS

Works listed in this section are somewhat similar to those in chapter 5, which are herbals and general works on herbs, but titles in this chapter have a more scientific slant. Many are intended for the research-level audience. There are several monumental works such as those by Flückiger and Hanbury, Morton, and Perry.

Books reviewed here make clear the fact that modern drugs have their origins in plant constituents. Medicinals are extracted from them; they provide intermediate chemicals for synthesizing drugs; and they have served as structural prototypes that have inspired chemists to synthesize analog drugs with even more desirable properties. Much scientific work remains to be done on medicinal plants, though. Botanical information, for instance, is much more complete and accurate than chemical or pharmacological knowledge.

A number of the works listed below cover medicinal plants of a certain geographical area only. Areas covered include: India, various regions of the U.S., Africa, West Pakistan, Great Britain, Spanish America, Iran and Iraq, China, east and southeast Asia, the Philippines, and Japan. There are also two books on medicines from the sea.

Unusual matters relating to medicinal plants are covered in some titles, for instance, the books by Iyengar and by Jackson and Snowdon deal with identification of powdered crude vegetable drugs. The book by Tétényi deals with the problem of variation in chemical composition among plants of the same species.

Some works discuss plants containing substances with potential for abuse, works such as those by Superweed, Norman Taylor, and Emboden.

A few of the titles could serve as field guides for identification of plants, but most books of this kind are listed in chapter 17.

* * * * *

392.   Ahuja, B. S. **Medicinal Plants of Saharanpur.** Hardwar, Survey of Medicinal Plants, Central Council of Ayurvedic Research, Gurukula Kangri Vishwavidyalaya, 1965. (Available from International Scholarly Books Services, Inc.). 95 p. illus. bibliog. index. $4.00pa.

This work was undertaken for the benefit of forest officers, research workers, and consumers, including medical practitioners. Collection of drug plants scattered in forests is troublesome and cost of collection is considerable. There was some concern at the time the book was written that a number of valuable species were being eradicated. The author discusses these problems in this book.

About 45 plants are listed. An illustration is included for each and the following information provided: general description of the plant, general distribution, local distribution, parts used, uses, collection, approximate quantity collected annually, macroscopic structure of the part used, folklore, preparations, and market sample.

393.   Altschul, Siri von Reis. **Drugs and Foods from Little-Known Plants: Notes in Harvard University Herbaria.** Cambridge, MA: Harvard University Press, 1973. 366p. illus. bibliog. index. $16.00. LC 72-85145. ISBN 0-674-21676-8.

This work is a compilation of unusual drug and food plants of which little is known. Its purpose is to bring to light little-known data about them. Plants included were drawn from specimens found in the combined collections of the Gray Herbarium and the Arnold Arboretum of Harvard University.

Many members of the Orchid family are lacking because information was unobtainable. Also missing are the gymnosperms, pteridophytes, bryophytes, fungi, and algae (because of the vastness of the undertaking and the feeling that these specimens would be of less interest), and specimens that were out on loan. Since this is a compilation of little-known plants, relatively well-known plants (about which information has been previously published) were generally eliminated unless additional information not previously known was noted. Most of these plants that were not included are found in *The Dictionary of Economic Plants* by Uphof (see entry 59). The emphasis of the compilation is on plants from eastern Asia, South America, and the South Pacific since the herbaria have specialized in collecting from those geographical areas.

There are about 5,000 plants included in the work. They are arranged in family groups, the authority being *Taxonomy of Vascular Plants* (G.H.M. Lawrence, Macmillan, 1955). Under each family group for each species is its entry number, Latin name, place of collection, collector's name and number, year collected, quotations of interest, common name (or names), dialect. The author says he has been faithful, as far as feasible, to the data as they appear on the herbarium labels, but that the researcher may want to go to the specimen itself for further information. There are three indexes—to families, genera, and medicinal uses.

394.   Angier, Bradford. **Field Guide to Medicinal Wild Plants.** Illustrations by Arthur J. Anderson. Harrisburg, PA: Stackpole Books, 1978. 320p. illus. (col.). index. $13.95. LC 78-19112. ISBAN 0-8117-2076-4.

This attractive book provides information for identifying about 100 wild native plants of North America that have traditional medicinal uses. Emphasis is on uses made by American Indians. The author advises strongly against any attempt at self-medication. Material is presented merely as an interesting history, which indeed it is.

The plants are listed alphabetically by common name. The following information is given for each: scientific name, plant family, other common names, characteristics, area found, and uses. There is, in addition, an attractive colored illustration for each plant. A good deal of historical information (perhaps a page or two) about the plants is given in each monograph. Material presented seems to be authentic and well researched, but no literature references have been provided. The author has also written a number of other books on related subjects.

395.   Ayensu, Edward S. **Medicinal Plants of West Africa.** Algonac, MI: Reference Publications, Inc. (218 St. Clair Dr., Algonac, MI 48001), 1978. 330p. illus. bibliog. index. $29.95. LC 78-3110. ISBN 0-917256-07-7.

The author of this work was born in Ghana, was educated in the United States and London, and is now Director of the Endangered Species Program at the Smithsonian Institution. He prepared this work to stimulate research interest in medicinal plants of West Africa and in response to many enquires about the subject.

Included are short monographs on 187 species of reported medicinal plants with illustrations of 127 of them. These are plants reported to be rather commonly used. They are listed by family, and each plant is listed by proper name as well as by its various colloquial names. Purported therapeutic properties are indicated. Also included are a glossary, a medicinal index, and an index to species. The work is probably most valuable as an introduction to medicinal plants of the area. The number of plants included is relatively small, as West Africa has an immense variety of drug plants. It is one of the few books in English to cover the whole of West Africa.

396. Baquar, Syed Riaz, and M. Tasnif. **Medicinal Plants of Southern West Pakistan.** Karachi, Pakistan: Botany Section, Central Laboratories, Pakistan Council of Scientific and Industrial Research, 1967. 108p. bibliog. index. (P.C.S.I.R. Bulletin/monograph No. 3).

This work represents a comprehensive survey of the taxonomic and phytochemical aspects of medicinal plants growing in southern West Pakistan. It was compiled as a first step in the development of drugs from natural sources by industry. The authors have collected and systematized available data so the plants may be collected, identified, and cultivated.

The main part of the work is a history of 263 plant species distributed over 59 families. Information provided for each includes vernacular names, part of plant used, flowering period, occurrence, distinguishing features, medicinal properties, and chemical work done on the plant. A bibliography, a glossary of medical terms, and indexes by chemical terms, scientific plant names, and vernacular and common names are included.

397. Bentley, Robert, and Henry Trimen. **Medicinal Plants: Being Descriptions with Original Figures of the Principal Plants Employed in Medicine and an Account of the Characters, Properties, and Uses of Their Parts and Products of Medicinal Value.** Plates by David Blair. London: J. and A. Churchill, 1880. 4v. illus. (part col.). bibliog. index.

This early work was designed originally to serve as an illustrated botanical guide to the *British Pharmacopoeia*, the *Pharmacopoeia of India*, and the *Pharmacopoeia of the United States of America*. It is illustrated with very fine hand-colored drawings of 306 species of medicinal plants.

Monographs on the plants are arranged by plant family. Treatment given to each species varies; some are discussed more completely than others, depending upon the attention given to the plant at the time. New remedies are given longer descriptions. Information given usually includes: synonymous names; derivation of plant name; sources were figures (illustrations) can be found; description; habitat; offical part and name; general characters and composition; medicinal properties and uses; description of the colored plate; and sometimes information is provided on collection, commerce, and substitutes.

398. Berry, James R. **Medicines from the Sea.** New York: a W. W. Norton book published by Grosset and Dunlap, Inc., 1972. 85p. illus. index. $4.95. LC 79-182008. ISBN 0-448-21427-X.

This is a somewhat elementary work, written by a science writer who has contributed to popular magazines. The author's view is that while folkloric remedies from the sea aren't new, scientific searching for remedies from marine plants and animals has just begun. The book discusses how research teams go about developing medicines from the sea, and it describes the sea creatures and plants that are objects of their interest. The following creatures and plants, among others, are considered: the hagfish, sponges, sea cucumbers, eels, clams, weever fish, puffer fish, stonefish, phytoplankton, giant kelp, barnacles, starfish, and jellyfish.

399.   Brain, K. R., and T. D. Turner. **The Practical Evaluation of Phytopharmaceuticals.** Bristol, U. K.: Wright-Scientechnica, 1975. 198p. illus. bibliog. index. £5.50pa. ISBN 0-85608-012-8.

Many drug plant products have been known and used for many centuries; others are still being isolated and evaluated. There is a good deal of variability in the products, and usable drugs should conform to certain specifications. This textbook is intended to present material on the methods and theoretical background of both traditional evaluative procedures and those of more recent origin. Included among the latter are optical micromeretics, chromatographic methods, ion-exchange systems, electrophoresis, and others.

The following areas are covered: identification and definition of new drug sources; assessment of quality of crude drugs for direct use or as a source of valuable constituents; and investigations of difficulties encountered in the extraction or use of a drug. The appendix includes tables of cytomorphological characters of common crude drugs.

The book is suitable for pharmacy students, food and drug analysts, forensic scientists, and cosmetic scientists. While it is too technical for the average reader, it shows an aspect of the subject not covered in ordinary herbals.

400.   Dymock, William, C. J. H. Warden, and David Hooper. **Pharmacographia Indica: A History of the Principal Drugs of Vegetable Origin Met with in British India.** Vol.1-3. London: Kegan Paul, Trench, Trübner and Co., Ltd., 1890-1893; repr. Karachi, Pakistan: Institute of Health and Tibbi Research under the auspices of Hamdard National Foundation, 1972. 546p. index. (Hamdard, the organ of the Institute of Health and Tibbi Research, V.15, Nos. 1-12, January-March 1972, Special Issue).

Because of the interest in plant drugs, it was decided to reprint the three volumes of *Pharmacographia Indica* in one reasonably priced volume. These 1890-1893 volumes still constitute the classical work of reference on medicinal plants of the Indo-Pakistan subcontinent.

Available information concerning drugs and medicinal plants of India was scattered through a number of books and periodicals in various languages. The authors of this work collected and verified the information and supplemented it when necessary. Plants of historical and mythological interest that were used in Indian medicine for superstitious reasons, though having little value, have been included with the others. The authors compared the empirical estimation of the drugs with information obtained by pharmacological research. References to scientific literature are made throughout. Information provided for each drug usually includes: scientific, vernacular, and synonymous names; habitat; history; uses; description; and chemical composition.

The work is considered a valuable compilation. Its title is similar to that of the work by Flückiger (see entry 404), but the latter, a historical classic, covers plants of virtually the whole world rather than those just in India.

401.   Emboden, William. **Narcotic Plants.** Rev. and enl. New York: Macmillan Publishing Co., 1979. 206p. illus. (part col.). bibliog. index. $15.95. LC 79-11758. ISBN 02-535480-9.

This is the second edition of a successful 1972 publication that was perhaps the first comprehensive book of its kind on psychoactive plants. It presents an overview of the historical and contemporaneous uses of psychactive drugs throughout the world. Botany, chemistry, anthropology, and archeology are integrated to explain the curious uses of the plants throughout history. The author, a Professor of Botany at California State University at Northridge and Research Associate in Botany at the Natural History Museum in Los Angeles, hopes the reader can learn something about narcotic plants and that the book will help clear up misconceptions, particularly so more-informed decisions can be made by legislators, teachers, and users of plant drugs.

Emboden presents in narrative form how drugs have been used in almost every civilization of the ancient and modern world, and how they have influenced the arts, religion, science, and medicine. Most ancient civilizations used them in magical and religious contexts, in foretelling the future, in communicating with the dead, and in withstanding the duress of harsh environments.

There are chapters on hypnotica (the sedatives and tranquilizers), tobacco (the enigmatic narcotic), hallucinogens, stimulants, and inebriants. In addition, two appendices cover a proposed structuring of some known mind-altering plant chemicals and a summation of the botany, geography, psychopharmacology and chemistry of narcotic plants. The latter is an abbreviated synopsis of the plants figured in the text. The following information is given about each: scientific name, common name(s), family, habitat, botanical description, primary narcotic effect, and active principle(s).

Emboden passes little judgment on individuals who use psychoactive drugs today. He points out that every civilization has had to decide whether use of a certain drug constitutes a socially acceptable pastime or violates a legal or social sanction.

The work is well done, and the illustrations, as in the original edition, are exceptionally fine.

402.   Fernie, William T. **Herbal Simples Approved for Modern Uses of Cure.** 2d ed. Philadelphia: Boericke & Tafel, 1897. 651p. index. (Reprinted edition available with the title: **Herbal Remedies Approved for Modern Uses of Cure.** New York, Gordon Press, 1977. $59.95. ISBN 0-8490-1940-0).

The term "herbal simple" was used in the past to describe a home remedy consisting of one ingredient only, that of a vegetable nature. This edition was revised and enlarged from an 1895 edition with the addition of about 50 herbs. It seeks to justify the use of herbal simples on what was considered a suitable scientific basis.

After a brief introduction, the book lists over 400 herbal plants alphabetically by common name. Each plant is usually discussed for several pages. Descriptions are given, as are quotations from literary and scientific works. Derivation of names are discussed, habitat and uses given, and scientific information that was known at the time of publication has been provided. The index lists diseases and indicates plants used as remedies.

This is a quaint, interesting old book that treats the subject fairly completely. The author was evidently an Englishman, but most of the plants are familiar in the United States.

403.   Flück, Hans. **Medicinal Plants and Their Uses: Medicinal Plants, Simply Described and Illustrated with Notes on Their Constituents, Actions and Uses, Their Collection, Cultivation and Preparations.** With the collaboration of Rita Jasperson-Schib; translated from the German by J. M. Rowson. London: W. Foulsham and Co., Ltd., 1976. 188p. illus. (col.). index. $11.95. ISBN 0-572-00903-8.

The author of this small book points out in the preface that many recent works about drug plants lack a critical approach, reportings, without serious checking, all uses attributed to them in both popular and scientific literature. He has attempted to compile a popular book based on scientific considerations.

About 150 plants are listed alphabetically by common name with a very attractive colored drawing illustrating each. The following information is provided: scientific name, common names, description, part used, habitat and collection, constituents and action, and usage.

The author has also provided special sections as follows: the use of medicinal plants; some important groups of active plant constituents and their mode of action; usage and methods of preparing medicinal plants; cultivation collection of medicinal plants; popular names of medicinal plants; calendar for collection of medicinal plants; teas from indigenous plants; lists of ailments and the plants used in their treatment; and a glossary.

The book is attractive and authoritative.

404.   Flückiger, Friedrich A., and Daniel Hanbury. **Pharmacographia: A History of the Principal Drugs of Vegetable Origin Met with in Great Britain and British India.** 2d ed. London, Macmillan and Co., 1879. 803p. bibliog. index.

This is the best known and most comprehensive work of its kind, and it has long been considered an authoritative classic. Later works have been based on it.

Drugs included are chiefly those that were commonly kept in pharmacies at the time and known in the spice market of London. A small number of drugs that belonged to the *Pharmacopoeia of India* have been included also, as have a few that were of little more than historical interest.

Material is arranged by family of the source plant. Each drug is headed by the Latin name, followed by synonyms, including those used in France and Germany as well as England. The botanical origin of the substance is discussed next, and the area of its growth or locale of its production is stated. Not much attempt is made to describe plants botanically, although sources for this information are quoted. Introduction of the substance into medicine is traced with careful documentation under the heading "history." Other information provided in the book includes method of preparation, production, commerce figures, description, microscopic structure, chemical composition, and uses. In some cases, information on adulteration and on substitutes is included. The work contains extensive bibliographic references and bibliographic notes relating to authors and books quoted in the text.

405.   Ford, Karen Cowan. **Las Yerbas de la Gente: A Study of Hispano-American Medicinal Plants.** Ann Arbor, MI: University of Michigan, 1975. 437p. bibliog. (Museum of Anthropology, University of Michigan. Anthropological papers. No.60). $5.00.

The author of this work says in her introduction that it may seem incongruous that folk cures are still popular in this day of modern medicine. There is still a place for herbal remedies, she thinks, and they should not be treated with indifference or condescension by the medical profession. They should instead be better understood and accepted as supplementary, complementary, or even substitute treatments. She also mentions the prevalent hobby interest in herbs.

The book contains little text material. Appendices make up the bulk of the work. Presented are tables of information on several collections of herbs. These include: 1) The Volney H. Jones Collection; 2) The Lundell and Whiting Collection; 3) The Leslie A. White Collection; 4) Juarez, Chihuaha Market Collection (Richard I. and Karen Cowan Ford); 5) Herb Collection, Roybal's Store; and 6) Glossary of Spanish-Named Medicinal Plants, (a miscellaneous collection including data from Appendices A-E). In each case

Spanish name, botanical name, location, literature reference, and uses are given. A Botanical Name Dictionary serves as an index to plants listed elsewhere in the volume by Spanish name.

406.   Hardin, James W. **North Carolina Drug Plants of Commercial Value.** Raleigh, NC: North Carolina State College, 1962. 34p. illus. bibliog. index. (North Carolina State College Agricultural Experiment Station. Bulletin no. 418).

This publication describes the most important commercial drug plants found in North Carolina, a state known as an important source of crude botanicals. About 25 plants are described in some detail with information included on their habitat, distribution, and relative demand. Some are illustrated with photographs. In addition, brief information is given on about 75 other plants of limited demand. Information on preparing plants for market has been provided for collectors. There are brief sections on cleaning, drying, packing, storing, and marketing.

407.   Harris, Ben Charles. **The Compleat Herbal: Being a Description of the Origins, the Lore, the Characteristics, the Types, and the Prescribed Uses of Medicinal Herbs, Including an Alphabetical Guide to All Common Medicinal Plants.** Barre, MA: Barre Publishers, 1972. 243p. bibliog. index. $6.95; $3.95pa. LC 77-185615. ISBN 8271-7211-7; 8271-7200-1pa.

The author of this work is favorably known for his books on herbs and edible plants. He is well qualified to write on the subject as he has been a pharmacist and a curator of economic botany at a museum of natural history. The subtitle of the book provides a good summary of its contents.

The presentation is in three parts. Part 1, "About Herbal Medicine," provides history of medicinal plants including material on superstitions and herb lore of the American Indian. Also presented is a section on the "Doctrine of Signatures," an early system of medicine based on the belief that medicinal uses of a plant could be determined by its fancied resemblance to normal or diseased organs. Part 2, "The Healing Herbs," provides instructions for collecting, drying, and preserving the plants, with uses for each given. Part 3, "Herbal Remedies," lists, identifies, and gives uses of about 200 common plants.

Harris disclaims any mystical properties or "cure-alls" for herbs, but points out that a great many medications found in drug stores were created from plants.

408.   **Herbs and Other Medicinal Plants.** With an Introduction by Jerry Cowhig. London: Orbis Books, 1972. 64p. illus. (part col.). bibliog. ISBN 0-85613-116-4.

More than half of this handsome book, printed on oversize pages, is made up of fine color photographs of herbal plants. The aim of the book is to describe plants that are and have been used as herbal remedies and to tell in what ways they have been used. No exaggerated claims for "natural" herbal remedies are made; the author of the introduction takes the view that herbal medicines have their place, but synthetic medicines do too. The matter is placed in perspective by pointing out that modern pharmacopeias have developed from ancient herbals just as modern chemistry owes its foundation to alchemy.

Using plants listed for home medication is discouraged because they can be dangerous since they contain powerful chemical agents.

Text material is brief and consists of the following sections: herbalism and medicine, the language of herbs, spices and drugs, collection and drying, drug preservation, active principles, types of medicine, how much to take (no dosages are given),

medicinal foods, wild and exotic plants, and not just for drugs (other uses for plants).
A glossary has been supplied.

The book would be difficult to use for ready references as there is no index.
Information about specific plants is, for the most part, given with the illustrations that
are apparently in random order.

409.   Hooper, David. **Useful Plants and Drugs of Iran and Iraq.** With notes by
Henry Field. Chicago, IL: Field Museum of Natural History, 1937. 170p. bibliog.
(Botanical Series, Field Museum of Natural History, v.IX, No.3, Publication 387).
LC 38-4074.

This work is a catalog of three collections of medicinal plants and drugs in
Iran and Iraq. One collection was made by Henry Field, who led the Field Museum
Anthropological Expedition to the Near East in 1934. Most of his specimens were
obtained from the markets of Tehran, Isfahan, and Baghdad, but some were gathered
from fields and gardens. Captain P. Johnston-Saint, of the Wellcome Historical Medical Museum in London, collected 200 vegetable, animal, and mineral medicines from
markets in Putrus and Tehran in 1933. The third collection was made in the spring of
1929 by Drs. J. M. Cowan and C. D. Darlington, who obtained the drugs from vegetables at markets in Tehran, Hamadan, and Kermanshah.

Plants are listed alphabetically by scientific name. Each entry includes: family name; local common names; references to other works; which collection the plant
came from; and a short description giving identification, English common names, uses,
and where found. There are also lists of drugs of mineral origin; drugs of animal origin;
prescriptions from Isfahan and Iran; and local names with their scientific equivalents.

The work provides an opportunity to study crude drugs and compare them
with names found in ancient literature of Iran and Iraq where the science of materia
medica developed early. The editors feared that the rapid westernization of these countries (in the 1930s) was causing primitive medical folklore to disappear.

410.   Iyengar, M. A. **Pharmacognosy of Powdered Crude Drugs.** Manipal, India:
The author (College of Pharmacy, Kasturba Medical College, Manipal 576119, Karna-
taka, India), 1974. 64p. illus. bibliog. Rs. 15.

The author says he wrote this book because no such publication existed for
Indian drugs (although some were available in Germany and other western countries).
He prepared it primarily for students, but researchers in the drug industries and government institutions, along with druggists dealing with Indian indigenous drugs, should
find it valuable. Specifically, it will assist with identification and analysis of plant drugs
in the powdered state.

Material is arranged on the basis of morphological classification. Following
are the headings: 1) Radix/Root Drugs; 2) Rhizoma/Rhizome Drugs; 3) Cortex/Bark
Drugs; 4) Lignum/Wood Drugs; 5) Folia/Leaf Drugs; 6) Flores/Flower Drugs; 7) Fructus/
Fruit Drugs; 8) Semen/Seed Drugs; 9) Herba/Herb Drugs; 10) Unorganized Drugs; and
11) Amylum/Starch. Under each grouping the drugs are dealt with in alphabetical
order. Included are Latin and common names, identifying characteristics, and drawings
of the particles.

411.   Jackson, Betty P., and Derek W. Snowdon. **Powdered Vegetable Drugs: An
Atlas of Microscopy for Use in the Identification and Authentication of Some Plant
Materials Employed as Medicinal Agents.** New York: American Elsevier Publishing
Co., 1968. 203p. illus. index. $19.50. LC 68-55656. ISBN 0-444-19903-9.

This work is intended to assist in identification of vegetable drugs in the powdered or much-broken condition, making use of the microscope to look at anatomical structures. There are few publications of this kind.

Substances are arranged in morphological groups and in alphabetical order by common name within the groups. Information given about each drug usually includes scientific and other names, description, diagnostic characters, and detailed line drawings of the powdered parts made at a magnification of 500 and reproduced at 300 times natural size. Groups included are: starches, wood, barks and galls, leaves and herbs, flowers, seeds, fruits, rhizomes and roots.

The book is intended primarily for the practicing analyst, but is useful also to pharmacognosists, pharmacy students, and others engaged in identification and authentication of plant materials.

412. Johnson, C. H. **Important Medicinal Plants of Florida.** Tallahassee, FL: Florida Department of Agriculture, 1961. 51p. illus. (Bulletin No. 14).

Written in response to continued interest of Floridians in growing and collecting medicinal plants for profit, this booklet furnishes sufficient information to enable interested people to recognize, collect, and prepare plants or plant parts as crude drugs or botanicals.

The introduction to the booklet discusses climatic features of Florida and the collection, gathering, drying, and culture of drug plants. The plants are then listed alphabetically by common names. Photographs are provided for many. About one-half page of information is provided about each plant. Scientific and synonymous names, a description, habitat, gathering season, uses, and possible demand for the plants are given. Also included is a list of minor medicinal plants native to Florida.

413. Keys, John D. **Chinese Herbs: Their Botany, Chemistry, and Pharmacodynamics.** Rutland, VT: Charles E. Tuttle Co., 1976. 388p. illus. bibliog. index. $15.00. LC 75-35399. ISBN 0-8048-1179-2.

There has been an upsurge of interest in Chinese medicine of late, so this compendium may be of interest to many, but particularly to the botanist, pharmaceutical scientist, and curiosity seeker. The listing of over 250 plants was a labor of love for the author and, while not a comprehensive collection, it includes herbs best known in the Western world. A few important drugs have been discovered as constitutents in botanicals from the folk medicine of China, and the author feels that the area should be more extensively studied.

Arrangement of the herbs is by division, class, order, family, and genera. The following information is given for most: scientific name, common English name, description, natural habitat, synonyms, pharmaceutical description (including physical description, taste, odor, and toxicity), phytochemical analysis, pharmacodynamic investigations, Chinese therapeutic use, dosage (from Chinese herbals), incompatible drugs, and related plants used for the same purpose. The book is illustrated with line drawings of most plants, and Chinese characters have been supplied.

There are several appendices as follows: 1) Supplementary botanical drugs (there was insufficient information for inclusion in the main section); 2) Mineral drugs; 3) Drugs of animal origin; 4) A collection of Chinese prescriptions; and 5) Table of toxic herbs. Also included is a glossary of botanical terms and a bibliography of 155 references, most from scientific journals.

Although the author does not seem to be a scientist, and most of the herbal medicines (particularly such substances as dried venom of the toad, hide of hedgehog, and red-spotted lizard tail) would not be used without considerable trepidation, the work is a carefully compiled compendium of interest.

414.   Kokwaro, J. O. **Medicinal Plants of East Africa.** Nairobi: East Africa Literature Bureau (P. O. Box 30022, Nairobi, Kenya), 1976. 354p. illus. bibliog. index. LC 77-980055.

The author of this work, a professor at the University of Nairobi, reports that herbal medicine men of East Africa will not like this book because it may deprive them of their profession once their secrets are revealed. Many were reluctant to show Kokwaro their drug plants when he was doing field research for the book. The art of native medicine in East Africa is passed on orally from one generation to the next. The knowledge is kept secret and confidential and is often not transmitted until a father, near death, passes the information on to a son.

The largest section of the book is a listing of plant species with diseases treated indicated. Some information is provided on how the herb is prepared for use. Material is arranged by botanical name of the plant, but vernacular names are given. Line drawings or photographs are provided for some plants. The second part of the book is a listing of diseases, specifying plant used for treatment. In addition to sections on common ailments, also covered are cancer, antidotes, aphrodisiacs, livestock and poultry diseases, witchcraft and psychosomatic diseases, and general medicinal plants.

A glossary of medical terms has been provided as have vernacular name and botanical name indexes.

415.   Krochmal, Arnold, and Connie Krochmal. **A Guide to the Medicinal Plants of the United States.** New York: Quadrangle/The New York Times Book Co. (330 Madison Ave., New York, NY 10017), 1973. 259p. illus. bibliog. index. $12.50. $5.95pa. LC 72-83289. ISBN 0-8129-0261-0; 0-8129-6264-8pa.

The 261 plants covered in this work were selected because they are "most likely to catch the eye and are simplest to identify." They are also "those plants that have been and still are used for the treatment of man's infirmities." The book appeals mostly to the lay public and could not be used as an authority for those seriously studying drug plants.

Covered briefly in introductory sections are the comparison of folklore and science, historical background of U.S. medicinal plants, plant identification, and drug plant sources.

In the guide to plants section, plants are arranged alphabetically by Latin name. Each description is numbered and headed by the most widely used common name. Preference was given to names recommended by the Subcommittee on Standardization of Common and Botanical Names of Weeds. Sections within each description are: other common names, plant description, where it grows, what is harvested and when, and uses. Each includes illustrations that are either photographs or simple line drawings or both. Appendix I is a brief list of sources of botanical supplies. Appendix II is a brief glossary of the meanings of scientific plant names.

416.   Krochmal, Arnold, Russell S. Walters, and Richard M. Doughty. **A Guide to Medicinal Plants of Appalachia.** Upper Darby, PA: Northeastern Forest Experiment Station, Forest Service, U.S. Department of Agriculture, 1969. 291p. illus. bibliog. index. (USDA Forest Service Research Paper NE-138).

This guide contains descriptions of 126 medicinal plants of the Appalachian region. In addition, there is information on collecting and processing the plants, collecting pollen, and a glossary of terms used. The guide section of the book lists plants alphabetically by scientific name with the following information given about each: common names, a description that will help identify the plant, information about when the plant flowers, its habitat, what part to harvest, and uses. A photograph or line drawing has been supplied also.

The Appalachian region is a principal American source of drug plant materials. The manual was prepared to assist collectors.

417.   Lewis, Walter H., and Memory P. F. Elvin-Lewis. **Medical Botany: Plants Affecting Man's Health.** A Wiley-Interscience publication. New York: John Wiley and Sons, 1977. 515p. illus. bibliog. index. $33.95. LC 76-44376. ISBN 0-471-53320-3.

The authors of this work, professors in biomedical areas, say they have designed this book to bring into perspective the massive knowledge known about plants that affect man's health. The book is directed to all concerned with the subject and should be useful to the physician and biologist and interesting to the lay public. It has been used by undergraduate students, particularly those planning medical or paramedical careers.

Material is presented in three sections: "Injurious" Plants, "Remedial" Plants, and "Psychoactive" Plants. The section on injurious plants includes chapters on internal poisons, allergy, and cell modifiers such as mutagens, teratogens and lectins that are mitogenic. The section on remedial plants covers cancer, the nervous system, heart and circulation, metabolism, special sensory organs (eye and ear), oral hygiene, gastrointestinal tract, respiratory system, urogenital system, skin, deterrents (antibiotics, antiseptics, and pesticides), and panaceas. Types of psychoactive plants discussed are stimulants, hallucinogens, and depressants.

Each chapter usually contains a historical introduction on a significant plant; a description of the function of the human system; how the plants are used in conventional medicine; a section on herbology describing how the plants are used in folk medicine in various parts of the world; and a bibliography of available research literature. Material is often presented in tabular form.

Appended is an outline classification of the plant kingdom, a glossary, and an exceptionally good bibliography of herbal medicine.

This is an outstanding work which presents a well-balanced view of the subject.

418.   Li, Shih-Chen. **Chinese Medicinal Herbs.** Translated and researched by F. Porter Smith and G. A. Stuart. San Francisco, CA: Georgetown Press, 1973. 467p. index. $5.95pa. LC 173494. ISBN 0-914558-00-5. (Translation of *Pen ts'ao kang mu*).

This is a newly compiled edition of a work translated from the Chinese. The author lived from 1518 to 1593. Translator Smith died in 1888, Stuart in 1911.

The work is essentially a dictionary of Chinese medicinal plants. Each plant is listed by its scientific name, Chinese name (both in Chinese and in transliterated form), and its common English name, if any. Entries usually include a description of the plant, its habitat, reported uses, and similar species of importance. Entires vary in length from a few lines to a few pages. Arrangement is alphabetical by botanical name, and there are indexes by common English name and botanical name. There is no indexing by Chinese name of medicinal uses of the plants.

The book has reference and research value for those interested in traditional Chinese herbal medicine.

419.   Marks, Geoffrey, and William K. Beatty. **The Medical Garden.** New York: Charles Scribner's Sons, 1971. 178p. illus. bibliog. index. $6.95. LC 74-167777. SBN 684-12383-5.

This is a history of the development of seven drugs, all derived from plants and all in wide use today. The drugs are: opium, cocaine, quinine, aspirin, colchicine, digitalis, and penicillin.

The accounts relate how each plant was originally used, the gradual growth of knowledge about its effectiveness, and the scientific work that led to the development of the modern medicine now used. Biographical material about the scientists involved is included.

The authors stress that these drugs should be used cautiously because all are dangerous, or even fatal, if used in uncontrolled doses.

Chapter headings are: 1) "The Plant of Good and Evil"—Opium; 2) The Divine Plant of the Incas—Cocaine; 3) The Powder of the Countess—Quinine; 4) The Remedy in Every Medicine Cabinet—Aspirin; 5) Calming a Swollen Toe—Colchicine; 6) A Cure for Dropsy—Digitalis; and 7) The Accidental Miracle—Penicillin.

The book is nicely done. The senior author is an editor and medical writer, the other a librarian and professor of medical bibliography.

420.   **Materia Medica.** St. Louis, MO: Luyties Pharmacal Co., 1977. 21p. illus.

Listed here are 31 homeopathic remedies. Most are plant drugs, and an illustration of the plant is included in such cases. Each listing includes synonymous names of the plant or drug, description, therapeutic use, and dosage.

421.   May, Lawrence A., ed. **Withering on the Foxglove and Other Classics in Pharmacology.** Oceanside, NY: Dabor Science Publications, 1977. 340p. $15.00. LC 77-16180. ISBN 0-89561-056-6.

This book reproduces a small collection of landmark articles in pharmacology that established the efficacy of certain medicines still used today. The most important contribution in the eighteenth century was *Withering's Account of Foxglove*, which is reprinted in facsimile. The other four monographs are shorter, of less interest, and do not involve plant drugs.

Withering's account explains how he began using foxglove for treating patients with edema. He recognized clinical implications of digitalis that are still accepted, chose an appropriate dose of the plant leaves, and appreciated the danger of digitalis toxicity.

The account provides an introduction to the subject; an examination of the plant; a large number of cases in which digitalis was given to patients at the direction of Withering; communications from correspondents; method of preparation and doses of foxglove; effects, rules, and cautions; and a description of the patient who can be helped by the drug.

422.   **Medicinal Plants: I.** Papers by Vimala Ramalingam, N. Singh, H. C. Mital, et al. New York: MSS Information Corporation, 1974. 161p. illus. bibliog. index. LC 74-10565. ISBN 0-8422-7240-2.

Medicinal agents extracted from plants are some of the most potent still used today, and plant species are still under scientific study. This work, the first of a three-volume set, is a collection of papers focusing on the chemical description and analysis of plant medicinal agents. Volume 2 is similar, and volume 3 focuses on the clinical and pharmacological effect of such substances.

This volume is divided into three parts; the first is on pharmacological investigation of new plant products, the second on structural studies on the chemistry of medicinal plant products, and the third on botanical classification of medicinal plants. Most papers deal with plants found in the Far East. The papers are scientific and technical. Plants studied include: motha, albizia gum, gingko leaves, cascara, Indian dill, Egyptian dill fruit, cassia, and catalpa seeds.

423.   Millspaugh, Charles F. **Medicinal Plants: An Illustrated and Descriptive Guide to Plants Indigenous to and Naturalized in the United States Which Are Used in Medicine, Their Description, Origin, History, Preparation, Chemistry, and Physiological Effects Fully Described.** Philadelphia, PA: J. C. Yorston and Co., 1892. 2v. illus. (col.). bibliog. index. (Available in reprinted edition with the title **American Medicinal Plants** with a new table of revised classification and nomenclature by E. S. Harrar. New York: Dover Publications, 1974. $10.00. LC 73-91487. ISBN 0-486-23034-1).

These handsome volumes list 1,000 medicinal plants with 180 full-page illustrations beautifully colored by the author. The plants are arranged in classified order. Information given about each includes scientific name, common names, description, history, habitat, part used, preparation, physiological action, and chemical constituents. Appended materials include a glossary, a bibliography, a bibliographic index, a general index, a therapeutic index, an index of French common names, an index of German common names, and a few additions.

424.   Moore, Michael. **Medicinal Plants of the Mountain West.** Santa Fe, NM: Museum of New Mexico Press (P. O. Box 2087, Santa Fe, NM 87503), 1979. 200p. illus. (part col.). bibliog. index. $6.95pa. LC 79-620000. ISBN 0-89013-104-X.

This work comprehensively discusses over 180 medicinal plants found in the "mountains, foothills, and upland areas of the American West." In truth, many of these plants are not limited to that area of the United States but may be found throughout the country. Ink drawings and several excellent color photographs illustrate the book.

Each plant discussion includes a descriptive statement of the plant's appearance; its other popular names; its habitat in the western United States; the useful part of the plant and how it is prepared for use; and, in some cases, how to cultivate it. Moore sometimes even includes a humorous note, for example, concerning the cultivation of cocklebur, "Avoid at all cost." Anyone familiar with cocklebur can certainly appreciate this advice. The most extensive part of each discussion concerns medicinal use of the plant. Exact preparation, dosages, possible toxicity, and, in some cases, the herb's active ingredients are included in each description.

The book ends with a good glossary, a therapeutic and use index, a plant classification table, a good list of references for further reading, and an index of common and Latin names for the plants discussed in the book.

The foreword states that the author has prepared this book from first-hand knowledge and experience. It has not been copied from earlier books or herbals as have many modern herbals. This appears to be true. The author says it is not strictly a botanical text, field guide, herb book, medical treatise, or a textbook of ethnobotany, pharmacognosy, or folk medicine. It is a bit of all of these, and it is quite well done.

425.   Morton, Julia F. **Atlas of Medicinal Plants of Middle America: Bahamas to Yucatan.** Springfield, IL: Charles C. Thomas, 1981. 1420p. illus. bibliog. index. About $100.00. LC 80-13503. ISBN 0-398-04036-2.

Large U.S. drug companies send agents about the world looking for plants to improve medical remedies, and researches are experimenting with native plants from distant places in their laboratories. The author of this monumental work has collected medicinal plants in Middle America (northern South America, the West Indies, the Bahamas, and Central America as far north as Yucatan), recording their uses by both botanical and vernacular names. She has assembled the data in tabular form in this book that covers more than 1,000 species.

Folk remedies employed in the area covered fall into about three classes: 1) well-known European medicinal plants introduced by the Spaniards and still cultivated; 2) indigenous wild and cultivated plants, the uses of which were learned from the Indians; and 3) ornamental or other plants of recent introduction, for which "curative" uses have evidently been invented without any historical bases. A possible fourth category of remedies includes some commonly available fruit, vegetable, or other natural product used for self-medication by middle and upper classes who shun the native "herb" markets.

After an introduction, the atlas consists of 985 pages that list the plants in tabular form. Plants are grouped by families and then arranged in natural order. Information given includes: vernacular names, plant descriptions, origin and distribution, medicinal uses, properties and effects (including toxicity), and food and other uses. Also included in the book are about 275 pages of illustrations, black and white photographs of many plants. There is a "Classified List of Medicinal Plants According to Principal Uses," a bibliography of 563 references, and scientific and vernacular name indexes.

The book should appeal mainly to scientists interested in folk medicine, botany, and phytochemistry. In addition, anthropologists, toxicologists, sociologists, epidemiologists, and related professionals will find material of interest.

426.   Morton, Julia F. **Major Medicinal Plants, Culture and Uses.** Springfield, IL: Charles C. Thomas, 1977. 431p. illus. (part col.). bibliog. index. $49.50. LC 77-3287. ISBN 0-398-03673-X.

The author of this work is Director of Morton Collectanea at the University of Miami, Carol Gables, Florida. She states that the book is not meant to be a textbook of pharmacognosy but was written to supplement such texts. Its aim is to provide information on the botany, culture, harvesting, and handling of medicinal plants. It emphasizes the botanical aspects of the subject, but also includes distribution, constituents, cultivation, uses, and toxicity of 58 major plants, and abbreviated information on over 100 more of lesser significance, the latter in tabular form.

The main part of the work consists of 28 chapters, one for each major plant family. The Latin name is given for each species along with the common name(s). For each is given: botanical description; origin and distribution; chemical constituents; propagation, cultivation, and harvesting; medicinal uses, toxicity; other uses if any; any related species; and an illustration. There are 16 colored illustrations following the main section of the book.

There are two appendices which include a table of "Medicinal Plants No Longer Official in the United States of America but Still Mentioned in the U.S. Dispensatory and/or American Textbooks on Pharmacognosy and Still in Use Abroad" and a table which lists "Plants which Serve as Pharmaceutical Aids or Adjuncts" (functioning as lubricants, vehicles, or flavors). Both tables give the Latin name, common name, and a brief mention of origin, distribution, part of plant used, chemical constituents, and former medicinal uses. The bibliography contains 636 references cited throughout the text.

Much information has been supplied in this attractive, comprehensive work. However, it is stronger on botanical aspects of the subject than on the chemical or medicinal.

427.   Perry, Lily M., comp. **Medicinal Plants of East and Southeast Asia: Attributed Properties and Uses.** With the assistance of Judith Metzger. Cambridge, MA: MIT Press, 1980. 620p. bibliog. index. $45.00. LC 79-25769. ISBN 0-262-16076-5.

Dr. Perry is a retired botanist formerly of the Arnold Arboretum of Harvard University. She is an acknowledged expert on the flora of Papua New Guinea, Indonesia, and north to the Philippines, China, and Korea. This work is a monumental achievement. It classifies more than 6,300 plant species in about 200 families. Also included are 900 references to literature from which the material comes.

Arrangement of entries is alphabetical by plant family, and genera and species are listed alphabetically under family. Each entry gives scientific name of the plant, its distribution, a description of its uses in different locales, chemical constituents, and references to literature and sources in herbaria. Five indexes are supplied: 1) Therapeutic properties ascribed to the plants; 2) Plants, listed according to attributed therapeutic properties; 3) Various disorders; 4) Plant remedies, listed according to disorders; and 5) Scientific names.

The book has been well received. It is a valuable reference book for physicians, phytochemists, pharmacologists, pharmacognosists, and research workers in anthropology, botany, ethnobotany, chemistry, and folk medicine. It is considered important today for underdeveloped countries with large populations of poor people to exploit native plants for medicinal purposes.

428.   Quisumbing, Eduardo. **Medicinal Plants of the Philippines.** Manila, Republic of the Philippines: Bureau of Printing, 1951. 1234p. bibliog. index. (Republic of the Philippines, Department of Agriculture and Natural Resources. Technical Bulletin 16).

During World War II the people of the Philippines were forced to rely on their own resources for drugs because imported ones were unavailable. This book was written to direct attention to Philippine medicinal herbs and their uses. It was felt that scientific cultivation of promising drug plants of that country had been neglected.

The introduction to the work reviews the history of the use of herbal medicines and mentions a number of publications of interest. The main part of the volume lists and provides information on 858 species of medicinal plants, of which 63 species are recognized in various pharmacopoeias. Arrangement is by families and genera. All available information on the species is provided: synonymous names, diagnostic descriptions of the species, edibility, economic importance, origin of the plant, geographic distribution, active constituents, pharmacologic action, therapeutic uses, general characteristics of the crude drug, feel, taste, smell, preparation, and dosage. Numerous literature references are included.

The bibliography lists 630 references, and there are several indexes as follows: therapeutic properties, specific diseases, local and common names, and scientific names.

429.   **Recent Advances in Phytochemistry.** v.9. Edited by V. C. Runeckles. New York: Plenum Press, 1975. 309p. illus. bibliog. index. LC 67-26242. ISBN 0-306-34709-1.

This volume of a well-known series deals with "Phytochemistry as Related to Disease and Medicine." It contains 11 papers presented at the 14th Annual Meeting of the Phytochemical Society of North America, held in August 1974.

It has been known for many centuries that plants affect the health of human beings in ways beyond their fundamental role as sources of food and energy. Some are harmful; others are useful as medicinal agents. Many medicinals are extracted from plant materials, and even more have served as structural prototypes that inspired chemists to synthesize analog drugs with even more desirable properties. Today's drugs have their origins in plant constituents. Papers presented here address this subject.

Following are titles of the papers: 1) Present knowledge of hallucinogenically used plants: a tabular study; 2) Recent advances in the chemistry and metabolism of the cannabinoids; 3) On the carcinogenicity of marijuana smoke; 4) Crop plant chemistry and folk medicine; 5) Contact allergy from plants; 6) Teratogenic constituents of potatoes; 7) Plant neurotoxins (lathyrogens and cyanogens); 8) Advances in the chemistry of tumor-inhibitory natural products; 9) Laboratory models for the biogenesis of indole alkaloids; 10) Antimicrobial agents from higher plants; and 11) Structure of the insect antifeedant azadirachtin. Most papers are highly scientific and aimed at the research audience. However, chapters 1 and 4 are suitable for general readers and would be of interest to them.

430.   Ross, M. S. F., and K. R. Brain. **An Introduction to Phytopharmacy.** Tunbridge Wells, Kent, England: Pitman Medical Publishing Co. Ltd., 1977. 305p. illus. bibliog. index. ISBN 0-272-00467-7.

The authors of this work introduce the term "phytopharmacy" to describe a subject that considers the reciprocal relationship between plants and drugs. It includes a study of plants that act as drugs and drugs that act on plants. Plant drugs constitute a large source of revenue to the pharmaceutical market as vegetable drugs, as sources of active constituents, as providers of intermediate chemicals, and as formulation aids.

This presentation, intended primarily as a textbook for pharmacy students, is in two parts. The first part deals with general principles, and the second takes up specific groups of materials. Chapter headings are as follows: 1) Introduction; 2) Plants and Their Constituents; 3) From Plant to Isolate; 4) Drug Variability; 5) The Search for Novel Plant Drugs; 6) Drugs Acting on the Central Nervous System; 7) Drugs Affecting the Mind; 8) Ophthalmic Drugs; 9) Drugs Acting on the Cardiovascular System; 10) Steroid Hormones; 11) Gastrintestinal Agents; 12) Drugs Affecting Respiration; 13) Vitamins; 14) Antibiosis; 15) Natural Toxic Agents; 16) Crop Protection Agents; and 17) Formulation Aids.

Diagrams of the chemical structures of plant substances are provided throughout the work.

431.   Schauenberg, Paul, and Ferdinand Paris. **Guide to Medicinal Plants.** From a translation by Maurice Pugh Jones. Color illustrations by Violette Niestle; line illustrations by Paul Schauenberg. Guildford and London: Lutterworth Press, 1977. 349p.+ 39 plates. illus. (part col.). index. ISBN 0-7188-2261-7.

This guide presents over 400 plants grouped according to active constituents. About 230 of them are shown in the color plate section, and there are line drawings throughout the text.

Chapter headings are: 1) Plants Containing Alkaloids; 2) Vitamins; 3) Antibiotics; 4) Sulphur Heterosides; 5) Cyanogenic Heterosides; 6) Simple Phenolic Heterosides; 7) Flavonoids; 8) Coumarin Heterosides; 9) Ranunculosides; 10) Anthracenosides; 11) Tannin; 12) Bitter Compounds; 13) Cardenolides; 14) Saponosides; 15) Essential Oils and Resins; 16) Acids; 17) Mucilages (glucides); 18) Inorganic Compounds; and 19) Plants from Other Continents. There is also a chapter on recipes for tisanes and compresses. In addition, there is a section on collection and use of medicinal plants, a section on famous figures in the history of medicine, a glossary of botanical terms and one of therapeutic terms, a list of abbreviations used in herbalism, and a list of maladies and treatments.

Each plant monograph provides the following: botanical, common English, French, and German names; habitat; description; flowering season; active constituents; properties; application; parts used; collecting season; toxicity (if any); and historical information.

This is a rather extensive and informative work, originally published in French.

432.   Schleiffer, Hedwig. **Narcotic Plants of the Old World Used in Everyday Life: An Anthology of Texts from Ancient Times to the Present.** Introduction by Richard Evans Schultes. Monticello, NY: Lubrecht and Cramer, 1979. 193p. illus. index. $12.50; $7.95pa. LC 79-66004. ISBN 0-934454-01-9; 0-934454-00-0pa.

This is a companion volume to the author's earlier work, *Scared Narcotic Plants of the New World Indians, An Anthology* (see entry 500). The term "narcotic" used in the title of the books is used in a broad, classical sense; many substances discussed are not usually considered narcotics. A great many are hallucinogens.

The book contains texts from classical literature which describe or refer to "narcotic" plants even though the author may have been unaware of the properties of the plant under discussion. Meaningful quotations have been culled from a wide range of literature—historical, anthropological, medical, botanical, and other. The following plants are discussed: mushrooms, canna, amaryllis, dogbane, hemp, heath, beach, mint, logania, nutmeg, poppy, pepper, nightshade, caltrop, and some unidentified ones. There is an index of authors quoted, as well as one of vernacular names of plants and plant products, and one of Latin names of genera and species.

The book is well done and provides an interesting glimpse of the history of some of the most important medicinal and toxic plants.

433.   Schultes, Richard Evans, and Albert Hofmann. **The Botany and Chemistry of Hallucinogens.** With a Foreword by Heinrich Klüver. Rev. and enl. 2d ed. Springfield, IL: Charles C. Thomas, 1980. illus. bibliog. index. (American Lecture Series, Publication No. 1025). $28.75. LC 78-27883. ISBN 0-398-03863-5.

This is the second edition of a work first published in 1973. The authors are authorities on the subject. Dr. Schultes is a Professor of Biology and Director and Curator of Economic Botany, Botanical Museum of Harvard University, and Dr. Hofmann is the discoverer of LSD. Recent advances made since the publication of the original work have been encompassed in this edition. The botany and chemistry of this class of plants has progressed rapidly since 1973.

The new edition contains a good deal of historical material, and a very thorough investigation of hallucinogenic plant chemistry has been made, using improved modern analytical methods. Ethnobotanical, pharmacological, and psychological aspects of hallucinogens are covered to some extent as well as the chemistry, botany, and history of the subject. Chapter headings are: 1) Hallucinogenic or Psychotomimetic Agents: What Are They?; 2) The Botanical Distribution of Hallucinogens; 3) The Structural Types of the Principal Plant Hallucinogens; 4) Plants of Hallucinogenic Use; 5) Plants of Possible of Suspected Hallucinogenic Use; and 6) Plants with Alleged Hallucinogenic Effects.

An extensive bibliography of more than 700 references has been provided, and illustrations in the work are outstanding. Most plants discussed are pictured, and views depicting preparation and use of the plants are included. Also included are photographs of scientists who have been involved with development of the field.

The first edition of the book was well received.

434.   Schwimmer, Morton, and David Schwimmer. **The Role of Algae and Plankton in Medicine.** New York: Grune and Stratton, 1955. 85p. bibliog. index. LC 55-11353.

The author of this book claims that although algae and plankton have been utilized as food sources, they have been neglected in the area of medicine. This work is a survey of the world literature on the subject. It could be considered an introductory overview. The author hopes that "such a compilation of background data, of current concepts, and of future potential might conceivably serve as a stimulus for wider activity in the field."

The book begins with a brief discussion on the definition and classification of algae and plankton. Seaweed (macroscopic algae) is considered. There are sections on its nutritional, medicinal, and miscellaneous uses. The section on plankton is divided into zooplankton and phytoplankton (microscopic algae). Beneficial aspects and toxic effects are discussed. The bibliography of 312 citations is referred to throughout the text.

435.   Superweed, Mary Jane. **Herbal Highs: A Guide to Natural and Legal Narcotics, Psychedelics, and Stimulants.** San Rafael, CA: Flash Mail Order (Dept. S, P. O. Box 240, San Rafael, CA 94902), 1970. 16p. illus.

An "underground" publication, the intent of this booklet is to "turn the reader on to herbs, cacti, mushrooms and other members of the vegetable kingdom which can get him high." Information is provided on dosage, methods of use, effects, aftereffects, and the chemical nature of the substances.

A monograph on each of the following plants is included: wild cucumber, lobelia, kava-kava, Hawaiian baby wood rose, morning glory, hydrangea, heliotrope, peyote, san pedro, doña ana, California poppy, mescal beans, colorines, wild lettuce, damiana, nutmeg, fly agaric, kola nuts, Syrian rue, camphor, yohimbe, areca nuts, hops, pipizintzintli, coleus, jimson weed, deadly nightshade, henbane, mandrake, catnip, Scotch broom, and Mexican calea. Little emphasis is given to the fact that some of these plants are poisonous.

436.   Swain, Tony, ed. **Plants in the Development of Modern Medicine.** Cambridge, MA: Harvard University Press, 1972. 367p. illus. bibliog. index. LC 79-169862. SBN 674-67330-1.

This work is the outgrowth of a symposium held May 8-10, 1968, in Cambridge, Massachusetts, sponsored by the Botanical Museum of Harvard University and the American Academy of Arts and Sciences. The symposium stressed the interdisciplinary outlook and drew from the fields of anthropology, botany, chemistry, pharmacy, and other pertinent areas. In addition, the historical outlook was heeded, recent discoveries reported, and the future or potential of plants as sources of new medicinal constituents emphasized.

The author of the introduction, Paul C. Mangelsdorf, writes that when he began teaching a course called "Plants and Human Affairs" in 1941 he was impressed with what then seemed to be a declining importance of medicinal drugs of plant origin. He predicted to his students that by the time he retired some 25 years later, medicinals of plant origin would be of little more than historical interest. Twenty-seven years later Mangelsdorf writes that he could scarcely have been more wrong. Today there is probably more interest in drugs derived from plants than any time in history.

The following papers, presented by international leaders, are included in the book: 1) The anthropological outlook for Amerindian medicinal plants, by S. Henry Wassén; 2) Magic and witchcraft in relation to plants and folk medicine, by John Mitchell Watt; 3) The future of plants as sources of new biodynamic compounds, by Richard Evans Schultes; 4) The significance of comparative phytochemistry in medical botany, by Tony Swain; 5) Medicinal plants and empirical drug research, by Rudolf Hänsel; 6) Biodynamic agents from microorganisms, by Nestor Bohonos; 7) Drugs from plants of the sea, by Ara Der Merderosian; 8) Ergot−a rich source of pharmacologically active substances, by Albert Hofmann; 9) Recent advances in the chemistry of tumor inhibitors of plant origin, by S. Morris Kupchan; 10) The phytochemistry and biological activity of *Catharanthus lanceus* (Apocynaceae), by Norman R. Farnsworth; and 11) The ordeal bean of Old Calabar: The pageant of *Physostigma venosum* in medicine, by Bo Holmstedt.

437.   Takatori, Jisuke. **Color Atlas, Medicinal Plants of Japan.** Tokyo: Hirokawa Publishing Co., 1966. 160p. illus. (col.).
The text accompanying the beautiful paintings that illustrate this book is in English and Japanese. The author (and illustrator) says he has taken 40 years to complete the illustrations for the 113 plants, shown in 80 different drawings. Plants included are chiefly of Japanese origin, but a few acclimated foreign species are also shown. Medicinal value as considered in old Chinese medicine is often quoted.
The book is large, with each full-size lovely illustration pasted to the recto pages; facing verso pages contain the text (in both languages). The text is brief and usually gives scientific name, Japanese name, habitat, description, use in medicine, and chemical constituents.
A second edition, published in 1980, is available at about $180.00.

438.   Taylor, Norman. **Narcotics, Nature's Dangerous Gifts.** Rev. ed. of **Flight from Reality.** New York: Dell Publishing Co., 1966. 222p. bibliog. index.
The author of this work, known for classic works in botany, in 1949 published an earlier edition of this book under the title *Flight from Reality.* The following chapters are presented: 1) The Pleasant Assassin: The Story of Marihuana; 2) The Abyss of Divine Enjoyment: The Story of Opium, Morphine and Heroin; 3) The Divine Plant of the Incas: The Story of Coca and Cocaine; 4) The Accident of Alcohol; 5) The Lively Image of Hell: The Story of Tobacco; 6) Come and Expel the Green Pain: The Story of Ololiuqui and Peyotl (mescaline); 7) Five Exotic Plants: The Stories of Pituri, Fly Agaric, Caapi, Kava and Betel; 8) Three Habit-Forming Beverages: The Stories of Coffee, Chocolate and Tea; and 9) A Boon or a Curse? The Story of LSD.
The viewpoint of the more recent work is a bit different from that of the earlier, which stressed that people never cease to look for things that offer respite from reality. This edition, as the title suggests, stresses that drugs are both a boon and a curse.

439.   Taylor, William I., and Norman R. Farnsworth, eds. **The Catharanthus Alkaloids: Botany, Chemistry, Pharmacology, and Clinical Use.** New York: Marcel Dekker, Inc., 1975. 323p. illus. bibliog. index. $44.75. LC 75-7710. ISBN 0-8247-6276-2.
Since plants have been a source of medicinal agents since the beginning of time, it is to be expected that present-day scientists will delve into the folkloric past in hope of discovering cures to disease. This work is a good example of a scientific publication reporting recent research into certain plant alkaloids. The research was undertaken because of reported folkloric use of the plants as medicinals. The genus *Catharanthus* is a member of the botanical family Apocynaceae. There are seven species native to Madagascar and one to India. The best known species, the Madagascar periwinkle, is an ornamental plant recently found to contain alkaloids with anticancer activity. The plant has stimulated much research for this reason.

The book contains eight scientific papers by various contributors who are experts in their fields. Most aspects of the *Catharanthus* class of substances are covered. The work is suitable for established researchers and for advanced graduates who are grounded well in organic chemistry, biochemistry, botany, pharmacology, and medicine.

440.   Taylor, William I., and Norman Fransworth, eds. **The Vinca Alkaloids: Botany, Chemistry, and Pharmacology.** New York: Marcel Dekker, Inc., 1973. 357p. illus. bibliog. index. LC 73-83859. ISBN 0-8247-6129-4.

This is a companion volume to the one listed above. Until recently, it was still debatable whether *Vinca* and *Catharanthus* were two different plant genera or the same. Scientific opinion now favors two genera. This work deals with the *Vinca* species; the other work covers *Catharanthus*.

The medical use of *Vinca* dates from the thirteenth century when it was used for nose bleeding and other ailments. In 1684 it was reportedly used for an inflamed chest. However, chemical investigation of the different *Vinca* species developed slowly, and thorough scientific investigation of the alkaloids did not get underway until the early 1950s. At present, about 80 alkaloids have been isolated from the different species, and this book presents a critical review of all aspects of their botany, phytochemistry, chemistry, and biological activities. It emphasizes the discovery and exploitation of biologically active substances from plants that have had an age-long reputation as folk medicines.

There are six chapters as follows: 1) A Synopsis of the Genus *Vinca* Including Its Taxonomic and Nomenclatural History; 2) The Phytochemistry of *Vinca* Species; 3) The Chemistry of the *Vinca* Alkaloids; 4) Chemotaxonomy of *Vinca* Species; 5) The Commercial Cultivation of *Vinca Minor*; and 6) The Pharmacology of *Vinca* Species and Their Alkaloids. Most material is highly scientific, suitable for the research audience.

441.   Tehon, Leo R. **The Drug Plants of Illinois.** Drawings by Kay H. Wadsworth. Urbana, IL: Illinois Natural History Survey Division, 1951. 135p. illus. index. (Illinois Natural History Survey Circular 44).

Although old, this is a very good compilation. The author estimates that about 900 plant species are used in the American drug trade. Some 350 of these are native or cultivated in the U.S., and about 300 grow wild or are cultivated in Illinois. A few of these are rare. The reported purpose of this publication is to encourage use of this natural resource by furnishing instructions for collecting, drying, packing, and marketing crude drugs and by listing, describing, and picturing the plants. The intent is that the plants will find their way into the commercial drug trade and not be used by individuals without a physician's direction.

The plant list is arranged alphabetically by scientific names of species. Common and family names are provided. A description is usually given (except for commonly cultivated plants), and mention is made of the part collected, the distribution in Illinois, medicinal contents, and use. An illustration is provided for each plant (a line drawing).

442.   Tétényi, Péter. **Infraspecific Chemical Taxa of Medicinal Plants.** New York: Chemical Publishing Co., Inc., 1970. 225p. bibliog. index.

Varieties of plants within species can differ in their chemistry, a fact that affects the breeding and production of medicinal plants. Those cultivating, collecting, or processing medicinal plants want varieties with an adequate quantity and quality of desired active substances. In this work, the term "medicinal plant" includes "all collected and cultivated plants whether employed directly for their curative power, or utilized as raw materials in pharmaceutical or essential oil industry, or used as spices."

The book is a critical review of the literature and is divided into two parts. The first part is a general discussion about causes of infraspecific differentiation (mainly chemical). According to the book, anything that alters the metabolic process alters chemical composition. These influences could be external, such as ecological-geographical factors; or they could be internal, such as vegetative stage as opposed to ripe fruit stage. Also covered are classification and nomenclature of infraspecific chemical taxa. The author feels that it is better to first classify species of medicinal plants by "chemical characteristics which are coupled with metabolism and then on the basis of the morphological characteristics." The second part of the work is a listing of groups of active substances of chemical taxa. Included are terpenes and related compounds, other compounds connected with acetate metabolism, derivatives of phenyl-propane and flavonoids, alkaloids, and isohodanidogenes. Listed under these groups are plants by family and then alphabetically by genus and species with infraspecific chemical taxa. Data are taken from literature cited. Included for each entry is a breakdown of the active substances and part of plant involved. About 750 species of medicinal plants are included in the list; however, the author realizes that the survey is not exhaustive and that "screening for further active principles of medicinal plant species will certainly lead to better and wider knowledge of this field."

443.   Trease, George Edward, and William Charles Evans. **Pharmacognosy.** 11th ed. London: Baillière Tindall; New York: Macmillan, 1978. 784p. illus. bibliog. index. $35.00. ISBN 0-02-859530-0.

Pharmacognosy is mainly concerned with physical characteristics and botanical sources of crude drugs. However, recent editions of this work have been broader in scope and include material on phytochemistry, genetics, chemotaxonomy, and newer laboratory techniques such as tissue culture methods, chromatography, spectrometry, and radiochemistry. Recent advances in the subject are covered.

There are eight chapters. The first four provide a detailed outline of plant constituents, their biochemistry, and possible synthetic pathways and basic plant morphology, anatomy, and taxonomy. The main part of the book deals with individual crude drugs and allied raw plant materials. The following is usually given about each plant source: common and scientific names, sources, collection, preparation, characteristics, constituents, uses, history, and a photograph or drawing. The last chapter deals with microscopical techniques and commercial fibers, the latter used in surgical dressings.

The book is the standard textbook on the subject in Great Britain. It is of wide interest, however, and is known for its comprehensiveness and modern approach to the subject.

444.   Tyler, Varro E., Lynn R. Brady, and James E. Robbers. **Pharmacognosy.** 8th ed. Philadelphia, PA: Lea and Febiger, 1981. 520p. illus. bibliog. index. $31.50. LC 81-8162. ISBN 0-8121-0793-4.

Intended primarily as a textbook for pharmacy students, this is a new edition of the standard text used in U.S. schools. It tells about plant and other crude drugs that enter commerce, their sources, their active ingredients, and uses. Older editions of the work generally contained more information about herbs than more recent ones, but this latest edition has been revised to reflect certain changes in the needs of pharmacists. Because of the increasing interest shown by consumers in herbal medicine, megadose vitamin therapy, and "health" foods, pharmacists are called upon to advise on the desirability of use of such substances. A new chapter on "Herbs and Health Foods" has been included in this edition at the end of the book. Most of the better-known remedies are covered with information on their safety and efficacy. Legality of sale, an explanation of how the terms "natural" and "organic" are misused, and an assessment of the value of "health" foods are provided. Appended literature references are listed under two headings: "Authoritative Literature" and "Advocacy Literature."

Other chapters included in the book are: 1) General Introduction; 2) Carbo-hydrates and Related Compounds; 3) Glycosides and Tannins; 4) Lipids; 5) Volatile Oils; 6) Resins and Resin Combinations; 7) Steroids; 8) Alkaloids; 9) Peptide Hormones and the Endocrine System; 10) Enzymes and Other Proteins; 11) Vitamins and Vitamin-Containing Drugs; 12) Antibiotics; 13) Biologics; 14) Allergens and Allergenic Prepara-tions; and 15) Poisonous Plants.

The book is of high quality, written by experts who hold academic positions in pharmacognosy. It makes a noteworthy contribution in the area of herbal medicine as well as in the scientific field of pharmacognosy. Particularly, it puts herbal medi-cine and "health" foods in proper perspective. Much material included, however, is too technical and scientific for the average reader.

445.   United Nations Industrial Development Organization. **Report of the Techni-cal Consultation on Production of Drugs from Medicinal Plants in Developing Countries.** Lucknow, India, 13-20 March 1978. Vienna: UNIDO, 1979. 45p. illus. bibliog. (ID/222; ID/WG.271/6).

Developing countries have frequently expressed a strong wish for promotion, development, and production of drugs derived from medicinal plants in order to utilize their own resources and become self-sufficient in pharmaceuticals. The United Nations Industrial Development Organization organized a workshop on the subject, and this publication reports on the meeting.

The first section provides a summary of the discussion. Part 2 contains sum-maries of technical papers, and part 3 presents summaries of activity in the field in the various countries. Several lists of medicinal plants are reproduced in annexes as follows: 1) Biologically active plants considered during the technical consultation; 2) Additional list of plants used mainly in traditional medicine in Africa, Asia and Latin America; 3) Important plant drugs suitable for production by developing countries; 4) Other plants of economic importance and export potential; 5) Biologically active plants for which drug development has reached an advanced stage; and 6) The important excipients. Facilities available in various countries are also listed.

446.   U.S. Department of Agriculture. **American Medicinal Plants of Commercial Importance.** By A. F. Sievers. Washington, DC: GPO, 1930. 74p. illus. index. (U.S. Department of Agriculture. Miscellaneous Publication No. 77).

This publication supersedes, to some extent, the one by Henkel listed below and several other bulletins of the Department. This publication was issued because of an interest shown in collecting medicinal plants for profit. Since it was difficult for persons without botanical training to identify the plants, the purpose of this publica-tion was to assist in, and provide other useful information in connection with, plant gathering.

After a brief section on collection and preparation of material, plants are list-ed alphabetically by the common name. Usually provided is scientific name, an illus-tration, synonyms names, habitat, range, description, part used, and a statement about demand.

Although old, the publication is of interest still because medicinal plants are being collected as curiosities and for home, if not commercial, use.

447.   U.S. Department of Agriculture. **Weeds Used in Medicine.** By Alice Henkel. Washington, DC: GPO, 1904. 47p. illus. (U.S. Department of Agriculture. Farmers' Bulletin No. 188).

This old bulletin is still of interest. The introduction states that farmers may be able to make a small profit out of some weeds. However, "the price paid for crude drugs from these sources is not great and would rarely tempt anyone to pursue this line of work as a business."

There are sections on collecting, curing, and disposing of drugs. Descriptions of plants are given, including burdock, dandelion, docks, couch grass, pokeweed, foxglove, mullein, lobelia, tansy, gum plant scaly grindelia, boneset, catnip, hoarhound, blessed thistle, yarrow, Canada fleabane, jimson weed, poison hemlock, American wormseed, and black and white mustard. Common names, range and habitat, description, parts used, and 1904 prices are given. The latter, indeed, seem quite low, only a few cents per pound.

448.   U.S. Department of Agriculture. Agriculture Research Service. **Drug and Condiment Plants.** By Louis O. Williams. Washington, DC: GPO, 1960. 37p. illus. bibliog. index. (Agriculture Handbook, No. 172).

The introduction to this pamphlet points out that there is a market for most plants discussed in this handbook. However, only a few would cause real concern to the national economy if the drug or condiment were not available. The suggestion is made that these crops could be grown on a trial basis to see if they provide a reasonable income.

About 60 plants are described. A common name for each plant is given, as are synonymous common names and the accepted botanical name. Other botanical names common in the literature (if any) are listed, and the name of the family indicated. A brief description of the plant follows and, if it is an "official" drug (from the *U.S. Pharmacopeia* or the *National Formulary*), the official description is quoted. History and constituents of the plant are sometimes provided, along with information on propagation, cultivation, and harvesting. Preparation of the crop for market is described when suitable. Most plants are illustrated with photographs. Warnings are given if the plant is toxic. A short glossary of drug terms has been included.

The booklet is nicely prepared and unique in that few publications include such valuable and reliable information on growing herbs for profit.

449.   Wagner, H., and P. Wolff, eds. **New Natural Products and Plant Drugs with Pharmacological, Biological or Therapeutical Activity.** Proceedings of the First International Congress on Medicinal Plant Research, Section A, held at the University of Munich, Germany, September 6-10, 1976. Berlin, Heidelberg, New York: Springer-Verlag, 1977. 286p. illus. bibliog. index. $35.50. LC 77-8846. ISBN 0-387-08292.

This publication stands in marked contrast to popular works on drug plants. The papers are highly scientific, and illustrations are mostly diagrams of chemical structures.

It seemed suitable to include the title in this bibliography, though, since there is much interest in medicine from natural sources. Many of these medicines and claims made for them are tinged with superstition, quackery, and mysticism. This book should throw light on the scientific aspects of the subject.

The book presents the text of 12 papers dealing with various aspects of the subject, including screening and evaluation of plants for medicinal use, reviews of anti-tumor agents and antibiotics, Indian medicinal plants, modification of natural substances in modern drug synthesis, and much more. The first paper covers problems associated with research into plants, such as the number of constituents present in a any one plant.

One author believes that the chances of discovering new drugs from old plant remedies is meager, but he also thinks chances of developing new drugs from synthetic compounds is meager. It may be worthwhile to continue investigation of plants believed to have medicinal value.

450.   Watt, John Mitchell, and Maria Gerdina Breyer-Brandwijk. **The Medicinal and Poisonous Plants of Southern and Eastern Africa.** 2d ed. Edinburgh and London: E. & S. Livingstone Ltd., 1962. 1457p. illus. (part col.). bibliog. index. $65.00. ISBN 0-443-00512-5.

The title page of this impressive scholarly work says it is an account of plants' medicinal and other uses, chemical composition, pharmacological effects, and toxicology in man and animal. In addition, material on folklore and charm uses has been included. Southern and Eastern Africa have a wealth and variety of plants and, through the centuries much information on popular remedies has accumulated, although the authors feared that folk medicine was disappearing at the time the book was written.

Material on the plants is arranged alphabetically according to botanical family, and within each family the genera and species are also listed alphabetically. The extensive bibliography is gathered into an appendix, each entry with a number referring to text material. In addition to a general index, there are lists of European names, vernacular names, and active principles of the plants. A great deal of information has been supplied about each plant. Included are descriptions, habitat, uses, toxicity data, effects on animals, chemical composition, notes on research studies, and folklore. The color plates are particularly nice.

The authors hope that the book will be of value to researchers in chemistry, pharmacology, and toxicology, and also to the medical practitioner, the pharmacist, the missionary, and the forensic worker.

451.   Wheelwright, Edith Grey. **The Physic Garden: Medicinal Plants and their History.** London: Jonathan Cape, 1934. 288p. illus. index. (A reprinted edition entitled **Medicinal Plants and their History** is available from Dover Publications, 1974. $3.00pa. LC 74-78815. ISBN 0-486-23103-8).

This work is a scholarly excursion into several aspects of the long association between man and his healing plants. Scientific, agricultural, artistic, literary, and historical features of the subject are covered.

The following chapters are presented: 1) Pre-history and early agricultural rites; climatic influences and migrations; disease among primitive races; poisonous plants, 2) Medicine among early races; drug plants of Mesopotamia, India and China, 3) Egyptian records; Greek medicine; Hippocrates, 4) The early Christian era; medicine in Rome; the rise of the Saracens, 5) European herbals; the organization of medicine from the Anglo-Saxon leechdom to the British Pharmacopoeia, 6) The English herbals; medicine in the sixteenth and seventeenth centuries, 7) Medicinal plants of the British flora, 8) The trade in medicinal herbs; European cultivation, and new enterprises, 9) Cultivation in England; the drug plants of the British Empire, and 10) The contents of the vegetable cell; essential oils; resins, etc.; bacteria. The book also includes a glossary of medical terms and a list of plants of the Indian materia medica. Although no formal bibliography is provided, numerous references to literature are found in the text.

The author concludes with the prophecy that "the slogan of 'back to the plant' is not impossible. . .never in the nature of things can the race outgrow its ultimate dependence upon the vegetable kingdom."

452.   Zaman, M. B., and Muhammad Shariq Khan. **Hundred Drug Plants of West Pakistan.** Peshawar: Pakistan Forest Institute, Medicinal Plant Branch, 1970. 106p. bibliog. index.

This work is the result of a research project sponsored by the United States Department of Agriculture, Agriculture Research Service. A need was felt for such a publication since there was no one source of information on West Pakistan medicinal plants, yet there is a growing interest in the subject. The business of medicinal plants is a major source of income for many local people in areas of West Pakistan. The work is not comprehensive; it covers about 100 plants of commercial importance.

The book begins with an account of the history and trade of medicinal plants of West Pakistan. The main body of the work is a listing of the plants by scientific name. Included with each are local names, English names, distribution, botanical description, constituents, actions, and uses. Appendices include a glossary of botanical terms and a glossary of medical terms. There are separate indices for families, scientific names, local names, and English names.

It should be understood that the plant principles that produce medicinal effects usually are poisons. In small amounts they may only stimulate, but in larger doses they produce stronger physiological reactions and may have effects worse than the illness they were intended to treat. They may prove extremely harmful, even fatal. It is not really surprising, then, that many plants listed in the poisonous plant books reviewed here are the same as those discussed in herbals and medicinal plant books. Some authors of poisonous plant books, such as Kingsbury, a noted expert (see entries 470-471) believe medicinal preparations should never be made from plants known to be poisonous. Herb books, however, tend to encourage such practice.

The recent back-to-nature movement and its emphasis on wild plants for food make it important that individuals interested in this movement learn to know dangerous species and avoid ingesting them. Many good books are listed in this chapter to assist in that endeavor. There has been some emphasis in recent books on mushroom poisoning, probably because a number of deadly species of mushrooms exist, and those sought for food may not be easily distinguished from dangerous ones. Hallucinogenic mushrooms are being sought because of their intoxicating properties. In addition to several titles included here, there are a number of field guides covering mushrooms listed in chapter 17.

Many books in this chapter give special attention to the poisoning of livestock and children by plants. Geographical areas specifically covered include virtually all parts of the United States, Venezuela, India, and Australia.

* * * * *

453.   Arena, Jay M. **Plants that Poison.** New York: Fischer Medical Publications, Inc., 1981. 19p. illus. (col.). (**Emergency Medicine: Common Emergencies in Daily Practice,** v.13, No.11, June 15, 1981, p.24-57).

Because poisonous plants are causing more and more trouble each year, a medical journal published this article and compendium to inform physicians about plants which are dangerous and how emergencies involving them can be handled. The author is a well-known toxicologist and pediatrician.

The article begins by pointing out that some widely cultivated flowers, vegetables, ornamental plants, and houseplants are among the few plants that are dangerous. They represent an enormous potential for poisoning, especially among small children. Also, a growing number of victims are outdoor enthusiasts who are ill-informed and eat wild plants. The author gives general rules for diagnosis of plant poisoning; then a long chart follows giving plant names, part of plant responsible for poisoning and the active principle, signs and symptoms of poisoning, and treatment. The next section lists the "Main Troublemakers" with a monograph of a paragraph or so on each. Longer monographs are given on a few plants, for instance, jimsonweed and mushrooms. Information provided includes plant description, habitat, symptoms of poisoning, treatment and prognosis.

This is a valuable article.

454.   Arnold, Robert E. **Poisonous Plants.** Jeffersontown, KY: Terra Publishing Inc. (Box 99103, Jeffersontown, KY), 1978. 51p. illus. (col.). bibliog. index. $5.95pa. LC 77-9240.

This book, written by a physician whose avocation is the study of hazardous poisons of nature, contains information about human poisoning from plants. The author's view is that people today know too little about this subject, and poisonous plants do not ordinarily carry labels of warning.

It is a concise book, listing 96 commonly known plants that are potentially poisonous. Most entries include a color photograph of the plant. The main arrangement is alphabetical by common name, but scientific names are also included. Dermatitis-producing and disease-producing plants are *not* discussed. Each entry gives a brief description, symptoms of poisoning, toxicity data, and treatment. The "numbering" systems used in the book are somewhat confusing, i.e., Contents references are to plant numbers; Index references are to page numbers; and text references are to photograph numbers that are easily confused with plant numbers. However, the book is effective as a quick reference book. The intended audience includes the gardener, the forager, and anyone who raises plants or has a yard.

The descriptions are interesting. For example, in regard to the poison hemlock, which was used to kill Socrates, the author writes: "This plant is very common in the United States and yet reported instances of severe poisoning are almost nonexistent. While it undoubtedly was used by the Greeks as a method of capital punishment, its capabilities seem to be exaggerated. After all, we don't know how many hemlock plants the Greeks used to make a lethal concoction."

It is of note that many plants listed in this book also appear in herb books because of their medicinal value.

455.   Baskin, Esther. **The Poppy and Other Deadly Plants.** Drawings by Leonard Baskin. New York: Delacorte Press, 1967. 73p. illus. $12.50. (A Seymour Lawrence Book). LC 66-15843.

The author of this work has woven together curious botanical facts and the legends, lore and history of a few common poisonous plants. The book is illustrated with fine drawings, and the text is full of references to literature and mythology. The work has a great deal of literary and artistic value, but little scientific information and no scientific documentation. About 15 poisonous plants are discussed in full with drawings provided. An addendum provides very brief notes on an additional 100 such plants.

456.   Blohm, Henrik. **Poisonous Plants of Venezuela.** Cambridge, MA: Harvard University Press, 1962. 136p. illus. (part col.). bibliog. index.

This valuable addition to books on poisonous plants is intended for specialists, students, and the lay public. It contains an especially valuable bibliography of about 400 literature references and a glossary. Slightly more than 100 plants are listed, although perhaps 250 poisonous species are known, according to the author. Plants were selected for listing because reliable information about them was available.

The introduction defines poisonous plants and classifies them according to the chemistry of the poisonous principles involved. Plants are listed according to species, genera, and families. Information on each plant includes description, range, toxicity or suspected toxicity, poisonous principle, condition of poisoning, symptoms, and treatment. Many photographs are included. Literature references and occasionally quotations are included with the monographs. A limitation of the work is that few common names have been provided in either the text or the index.

457.   Childers, Norman Franklin, and Gerard M. Russo, eds. **Nightshades and Health.** Somerville, NJ: Somerset Press (Horticultural Publications, Somerset Press, Inc., Sommerville, NJ 08876), 1977. 189p. illus. bibliog. index. $20.00. LC 77-80822.

The nightshade family of plants includes a number that are used as food and also some that are poisons because of the alkaloids they contain. Many are considered herbs.

The point of view taken in this work is that nightshade plants (Solanaceae species) are the main causes of several diseases. The nightshade plants considered in the study are the white potato, tomato, ground cherry (or husk tomato), garden peppers (of all colors), eggplant, and tobacco. It is suggested that these plants and any products containing them are major causes of arthritis, dental caries, osteoporosis, diverticulitis, several other degenerative and chronic diseases, and even libido problems.

The eight chapters of the book, by various authors, are as follows: 1) Introduction; 2) The Diet; 3) Case Histories, Comments; 4) Steroids and Capsaicinoids of Solanaceous Food Plants; 5) Tobacco and Tobacco Smoke; 6) Effects of a Nightshade on Livestock and Calcium Metabolism; 7) Literature Abstracts; and 8) Some Common Toxic Plants. Chapter 4 is rather technical. Chapter 3 contains nearly 10 pages of case histories of "cooperators" who have eliminated nightshade products from their diets. Chapter 8 presents long tables of toxic plants, indicating common names, botanical name, habits, toxic parts, severity of toxicity, and symptoms of poisoning.

The authors of the material are, for the most part, in academic positions, and the book is well documented. If their suggestions were taken seriously, the eating habits of the population would be drastically altered.

458.   Chopra, R. N., R. L. Badhwar, and S. Ghosh. **Poisonous Plants of India.** 2d rev. and enl. ed. New Delhi: Indian Council of Agricultural Research, 1965. 2v. illus. bibliog. index.

Volume 1 of this work was first published in 1949 as Monograph 17 of the Indian Council of Agricultural Research. Volume 2 contains material not previously published.

Introductory material includes sections on the toxic constituents of plants, the actions of poisons, symptoms and diagnosis of plant poisoning, prognosis and treatment, factors determining the toxicity of plants, economic and toxicological aspects, and classification of poisonous plants. The remainder of the two volumes lists poisonous plants of India arranged by plant family. There is a general discussion of the plants of each family and a key to the genera. About each species is usually given: common names including the regional, distribution, botanical characters, uses and properties, constituents, symptoms of poisoning, and treatment. Also given in some instances are economic aspects of the plant and miscellaneous information. Numerous literature references are provided, some to older, obscure Indian literature. A glossary of botanical terms is appended. Illustrations are mostly line drawings of reasonably good quality.

This is comprehensive work of quality that provides much information. About 700 plants are dealt with in volume 1, and about 150 in volume 2. The publication serves as a reference work for physicians and veterinarians who deal with practical problems caused by poisonous plants and as a source of literature references on toxic plants of India.

459.　　Creekmore, Hubert. **Daffodils Are Dangerous: The Poisonous Plants in Your Garden.** Illustrations by Helen Spence. New York: Walker and Co., 1966. 258p. illus. bibliog. LC 66-17224.

　　The author of this work, an amateur gardener and literary critic, has written the book in the hope of arousing more serious interest in poisonous plants and drawing attention to the problem they create, especially where children and livestock are concerned.

　　The plants are discussed under the following headings: the garden plants, intruders (weeds), the indoor garden plants, and miscellany. Plants are described, and their toxic properties and effects discussed. Many episodes of literature and history are presented. In addition, there are many text references to authoritative works.

　　Some of the plants discussed are as follows: the daffodil family, autumn crocus, black locust tree, bleeding heart, box hedge, castor bean plant, cherry laurel, chinaberry tree, Christmas rose, daphne, English ivy, foxglove, gingko tree, golden chain tree, larkspur, lillies, lily of the valley, monkshood, mountain laurel, rhododendron, narcissus, jonquil, oleander, poppy, privet, snow-on-the-mountain, star-of-Bethlehem, tobacco, yew, deadly nightshade, Indian hemp, hemlock, henbane, jimsonweed, mandrake, mushrooms, poison ivy, pokeweed, night-blooming cereus, poinsettia, holly, mistletoe, sweet pea, and mock orange. A number of these plants have medicinal value, but more surprising is the fact that so many are common, popular ornamental plants. The book is interesting and well-written, and illustrations are attractive.

460.　　Ellis, Michael D., ed. **Dangerous Plants, Snakes, Arthropods and Marine Life: Toxicity and Treatment with Special Reference to the State of Texas.** Hamilton, IL: Drug Intelligence Publications, 1978. 277p. illus. (col.). bibliog. index. $18.00. LC 78-50198. ISBN 0-914768-32-8. (A reissue of a 1975 publication entitled **Dangerous Plants, Snakes, Anthropods and Marine Life of Texas**).

　　Since there are many and diverse plants and animals found in the United States, it is likely that man will from time to time come into contact with dangerous organisms and suffer from the encounter. It is hoped that this volume will be of assistance to those who treat such problems. It is necessary that symptoms and treatments be known and that identification of the plant or animal be established. The book should be of considerable assistance in these endeavors.

　　The presentation is in four parts: 1) Poisonous plants; 2) Venomous and non-venomous snakes; 3) Dangerous arthropods; and 4) Dangerous marine life. The section on plants makes up about half the book. It is divided into further sections on cultivated house and garden plants and on wild plants of the woods and/or meadows. Information given includes common names, scientific names, descriptions, general information on toxicity, symptomatology, pathology, and treatment. Chemical formulas for active constituents are often provided, as are literature references. Excellent color photographs are included.

　　The other sections of the book are similar to, although shorter than, the section on plants.

461.　　Eshleman, Alan. **Poison Plants.** With original illustrations by Kristin Jakob. Boston, MA: Houghton Mifflin Co., 1977. 188p. illus. bibliog. $6.95. LC 77-14176. ISBN 0-395-25298-9.

　　This is an introductory work on poisonous plants, perhaps intended primarily for the young person. However, it is quite well done and should be of interest to a much wider group. The history, importance in the modern world, and descriptions of about 30 poisonous plants are provided. There are about 700 known poisonous plants, and those discussed in this book are ones the author considers most intriguing and that illustrate the many different kinds of plant poisons.

The first section of the book includes chapters on history, an explanation of how poisons work, and information on the plant kingdom. Part II begins with a chapter "Poisonous Plants in the United States" and includes a table of "The Twenty-Five Most Frequently Mentioned Poisonous Plants from 1974 National Clearinghouse for Poison Control Centers Reports." Then follows the main part of the book, plant monographs grouped under the following headings: fungi, algae, gymnosperms, flowering plants, and flowering plants (trees). An additional section, "Poisonous Plants around the World" contains monographs on such plants as nutmeg, curare poison, cashew nut, opium poppy, and mandrake. Each monograph is about two pages in length. The plants are illustrated with excellent line drawings. Information given about each plant includes common names, scientific name, description, location, how it poisons, and general information about the plant and its history.

462. Everist, Selwyn L. **Poisonous Plants of Australia.** Sydney: Angus and Robertson Publishers, 1974. 684p. illus. (part col.). bibliog. index. ISBN 0-207-12773-5.

The purpose of this substantial book is to describe Australian plants that are known to cause poisoning in livestock or man, to summarize their distribution and properties, to assist in diagnosis, and to outline measures that may prevent poisoning or treat it in animals. Most plants listed are native to Australia, but a few garden plants also are included. The intended audience is graziers, farmers, students, and professionals.

The book is in two parts. The first, general considerations, covers economic importance of plant poisoning, history of plant poisoning, influence of land use, evidence of toxicity, factors affecting toxicity, methods of investigation, toxic substances in plants, and prevention and treatment. The second and largest part of the book contains individual descriptions of the poisonous plants. They are arranged in three groups: seed-bearing plants, ferns and fern allies, and other plants. Information given about each plant includes names (common and scientific); description; distribution and habitat; toxicity, symptoms, and lesions; and prevention and treatment. The author says he has drawn heavily for his information on standard works from other countries. Many plants are illustrated with good photographs, some in color. There are three appendices: 1) Distribution of poisonous plants (a chart); 2) Poisonous plants grouped by symptoms (a chart); and 3) Toxic principles in Australian plants (a chart).

Many of the plants are familiar. The reader will be impressed that there are a great many poisonous plants. The work is well done.

463. Evers, Robert A., and Roger P. Link. **Poisonous Plants of the Midwest and Their Effects on Livestock.** Urbana, IL: University of Illinois, 1972. 165p. illus. (part col.). index. (University of Illinois, College of Agriculture Special Publication 24).

Written for the general reader as well as for students, teachers, livestock owners, veterinarians, and botanists, this book presents information about poisonous plants in the United States, particularly those found in the Midwest. The descriptions and illustrations help to identify about 70 plants. In addition to specific plant monographs, general information about protecting animals from dangerous plants is provided with tips about how to recognize problems. A glossary of botanical terms is included, and two indexes, of common and botanical names, are provided.

Plants are listed under the following headings: 1) Plants usually found in dry, open pastures and meadows; 2) Plants usually found in moist, open pastures and meadows; 3) Plants of wooded and old woodland pastures; 4) Plants of fencerows, roadsides, barnyards, fields, and waste places; 5) Plants of streams, ditches, ponds, springs, and swampy meadows; and 6) Plants found in hay and grain. Each monograph usually includes an illustration, description, occurrence, conditions of poisoning, control, toxic principle, clinical signs, necropsy, and treatment. Most plants listed are the same as those included in books on plants dangerous to people, and many are discussed in herbals.

464.   Francis, D. F., and R. V. Southcott. **Plants Harmful to Man in Australia.** Adelaide, South Australia: Board of Governors, Botanic Garden Adelaide, 1967. 53p. illus. bibliog. index. (Botanic Garden Adelaide, Miscellaneous Bulletin No.1).

Information published here was presented at the Third Convention of the Australian College of General Practitioners in Adelaide in 1966. Higher plants and fungi are included in the discussion, which is directed toward physicians rather than botanists.

After general introductory material on plant injuries, harmful plants are listed alphabetically by scientific name. About each is given: common names, description, symptoms, poisonous principle, and treatment. In the section on harmful fungi, hallucinogenesis is discussed. Line drawings are provided for some plants.

Although the work is brief, a good deal of succinct information of high quality is provided.

465.   Gadd, Laurence. **Deadly Beautiful: The World's Most Poisonous Animals and Plants.** New York: Macmillan Publishing Co., 1980. 208p. illus. (part col.). index. $17.95. LC 79-27747. ISBN 0-02-542090-9.

This book emphasizes the beauty of many poisonous plants and animals. It contains 200 exquisite color and black-and-white photographs of deadly species. It is not a scientific work as much as it is one that encourages appreciation of nature, but with caution.

The presentation is in three parts. The first is on venomous animals, the second on poisonous plants, and the third is a long table showing the world distribution of venomous animals and poisonous plants. The first and second sections provide general discussions and then present lethal species, including descriptions, toxic symptoms, and the like. Plants included are: panther amanita, fly amanita, death cap, poison pie, ink coprinus, false morel, iris family, elder, stinging nettle, milkweed, windflower or pasqueflower, buckeye or horsechestnut, deadly nightshade, bleeding heart, rock poppy, baneberry, hellebore, mayapple or mandrake, rhododendron, buttercup, monkshood, foxglove, marsh marigold, columbine, death comas, jack-in-the-pulpit, lily of the valley, and bloodroot.

466.   Hardin, James W., and Jay M. Arena. **Human Poisoning from Native and Cultivated Plants.** 2d ed. Durham, NC: Duke University Press, 1974. 194p. illus. (part col.). bibliog. index. $7.95. LC 73-76174. ISBN 8223-0303-5.

The authors felt there was need for this authoritative work because most existing literature on poisonous plants deals with plants poisonous to livestock. This book was written for physicians, health officers, nurses, scout leaders, camp counselors, teachers, parents, and others who work with children and who should know dangerous plants of their area and have a ready reference book in case of an emergency. The book has been well received.

The primary material is arranged under the following headings: allergies, dermatitis, and internal poisoning (the largest section). There is an introductory section which lists 14 ways to avoid plant poisoning and also contains a list of dangerous plants. There is, in addition, a short chapter on poisoning of pets and a glossary. The bibliography includes a list of poisonous plant manuals by state. The main sections contain text material to introduce each part, suggest first aid measures in case of poisoning, and list the common poisonous plants with illustrations, descriptions, habitat, symptoms of poisoning, and suggestions to the physician.

467.   Hulbert, Lloyd C., and Frederick W. Oehme. **Plants Poisonous to Livestock: Selected Plants of the United States and Canada of Importance to Veterinarians.** 3d ed. Manhattan, KS: Kansas State University Printing Service, 1968. 138p. illus. bibliog. index. $6.25pa.

This manual was originally prepared for use in a course on toxicology at the College of Veterinary Medicine, Kansas State University. It presents a listing of plants the authors consider most important to a veterinary student preparing for practice in the U.S. or Canada.

Preliminary sections are on the ecology of livestock poisoning by plants and on plant identification. The plant monographs are arranged in classified order. The following information is usually provided for each plant: distinguishing features, range, occurrence of plants, toxic principle, occurrence of poisoning, clinical signs, necropsy, treatment, and remarks. Line drawings of the plants and maps showing range are included as are extensive literature references. A glossary is appended.

468.   Jenkins, David T. **A Taxonomic and Nomenclatural Study of the Genus** *Amanita* **Section** *Amanita* **for North America.** Vaduz: J. Cramer, 1977. 126p. illus. (part col.). bibliog. (Bibliotheca Mycologica. Bd. 57). $20.00pa. ISBN 3-7682-1132-0.

This publication presents material on the Genus *Amanita*, mushrooms of which many of the species are toxic and/or hallucinogenic. It is a scholarly, scientific treatment, suitable for mushroom experts. The presentation is introduced with historical background material; then general toxonomic characteristics are outlined. Next each taxa is described, and lastly, there is a section of type studies. In the descriptions there is information on habitat and distribution, collections examined, and observational remarks.

469.   Kinghorn, A. Douglas, ed. **Toxic Plants.** New York: Columbia University Press, 1979. 195p. bibliog. index. $20.00. LC 79-16180. ISBN 0-231-04686-3.

This publication contains eight papers presented at the 18th Annual Meeting of the Society for Economic Botany, Symposium on "Toxic Plants," June 11-15, 1977, at the University of Miami. Emphasis is on plants that are lethal or that cause suffering for humans. Chemical, biochemical, and toxicological information is included on selected toxic plants that have been inadequately documented in other texts and about which recent advances have been made in understanding their chemical and toxic nature.

The first paper is an overview of the problem of poisonous plants; the second is a 50-page chapter on toxic mushrooms. The latter is an important paper because the collection of wild mushrooms for food and for hallucinogenic "trips" is growing in popularity. The third paper is on toxins and teratogens of the lily and nightshade family; tobacco, jimsonweed, and henbane are among plants discussed. Other papers discuss pokeweed and other lymphocyte mitogens (seed proteins which are very toxic) and toxic house plants. The final three papers focus on plants that are externally toxic to the skin and eyes, such as poison ivy, poison oak, and others.

The book is written for the research audience, but those interested in the use of herbs should also be more aware of the dangers of poisonous plants and may find the book helpful. Many plants listed in herbals contain toxic constituents that are dangerous, and the books often contain no up-to-date information on these substances and little warning.

470.   Kingsbury, John M. **Deadly Harvest: A Guide to Common Poisonous Plants.** New York: Holt, Rinehart and Winston, 1965. 128p. illus. index. $2.95pa. LC 65-14441. ISBN 0-03-0914795.

Kingsbury mounts a small campaign for better understanding of poisonous plants in this book. He feels the public should be better informed so poisonings will occur less frequently. He also wants to encourage more significant research on the subject.

In this small book, Kingsbury has selected interesting and instructive stories about the poisonous nature of plants, and has included those most likely to cause trouble for human beings.

Chapter headings are as follows: 1) Introducing Poisonous Plants; 2) History; 3) Where is Toxicity?; 4) How Plants Are Toxic; 5) Plants Everyone Should Recognize as Dangerous; and 6) What to Do about Poisonous Plants.

In summary, Kingsbury advises the public to learn the poisonous plants of the neighborhood; know the scientific name; never eat or allow children to eat any unknown or wild plant, herb, shrub, or tree; never make medicinal preparations from them; keep prunnings and clippings away from animals; in case of poisoning or suspected poisoning call a physician or take the patient to the hospital; and save evidence that may help identify the plant.

471.   Kingsbury, John M. **Poisonous Plants of the United States and Canada.** Englewood Cliffs, NJ: Prentice-Hall, Inc., 1964. 626p. illus. (part col.). bibliog. index. $23.95. LC 64-14394.

Intended primarily as a reference book for the physician and veterinarian who deal with practical problems caused by poisonous plants, this work is also suitable as a textbook for students and as an introduction to the literature of the field for all who are interested. It is of value also to those interested in the physiologically active compounds in plants.

The first section reviews the subject. Foundations in Western tradition, early European publications dealing with poisonous plants, other early literature, and investigations on poisonous plants are covered. The next section is a scientific discussion on poisonous principles in plants. The bulk of the work, however, is made up of autonomous descriptions of individual poisonous plants arranged alphabetically by scientific name, within families taxonomically arranged. Each entry usually gives scientific name, common names, description, distribution and habitat, poisonous principle, toxicity, symptoms and lesions, and conditions of poisoning. Since antidotal agents for plant poisoning are not usually available, only limited attention has been given to them.

Most illustrations are line drawings, although a few color plates and photographs of plants are included. A bibliography of 1,715 references is provided.

The work is a standard, classical reference book of the field.

472.   Liener, Irvin E., ed. **Toxic Constituents of Plant Foodstuffs.** 2d ed. New York: Academic Press, 1980. 502p. illus. bibliog. index. (Food Science and Technology: A Series of Monographs). $39.50. LC 79-51681. ISBN 0-12-449960-0.

This work is far more scientific and technical than most books in this bibliography. It is included because it stands as a reminder that many plants contain toxic substances and that plant constituents are far more complicated than the lay public generally realizes.

The subject matter of the book has grown in importance since the appearance of the first edition about 10 years ago. The main reasons for this interest are: 1) that more plant proteins are needed to feed a growing world population; 2) there is evidence of a link between excessive consumption of animal fat and heart disease; and 3) there is believed to be a beneficial effect of crude plant fiber in the prevention of colon cancer. These positive effects, though, must be weighed against the fact that plants contain toxic materials that may limit their use unless the poisons are eliminated by processing techniques. Man has heretofore learned by trial and error which foods to avoid and which require some form of processing to make them safe for consumption.

Following are the chapters presented: 1) Introduction; 2) Protease Inhibitors; 3) Hemagglutinins (Lectins); 4) Glucosinolates; 5) Cyanogens; 6) Saponins; 7) Gossypol; 8) Lathyrogens; 9) Favism; 10) Allergens; 11) Naturally Occurring Carcinogens; 12) Toxic Factors Induced by Processing; and 13) Miscellaneous Toxic Factors.

473.   Menser, Gary P. **Hallucinogenic and Poisonous Mushroom Field Guide.** Berkeley, CA: And/Or Press, 1977. 140p. illus. (part col.). bibliog. $5.95pa. ISBN 0-915904-28-4.

This book is intended as a field guide for identification of various genera and species of psychoactive and lethal wild mushrooms of the western half of North America, excluding Mexico. Some species share similar characteristics and some can only be identified through chemical analysis or expert microscopic evaluation. Confusing species may have lethal results, it is noted in the book.

The following sections are presented: 1) Introduction; 2) What are mushrooms?; 3) How to collect, identify and dry; 4) Chemical qualities; 5) Key of macroscopic characteristics; 6) Genus and species information, with taxonomy and drawings; 7) Glossaries; and 8) Bibliography and selected readings. The genus and species information section, which makes up about half the book, describes 24 species that are hallucinogenic. Eight species, which are lethal and which may be confused with the others, are also described.

474.   Mitchell, John, and Arthur Rook. **Botanical Dermatology: Plants and Plant Products Injurious to the Skin.** Vancouver, British Columbia, Canada: Greenglass Ltd., 1979. 787p. bibliog. index. $39.50. ISBN 0-88978-047-1.

The authors of this work are dermatologists. They have located and analyzed reports of skin injuries caused by 248 families of plants, comprising about 1,400 genera and thousands of species. The authors hope that this reference work will save interested persons many hours of work searching the literature in an attempt to identify offending plants, to recognize the skin lesions they produce, and to learn how to avoid such exposure.

The first part of the book is made up of relatively short sections on the history of contact dermatitis from plants, the history of epicutaneous testing to plants and plant products, reports of adverse contact skin reactions to plants to 1900 (a 12-page table with literature references), mechanical injury by plants, patch testing with plants and plant products, plant allergens, and hyposensitization. The main part of the book is an "Alphabetical Listing of Irritant and Allergic Plants." A paragraph or so about the genus is given, then a substantial list of literature references. Many references are repeated under other plant headings as many will cover a number of plants. The last section of the book provides sections on perfume, flavoring and essential oil dermatitis; ill-effects to the eye; respiratory ill-effects; hayfever plants; tree-wood, sawdust dermatitis; weed dermatitis; phytophotodermatitis; contact urticaria; agricultural chemicals, and pesticides; and minerals in foods.

Although the work has been criticized because the authors have not always brought the plant nomenclature up-to-date and noted changes in scientific names, it is a very substantial and useful book.

475.   Morton, Julia F. **Plants Poisonous to People in Florida and Other Warm Areas.** Miami, FL: Hurricane House (14301 S. W. 87th Ave., Miami, FL 33158), 1971. 116p. illus. (col.). index. LC 71-156872.

This work begins with a discussion of plants with poisonous and/or irritant properties. Emphasis is placed on plants growing in Florida, although many of those mentioned grow elsewhere.

The main section lists the plants divided into these categories: 1) Plants causing primarily internal poisoning; 2) Plants causing primarily skin and respiratory irritation; and 3) Some other potentially hazardous plants. Provided are 48 good color photographs. The following information is given for each plant: scientific and common names, type of plant (tree, shrub), description, habitat, toxicity, and cases of poisoning. Some plants listed are: oleander, pokeweed, lantana, chinaberry, coral plant, castor bean, chili pepper, century plant, poison ivy, and mango.

476.   Muenscher, Walter Conrad. **Poisonous Plants of the United States.** Rev. ed. New York: Macmillan, 1951. 277p. illus. bibliog. index. $6.95.

The subject of this work is of vital interest to everyone who is attempting to use native plants. The book has been widely used. The author was a professor of botany at Cornell University.

The first part of the work contains three sections as follows: 1) Nature and classification of poisonous plants; 2) The classification of poisonous plants; and 3) Plants poisonous or injurious under special conditions. The second part contains monographs on poisonous plants arranged according to family. There is an index of botanical and common names. In addition, the text is illustrated by many drawings to aid in identification of various plants.

The following information is usually given about each plant: description, distribution and habitat, conditions of poisoning, symptoms, and treatment.

The following comment is found in a preliminary page of the book: "Many hypotheses have been advanced to explain the significance of toxic substances produced in plants, as, that they are developed to protect the plant against herbivorous animals, are waste products, are stages in the process of metabolism. Of these suggestions the first appears the least acceptable and the last the most plausible."

477.   **Poisonous Plants.** Jamaica Plain, MA: Arnold Arboretum of Harvard University, 1974. 41-96p. illus. bibliog. index. $1.00. (Reprinted from **Arnoldia**, Vol. 34, No.2, Mar./Apr., 1974).

The first part of this presentation is an essay on "Living with Poisonous Plants" by Richard A. Howard. The pamphlet is "a guide to the most common plants of woodlands, gardens, and homes which are potentially dangerous if misused." Safety rules are laid down and information is provided on what to do if poisoning is suspect-ed. Emphasis throughout the work is on protecting children from plant poisons.

The second part of the booklet is a "Guide to Potentially Dangerous Plants" by Gordon P. De Wolf, Jr. Approximately 45 plants are shown, including some com-mon ones, such as dumbcane, English ivy, privet, rhubarb, potato, and poison ivy. No mushrooms, toadstools, or fungi are listed. Arrangement is alphabetical by scientific name, with one plant per page, plus a black-and-white photograph or an ink drawing. Information on each plant includes a short description of poisonous parts, symptoms of poisoning (including some reaction times), and where the plant is commonly found

The index includes common names of the plants. A guide to Poison Control Centers in Massachusetts is also included. This is a concise, useful little guide to poison-ous plants of the northeastern United States and the Midwest. It is noteworthy that the plants listed are quite common, although it may not be generally known that they are potentially dangerous if misused. Most plants listed in this book can be found in herbals; fortunately, warnings often accompany the text.

478.   Ricciuti, Edward R. **The Devil's Garden: Facts and Folklore of Perilous Plants.** New York: Walker and Co., 1978. 172p. illus. index. $9.95. LC 77-79624. ISBN 0-8027-0581-2.

The author of this work, who has written a number of natural history books for children, has produced a non-technical, interesting, and attractive publication on intoxicating and harmful plants. He states that the trend toward "getting back to nature" has inspired a new interest in gardening, house plants, and wild foods. While this may encourage an appreciation of nature, many individuals believe that "natural" means "beneficial," which is an unwarranted and dangerous assumption when applied to plants.

The book begins with a historical look at how certain plants have been asso-ciated with death and occult arts. Present-day abuse of intoxicating and hallucinogenic plants is then discussed, focusing on commonly abused drugs as well as other sub-stances. Harmful and dangerous effects of drug plants are stressed.

The book has a dual aim. It warns the reader of the dangers of common toxic plants such as yews, castor beans, oleander, and the nightshade; it also points out the dan-gers of drugs of abuse such as cocaine, opiates, marihuana, and hallucinogenic mushrooms.

While there are many references in the text to various historical events and scientific studies concerning dangerous plants (which seem to be authentic), no formal bibliography has been included.

479.   Rumack, Barry H., and Emanuel Salzman, eds. **Mushroom Poisoning: Diag-nosis and Treatment.** West Palm Beach, FL: CRC Press, 1978. 263p. illus. (part col.). bibliog. index. $62.95. LC 77-21633. ISBN 0-8493-5185-5.

This publication is an outgrowth of the annual Aspen Mushroom Conference. The purpose of these conferences has been to coordinate activity and facilitate exchange of information between mycologists and physicians who treat poisoned patients, the aim being to improve treatment of poisoned victims. The book should interest those who use wild foods because it points out the dangerous effects of consuming poison-ous mushrooms.

The book contains 15 chapters divided into three sections: (1) Mushroom identification; (2) Mushroom toxicology; and (3) Mushroom hallucination. Chapter headings are: 1) Principles of Mushroom Identification; 2) Identification of Common Poisonous Mushrooms; 3) Poisonous Mushrooms: Their Habitats, Geographic Distri-bution, and Physiological Variation within Species; 4) The Diagnoses of Mushroom

Orders and Families; 5) Amateur Opportunity; 6) Chemistry and Mode of Action of
Mushroom Toxins; 7) Pharmacology and Therapy of Mushroom Intoxications;
8) Symptomatic Diagnosis and Treatment of Mushroom Poisoning; 9) The Disulfiram-
Like Effects of *Coprinus Atramentarius* and Related Mushrooms; 10) Respiratory Dis-
ease Due to Mushrooms: Mushroom Worker's Lung; 11) Acute Encephalopathy in
Children after Eating Wild Mushrooms; 12) Hallucinogenic Mushrooms; 13) The Present
Status of Soma: The Effects of California *Amanita Muscaria* on Normal Human Volun-
teers; 14) The Abuse of Drug Terminology; and 15) Recreational Use of Hallucinogenic
Mushrooms in the United States.

The extensively documented chapters are by well-known authorities. The
book has some popular appeal, but it is rather scientific and technical.

480.　　Schmutz, Ervin M., and Lucretia Breazeale Hamilton. **Plants that Poison: An
Illustrated Guide for the American Southwest.** Illustrations by Lucretia Breazeale
Hamilton. Flagstaff, AZ: Northland Press, 1979. 241p. illus. bibliog. index. $7.50pa.
LC 78-74037. ISBN 0-87358-193-8.

The potential for accidental poisoning has grown in recent years, largely due
to the "back-to-nature" movement and its involvement with plants as "natural" foods.
Plants are being used as drugs in the practice of ethnic and "do-it-yourself" medicine,
and, in addition, they have become popular as ornamentation. Certain plants, mushrooms and cacti, are being sought for their hallucinogenic effects.

Plants included in this book are native and introduced wild plants, cultivated
crops, ornamental and garden plants, and house plants. They all grow in the southwestern U.S. and northwestern Mexico, and they contain poisonous substances that
cause toxic reactions, illness, or death. A few relatively nontoxic plants with poisonous
reputations have been included for clarification.

The plants are arranged alphabetically by common name. Information given
includes: scientific name, synonymous names, description and distribution, toxic parts,
poisonous principles, symptoms of poisoning, and miscellaneous comments. Line drawings are included for most species, and there are general sections on prevention and
treatment. A short glossary is appended.

As the authors point out, many plants listed are used for medicinal purposes,
and proper amounts are not dangerous. However, they should always be used with
caution. It is also of note that many of the plants are common food plants. Ordinarily,
according to the book, the part of the plant eaten is not poisonous, but the seeds of many
fruits (peaches, plums, cherries), the leaves of such plants as rhubarb and spinach, and the
sprouts of potatoes are poisonous.

This is a high quality book, clearly written. It is of general interest, too, because
a large number of the plants listed grow elsewhere than Southwestern United States.

481.　　Schmutz, Ervin M., Barry N. Freeman, and Raymond E. Reed. **Livestock-
Poisoning Plants of Arizona.** Tucson, AZ: University of Arizona Press, 1968. 176p.
illus. bibliog. index. $5.95pa. LC 67-30669. ISBN 0-8165-0502-0.

The annual loss of livestock from poisonous plants in the western United
States is high; few other causes of death exceed those from consumption of such plants.
This book explains the extent of the problem, helps to identify dangerous plants, and
summarizes important information known about the various plants. Nearly 300
suspected or known poisonous plants found in Arizona are listed and described.

The introductory section of the book names the types of poisons found in the
plants, provides general information on treatment of the poisoned animals, and discusses how to determine the poison ingested. In addition, management to prevent such

losses and control of poisonous plants are covered. Section 2 lists major poisonous range plants. About each is given: a description, growth and distribution, poisonous principle, symptoms and treatment, and management and control. Common and scientific names are given. In addition, a good line drawing is provided for each plant. Section 3 lists secondary poisonous range plants and provides similar information. Section 4 presents a long table of rarely poisonous and suspected poisonous range plants. Some illustrations are provided. Section 5 is another table, on poisonous cropland and garden plants, with some illustrations. There is a glossary, and the index lists common and scientific names.

It is of note that most plants listed are common, even in places other than Arizona. Many are considered medicinal herbs.

482. Stephens, H. A. **Poisonous Plants of the Central United States.** Lawrence, KS: Regents Press of Kansas, 1980. 165p. illus. bibliog. index. $16.00; $9.95pa. LC 79-28161. ISBN 0-7006-0202-X; 0-7006-0204-6pa.

Intended to be of practical use to physicians, nurses, veterinarians, ranchers, parents of small children, teachers, camp directors, and sportsmen, this book provides ready information about poisonous plants of the central United States. Only vascular plants are included. Listed are plants that cause chemical poisoning, photosensitization, mechanical injury, dermatitis, and hay fever. Many, if not most, of the plants are familiar, and they include garden vegetables, flowers, and house plants. Many are considered herbs or medicinal plants.

The first section of the book is a glossary. The second section (most of the book) lists about 300 plants. About each is given: a description, habitat, range, toxicity information, symptoms of poisoning (in both humans and livestock), and several illustrations of various parts of the plant. The last section lists the poisonous plants by toxic principle. The toxin is named, scientific and common names listed, and the toxic part of the plant indicated.

The book has been criticized because it emphasizes livestock poisoning more than human and does not contain much information on the effects of the poisonous compounds. Some reviewers feel recent literature on the subject could have been covered better.

483. Tampion, John. **Dangerous Plants.** New York: Universe Books, 1977. 176p. illus. bibliog. index. $12.50. LC 76-55116. ISBN 0-87663-280-0.

This book is similar to the pamphlet *Poisonous Plants* reprinted from *Arnoldia* (see entry 477), except that it lists about twice as many plants, includes mushrooms, and provides a bit more information. Illustrations in the pamphlet look more realistic, however.

After an introductory chapter, "The Problem and the Solution," dangerous plants are listed in three categories: commonly cultivated, frequently growing wild, and fungi. Each entry includes a line drawing and a description, along with information about distribution and habitat, dangers, and related plants. Scientific and common names are provided.

The book also contains chapters on plant poisons, allergies, and harmful substances in food. Appendix 1 is a list of plants reported as poisonous to man, and appendix 2 is a list of plants causing dermatitis. A short glossary (illustrated) is provided in the section on plant descriptions.

The book has been well recommended for the nonprofessional botanist and the lay public. The professional, however, would require more specific documentation about poisoning and deaths.

484.   Tichy, William. **Poisons: Antidotes and Anecdotes.** New York: Sterling
Publishing Co., 1977. 192p. illus. index. $7.95. LC 76-51188. ISBN 0-8069-3738-6.
    This popularly written book provides historical and recent material on poisons
and poisonings and includes numerous anecdotes about them. Despite the title there
are few, if any, real poison antidotes, although people have sought them since primitive
times.
    Contents of the book is as follows: 1) Poison fundamentals; 2) Poison myster-
ies and madness through the ages; 3) Poisons and modern biology; 4) Exotic poisons
of nature: deadly beasts of the world; 5) Exotic poisons of nature: poisonous plants
of the world; 6) Exotic poisons of nature: deadly minerals and chemical creations;
7) Protecting the public from poisons; 8) Antidotes, action and treatment. The last
chapter provides a table that lists common household products, giving special instructions on how to treat victims of such poisoning. Also provided is a Table of Chemical
Poisons with signs, symptoms, and emergency treatment outlined, and a similar table
for poisonous plants. A final section contains brief information about poisonous
animals and how to deal with poisoning by them.

485.   U.S. Public Health Service, Division of Accident Prevention; Rhode Island
Department of Health, Division of Health Education and Information; and the University of Rhode Island. **Common Poisonous Plants of New England.** Prepared by Heber
W. Youngken, Jr., and others. Washington, DC: GPO, 1964. 23p. illus. (col.). index.
(U.S. Public Health Service Publication No. 1220).
    This booklet was prepared because of many inquiries regarding toxic plants,
berries, and flowers. The intent is to aid families in planning safe gardens, to provide
fuller knowledge about wild plants, and, in the case of accidental ingestion, to provide
assistance in identifying the plant. A little basic information about treatment is also
included. Twenty common toxic plants are pictured in color and described. Poisonous
parts are identified, and antidotes or treatments are suggested. In addition to the 20
common plants, other toxic plants of the same family or genus are mentioned. Poison
Control Centers of New England are listed in an appendix.

13
MAGIC, WITCHCRAFT, SUPERSTITION, AND SACRED PLANTS

Some unusual, fascinating, and occasionally even amusing books, are listed here. They are similar to the materials in chapter 9 on folk medicine, but they emphasize the more bizarre and mysterious aspects of plants.

Since problems of the modern day are so complex, and often insoluble, there has been a tendency to turn to less rational ways of knowing, and the occult and the pseudosciences are making a comeback, as can be seen in some of the works listed below. A number, however, present the material as lore and historical information only.

There are several books included on the use of sacred plants, usually hallucinogens; for instance, see the titles by the Church of the Tree of Life Staff, Furst, Harner, Schultes, and Wasson.

For those who think plant substances are mysterious, a look at a truly scientific book or journal on the subject should convince them that this is indeed true, but not in the way suggested in magic, occult, and witchcraft books. The medicinal plant field is highly developed scientifically.

* * * * *

486.   Baker, Margaret. **Gardener's Magic and Folklore.** New York: Universe Books, 1978. 181p. illus. bibliog. index. $12.50. LC 77-73799. ISBN 0-87663-299-1.

This book is a collection of folklore regarding gardening. The author feels that old customs and old wives' tales may contain some truth and should not be buried in oblivion. Many superstitions mentioned in the book have to do with growing plants, but other aspects are also treated, such as plants for medicinal use and witchcraft and curses involving plants.

Contents of the book is as follows: 1) Moon, sun and stars (includes a discussion of almanacs, the zodiac, and planting by the signs); 2) Growing magic (discusses way plants have evidently been improved by the use of magic); 3) Seasons and Saints' Days: the rolling year (special days of the year are discussed); 4) Witchcraft and the supernatural (a discussion of curses, spells, and signs); 5) Plants, personalities and predictions (such matters as "green thumbs"; talking to plants; plants responsive to music, touch, and praying; and responses to personality covered); 6) Traditional receipts (includes insect and pest repellants from plants, medicines from plants, and plants for bees and butterflies); and 7) Companion planting (discussion of herbs as companions to other plants and garden plants that thrive together).

487.   Camp, John. **Magic, Myth and Medicine.** New York: Taplinger Publishing Co., 1974. 192p. illus. bibliog. index. $8.50. LC 73-18793. ISBN 0-8008-5046-7.

The instinct for survival, according to the author of this work, shows itself in many ways. When it is not possible to flee or face the aggressor, man will turn to divine providence for assistance. Camp examines the folk medicine of a number of countries, traces its origins and development, and discusses its survival. He believes that many folk "cures" have a surprisingly scientific basis and may be far more valuable than might be supposed considering the beliefs on which they appear to be founded.

Chapter titles are: 1) The Instinct for Survival; 2) Fertility and Birth; 3) Contraception and Abortion; 4) Folklore of Infancy; 5) Household Cures and Self-Medication; 6) Herbal Remedies; 7) Quacks and Their Cures; 8) Faith and Healing; 9) Sickness and Superstition; 10) Fringe Medicine (includes homeopathy, acupuncture, osteopathy, chiropractic, and various psychiatric techniques); 11) Taking the Cure (by way of spas and watering places); 12) Death and Superstition; and 13) The Survival of Superstition.

In conclusion, the author remarks that mankind is largely ignorant, but long of memory. He thinks superstition will continue to flourish along with scientific progress. He believes it is just as well because it may act as a safety-valve and an escape route from the full realization of what the future may hold for us.

488.   Church of the Tree of Life Staff. **The First Book of Sacraments of the Church of the Tree of Life: A Guide for the Religious Use of Legal Mind Alterants.** Edited by John Mann. San Francisco, CA: Tree of Life Press (451 Columbus Ave., San Francisco, CA 94133), 1972. 32p. illus. bibliog.

The most fundamental belief of the Church of the Tree of Life is said to be that every person has the right to do with himself whatever he pleases as long as his actions do not interfere with the rights of others. Consequently, the members of this group believe that a person may treat ailments with any medicine he chooses and alter his consciousness with any psychoactive agent he wishes to use. Many of the "gifts of God" (herbs and psychedelic agents) have been outlawed in the U.S. and other places. The church has proclaimed as its sacraments all substances not illegal at the present time.

This publication, which deals primarily with the ritual use of legal mind-altering sacraments, imparts to the reader basic information necessary to use the sacraments successfully. It is of note that some of the substances listed are of doubtful legality.

There are short monographs of about a page on the following substances: areca (betel nut), calamus, calea, Canary island broom, ginseng, goldenseal, kava, nutmeg, ololuique, peyote, pipilzintzintli, psilocybe mushrooms, san pedro. sinicuichi, soma (*Amanita muscaria*), yohimbe. Also provided are sections on the use of sacraments, the value of ritual, the use of mind alterants, suppliers of sacraments, the future of freedom, sacraments and magic, a good bibliography, and a "Table of Sympathetic Correspondences of Mind-Altering Sacraments."

The following information is usually given in the monographs on the plants: what the sacrament is for (e.g., divination and healing), scientific and other names, effects of the active constituents, historical use, habitat, description, preparation for use, and some toxicity information.

489.   Emboden, William A. **Bizarre Plants: Magical, Monstrous, Mythical.** New York: Macmillan, 1974. 214p. illus. bibliog. index. $10.95. LC 73-2749.

This book discusses some of the oddities of the plant kingdom and the lore and superstitions connected with them. The author, an authority on the chemistry and pharmacology of plants, also provides information on how the plants are currently used in medicine.

Contents of the book is as follows: 1) Monstrous plants; 2) Orchids in witchcraft and medicine; 3) Satan's simples: the herbs of black magic; 4) Herbs of grace: witches and warlocks undone; 5) Dragon's blood; 6) The fabulous Coco-de-Mer; 7) Plants that eat animals; 8) The hand of glory—mandragora; 9) Ginseng—wonder of the world; 10) Fungal fantasies; and 11) Plants that never were: a floral "talepiece."

Plants discussed include the baobab tree that appears to be upside down with roots at the top; the *Rafflesia arnoldii*, the world's largest flower (three foot in diameter); the *Amorphophallus titanium*, also very large; henbane (or the Devil's eye); the mandrake; ginseng; orchids; dragon-blood tree; pitcher plants; Venus flytrap (which entraps insects); the truffle; the mushroom "fly agaric" (*Amanita muscaria*); and some mythological plants such as the "barnacle tree," "the tree of life," and "the tree of knowledge."

This is a fascinating book.

490.   Furst, Peter T. **Hallucinogens and Culture.** San Francisco, CA: Chandler & Sharp Publishers, Inc., 1976. 194p. illus. bibliog. index. (Chandler and Sharp Series in Cross-Cultural Themes). $4.95pa. LC 75-25442. ISBN 0-88316-517-1.

Written by a professor of anthropology, this work serves as an introduction to some hallucinogenic drugs in a cultural and historical setting. It stresses their role in religious, healing, and magical ceremonies. Various cultures in the world, both historical and modern, are explored.

The following chapters are presented: 1) "Idolatry," Hallucinogens, and Cultural Survival; 2) Tobacco: "Proper Food of the Gods"; 3) Cannabis (spp.) and Nutmeg Derivatives; 4) Ibogaine and the Vine of Souls: From Tropical Forest Ritual to Psychotherapy; 5) Hallucinogens and "Archetypes"; 6) LSD and the Sacred Morning Glories of Indian Mexico; 7) The Sacred Mushrooms: Rediscovery in Mexico; 8) The Fly-Agaric: "Mushroom of Immortality"; 9) R. Gordon Wasson and the Identification of the Divine Soma; 10) The "Diabolic Root"; 11) "To Find Our Life": Peyote Hunt of the Huichols of Mexico; 12) Datura: A Hallucinogen That Can Kill; 13) Hallucinogenic Snuffs and Animal Symbolism; 14) The Toad as Earth Mother: A Problem in Symbolism and Psychopharmacology; and 15) Hallucinogens and the Sacred Deer.

The subject of this book is of growing interest because new or long-forgotten naturally occurring psychoactive substances are now being discovered and scientifically described and tested. The identity of every species presently used by natives is not known.

491.   Gimlette, John D. **Malay Poisons and Charm Cures.** 3d ed. London: J. and A. Churchill, 1929. 301p. illus. bibliog. index. (A reprinted second edition, published in 1923 is available from AMS Press. $22.00. LC 77-87027. ISBN 0-404-16821-3).

The author of this unusual book was a surgeon who gathered material for it while in the service of the government of the Federated Malay States. He made his observations from consultation with friendly "medicine-men" and "witch-doctors" and from actual acquaintance with the individual drugs mentioned.

The first chapter begins with the statement that the Malay used poison to get vengeance. The intent often was to cause annoyance or injury rather than death. Obviously, charms and antidotes were important.

Contents of the book is as follows: 1) Methods of poisoning and Malay charms in general; 2) The work of the bomor (person who practices the healing art by utilizing magic) in relation to clinical medicine; 3) Charms and amulets; 4) Black art in

Malay medicine; 5) Spells and soothsaying; 6) Poisons obtained by Malays from fish; 7) Other poisons obtained by Malays from the animal kingdom (tortoises, snakes, frogs, warms); 8) Poisons obtained by Malays from jungle plants; 9) Other poisons of vegetable origin (includes the familiar papaya, pepper, datura, and pineapple); 10) Poisons from inorganic sources used by Malays (arsenic, cyanide of potassium, mercury, pounded glass, sand, and quicklime). There are three appendices, spells and charms transcribed into Romanized Malay, classification in natural orders of the poisonous plants, and a list of poisons.

492. Goran, Morris. **Fact, Fraud, and Fantasy: The Occult and Pseudosciences.** South Brunswick and New York: A. S. Barnes and Co., 1979. 189p. bibliog. index. $8.95. LC 77-84569. ISBN 0-498-2122-X.

The author of this book believes that problems faced by individuals today may seem difficult, perhaps insoluble. Consequently confidence in human reason is eroding, and other less rational ways of knowing are becoming appealing. The occult and pseudosciences have become replacements for the use of the human brain. The aim of the book is to analyze the pseudo- and occult sciences to gain a more objective view of them. Goran feels that understanding these topics in proper context is educational and entertaining. (The book is interesting as well as educational.) The book also tries to show how some characteristics of science can be found in the occult and pseudosciences, but differences are delineated.

Contents of the book is as follows: 1) Correlations (phrenology, pyramidology, palmistry, numerology, I Ching, Tarot cards); 2) Periodicity (astrology, biorhythm); 3) Analogy (alchemy); 4) Revolutionists (Donnelly, Hörbiger, Fort, Velikovsky, von Däniken); 5) Gadgets (dowsers, medical boxes, Kirlian photography); 6) Imponderables (scientology); 7) Control (witchcraft, magic, mesmerism and hypnotism, psychic healing, spiritualism); 8) Show time (clairvoyance, precognition, telepathy, psychokinesis); 9) Futurists; and 10) Detection.

Goran stresses keeping an open mind to all ideas, unless, of course, they bring harm such as illness or death. Since science does not pretend to have all the answers, the average person with a nonscientific frame of mind may turn to the occult. The tendency may stem from disillusionment with the supposed failure of traditional values and systems. Younger people are the customers for paperbacks about flying saucers, magic, and witchcraft. Perhaps the popularity of this kind of material will wane. However, as Goran says, those seeking certainty and ego-building will continue to be interested in these topics, as will the individual seeking entertainment.

493. Grillot de Givry, Emile **Witchcraft, Magic, and Alchemy.** Translated by J. Courtenay Locke. New York: Houghton Mifflin, 1931; repr. Dover, 1971. 395p. illus. index. $6.00pa. LC 78-142878. ISBN 0-486-22493-7.

This unique work provides a great deal of material on witches, sorcerers, magicians, alchemists, ghosts, demons, and the like. The author has collected and explained more than 350 pictures, chosen from curious and rare works on these subjects, including works in manuscript and incunabula form. Dates covered range from the Middle Ages to the beginning of the nineteenth century.

The book is in three parts: Sorcerers, Magicians, and Alchemists. Chapter headings are: Part I, 1) The World of Shadows as Rival of the World of Light; 2) Sacerdotal Representation of the Dark World; 3) Diabolic Manifestations in the Religious Life; 4) The Sorcerer as Priest of the Demoniacal Church; 5) The Preparation for the Sabbath; 6) The Sabbath; 7) The Evocation of Demons; 8) The Books of the Sorcerers; 9) Pacts with Demons; 10) Some Concrete Notions about Demons Furnished by Old

Authors; 11) Involuntary Demoniacs; 12) Possession by Demons; 13) Necromancy, or the Evocation of the Dead; 14) Spells; 15) Philtres and Death-Spells; and 16) The Punishment of Sorcerers. Part II, 1) The Jewish and Christian Cabbalists; 2) Astrology and the Macrocosm; 3) Astrology and the Microcosm; 4) Metoposcopy, or the Science of the Frontal Lines; 5) Physiognomy; 6) Cheiromancy; 7) Cartomancy and the Tarot; 8) The Divinatory Arts; 9) Rhabdomancy, or the Art of Using the Divining-Rod; 10) The Mystery of Sleep and Clairvoyance; 11) Curative Virtues of the Invisible Forces; and 12) Talismans. Part III, 1) The Secret Doctrine; 2) The Alchemic Material and the Operations of the Work; and 3) The Laboratory of the Alchemists and of the Puffers.

No formal bibliography is included, but works cited are identified in the text, and names and titles appear in the index. This is a fascinating book.

494.   Haggard, Howard W. **Mystery, Magic and Medicine: The Rise of Medicine from Superstition to Science.** Garden City, NY: Doubleday, Doran and Co., 1933; repr. Folcroft, PA: Folcroft Library Editions, 1978. 192p. illus. $10.00. ISBN 0-8414-4788-8.

Although this book was written in 1933, the physician-author says much that is still relevant today. This is basically a chronological history of medicine, focusing heavily on the contributions of great men of the past. It tells of the rise of scientific medicine from its beginning in mystery and superstition and of the ignorance and quackery that encumbered its progress. It is interesting that the book is dedicated to Dr. E. R. Squibb (1819-1888), founder of the pharmaceutical firm that still leads in scientific research. Appended is a substantial "Glossary of Proper Names and Medical Terms" which includes short biographies of the scientists.

The most noteworthy aspects of the book are the author's views and philosophy. For example, Haggard points out that the basic philosophy of primitive medicine was that supernatural forces caused disease; ceremonies were developed to overcome these forces. Although these practices were not superstitions then, they seem so now because of knowledge gained through scientific study.

Haggard says some interesting things about plant medicine: "Almost literally every plant substance that has grown upon the face of the earth has been used in treating disease. . . . The great majority have no virtue. . .but the old herb remedies have been carried down even into modern times." (Indeed, we have had a resurgence of herbal treatments in the nearly half a century since this book was written.) Haggard points out that plant remedies espoused by Galen fell into disuse when Paracelsus during the Renaissance founded the "chemical school" and substituted such strong mineral medications as mercury, lead, sulphur, iron, and arsenic. "This precipitated a controversy that was to last for three centuries." The herbal remedies were safer than the mineral treatments, but were more often useless. Although the minerals were beneficial in some instances, in the large doses of early days they were often harmful. Modern medicines, of course, make use of both types of substances. The three-century controversy has not ended for everybody; many people today believe that "natural" plant materials are superior to modern chemical pharmaceuticals, notwithstanding the fact that many of the latter are of plant origin, and that many of the former are perhaps harmful as well as useless for the intended purposes.

Haggard mentions some "systems," such as that advanced by John Brown (1735-1788) which for a time enjoyed great vogue. All disease fell into one of two categories: those in which there was too much bodily excitement or those in which there was too little. Opium or alcohol respectively could correct these conditions. Brown died of the abuse of the two therapeutic agents he advanced. Many of the more recent "systems" are no better.

495.   Hansen, Harold A. **The Witch's Garden.** Translated from Danish by Muriel Crofts. Santa Cruz, CA: Unity Press-Michael Kesend (113 New St., Santa Cruz, CA 95060), 1978. 128p. illus. bibliog. index. $4.95pa. LC 78-5469. ISBN 0-913300-47-0.

This book takes up the role that hallucinogenic, poisonous, and narcotic plants have played in witchcraft and demonology. A chapter is devoted to each of seven plants that have played a part in the history of European witchcraft and superstition, each illustrated with nicely done medieval woodcuts. Plants considered are mandrake, henbane, deadly nightshade, thornapple, hemlock, water hemlock, and monkshood. In addition, there is a chapter on "The Witches' Flying Ointments." Witches of antiquity, it has been written, smeared themselves with an ointment and were able to fly over rooftops. It is presumed that the ointments contained a hallucinogenic ingredient that produced the feeling of flying. Some of the plants mentioned in old recipes are identified.

Appended is an essay on "The Witches' Brew in Macbeth." Shakespeare, who always showed knowledge of the superstitions of his contemporaries, was aware of what many people imagined witches put in to their brews. Hansen identifies some of the ingredients mentioned.

The book has general as well as scholarly appeal. Those interested in religious, social, and cultural development of the West and those concerned with drug plants and psychopharmacology will enjoy it. It is well done.

496.   Harner, Michael J., ed. **Hallucinogens and Shamanism.** New York: Oxford University Press, 1973. 200p. illus. bibliog. index. $8.50. LC 72-92292.

These 10 field studies by anthropologists explore the use of hallucinogens in shamanism, the ancient practice of invoking a trance by using a hallucinogenic plant in order to perceive and manipulate the supernatural. The varieties of drug-induced shamanism are presented in the following sections: 1) In the primitive world: the upper Amazon; 2) In cultures undergoing Westernization; 3) In the traditional Western world; and 4) Hallucinogens and shamanism: the question of a trans-cultural experience. Section 1 deals with primitive people; section 2 with such groups as the North American Indian and urban slum-dwellers; section 3 with the role of hallucinogens in medieval European witchcraft; and section 4 with two very different cultures, the South American Indians and 35 white urban volunteers who used a hallucinogenic drug in a laboratory setting. The latter two groups had similar visions, showing that local tradition did not have as much influence as the state induced by the drug.

The editor hopes that this book will focus attention on native hallucinogens that have been relatively neglected by anthropologists.

497.   Jacob, Dorothy. **Cures and Curses.** New York: Taplinger Publishing Co., 1967. bibliog. $5.50. LC 66-22031. ISBN 0-8008-2100-9.

This is a companion volume to another work by Jacob, *A Witch's Guide to Gardening.* The cures and curses related in the book have been taken from ancient works on witchcraft and from old herbals. The material is rather light and entertaining; the author says serious students of necromancy can find gruesome prescriptions and uninhibited details in books in libraries, some of which are listed in the bibliography.

Chapter headings are: 1) M.D. or Witch?; 2) Doctors' Dilemmas; 3) The Dietician; 4) Cradle and Coffin; 5) Hushaby-Baby; 6) Thy Servant a Dog; 7) Household Hygiene; and 8) Spellbound.

Following is an example of a recipe given for preserving and thickening hair: "Take one quart of white wine, put in one handful of rosemary flowers, half a pound of honey, distil them together; then add a quarter of a pint of oil of sweet almonds, shake it very well together, put a little of it into a cup, warm it blood-warm, rub it well on your head and comb it dry." And here is an example of a simple spoken charm to cure hiccups: "Hiccup, hiccup,/Rise up right up,/Three drops in a cup/Are good for the hiccup."

498.   Leek, Sybil. **Herbs: Medicine and Mysticism.** Chicago, IL: Henry Regnery Co., 1975. 255p. $8.95. LC 74-30262. ISBN 0-8092-8431-6.

In his classic work on herbs, Culpeper (see entry 139) included astrological material, relating signs of the zodiac and herbal medicine. The author of this work attempts to extend this material and "bridge the gap between Culpeper's astrological classification and the escalating interest in both astrology and herbs that we are undergoing today." The medicinal, culinary, and astrological significance of herbs of the Western Hemisphere is analyzed. The herbs are classified by planet and astrological sign, and a discussion is given of those considered most beneficial to members of each sign.

The first chapter, "The Indestructible Herbs," is mainly a review of early works on herbal medicine. Chapter 2 is on the Hopi Indians and their herbs. Chapter 3, "Passionate Herbs," deals with love philtres and aphrodisiacs. A classification of herbs by astrology and a chapter on herbs and the zodiac, are included. The reader can find under his sign where the vulnerable areas of his body are and what herbal remedies can be used to strengthen the areas. The sixth and longest chapter contains a lexicon of herbal medical terms and an "Encyclopedia of Herbs" of more than 150 pages. Herbs in the encyclopedia are listed alphabetically and described as follows: botanical name, synonyms, habitat, physical description, action, medicinal uses, method of preparation, dosage, and culinary uses. The last section is a list of herb suppliers arranged by state.

The book contains interesting lore, but the astrology included and many suggested remedies can hardly be taken seriously.

499.   Middleton, John, ed. **Magic, Witchcraft, and Curing.** Austin, TX: University of Texas Press, 1967. 346p. bibliog. index. (Texas Press Sourcebooks in Anthropology, No. 7). $6.95pa. LC 75-44038. ISBN 0-292-75031-5.

Readings collected in this work report on the role of magic, including witchcraft, sorcery, divination, and curing, in the lives of primitive people. The editor is an anthropologist who has taught at several academic institutions. He says all contributors to the book have placed their analyses in a social context. Articles describe beliefs held by people who apply them in their everyday lives.

Following are the titles of the readings: 1) The morphology and function of magic: a comparative study of Trobriand and Zande ritual and spells; 2) The sorcerer and his magic; 3) Miching Mallecho, that means witchcraft; 4) The concept of "bewitching" in Lugbara; 5) Nagual, witch, and sorcerer in a Quiché village; 6) The sociology of sorcery in a central African tribe; 7) Witchcraft as social process in a Tzeltal community; 8) A sociological analysis of witch beliefs in a Mysore village; 9) Konkomba sorcery; 10) Dreams and the wishes of the soul: a type of psychoanalytic theory among the seventeenth century Iroquois; 11) Shamanistic behavior among the Netsilik Eskimos; 12) Divination in Bunyoro, Uganda; 13) Divination and its social contexts; 14) Witchcraft and clanship in Cochiti therapy; 15) Group therapy and social status in the Zar cult of Ethiopia; and 16) Spirit possession as illness in a north Indian village.

500.   Schleiffer, Hedwig. **Sacred Narcotic Plants of the New World Indians: An Anthology of Texts from the 16th Century to Date.** Riverside, NJ: Hafner Press, 1974. 160p. illus. index. $5.95pa. ISBN 0-02-0851780-6.

Many selections included here are from material that is scarce or unobtainable in libraries today. The anthology preserves a culturally and historically balanced sampling of diverse points of view, since hallucinogens have been both praised and condemned in the past. The earliest selections date back to the Europeans who first encountered these plants; other items cover the cultural disruptions brought upon the American Indians by European civilization; finally, selections reflect today's resurgence of interest in hallucinogens.

The book is probably of most interest to the general reader, but students, teachers, and research workers in anthropology, botany, ethnobotany, pharmacology, psychology, and medicine may also benefit from reading it. The two indexes, one of Latin names of genera and species of plants and another listing vernacular names of plants and plant products, give the work some reference value.

501.   Schultes, Richard Evans, and Albert Hofmann. **Plants of the Gods: Origins of Hallucinogenic Use.** New York: McGraw-Hill Book Co., 1979. 192p. illus. (part col.). bibliog. index. $34.95. LC 79-13382. ISBN 0-07-056089-7.

The primary intent of this book seems to be to promote a better understanding of the role of hallucinogenic plants in the cultural development of man in various societies through the centuries. Some scientific information also is offered, however. The authors are noted authorities on the subject, and they have brought together a large number of illustrations, including photographs, drawings, and artistic reproductions from other works to illustrate the text. The book is attractive although perhaps lacking in organization. Information is scattered throughout, with text dividing reference sections that are located in the center of the book.

Hallucinogenic drugs are of interest for several reasons. They have been used to attain "the mystic experience" in religions and as aids in hedonistic adventure. A more thorough understanding of their chemical composition may lead to new pharmaceutical products for psychiatric treatment and/or experimentation. The use of such drugs in psychoanalysis, the authors say, is based on effects which are opposite to those of tranquilizers. The latter suppress the patient's problems; hallucinogens bring conflicts to the surface making them more intense, and therefore more clearly recognizable and treatable. Hallucinogenic drug use was brought dramatically to the public eye in the 1960s. The controversial nature of the subject has slowed scientific research. However, scientific interest has continued, and the authors feel the public should be informed about the drugs.

The main contents of the book, in order of presentation, is as follows: 1) What are plant hallucinogens?; 2) The plant kingdom (the extent and botanical relationship of hallucinogenic plants); 3) Phytochemical research on sacred plants; 4) Geography and usage and botanical range; 5) Plant lexicon (color illustrations and botanical description of 91 plants with psychoactive properties); 6) Users of hallucinogenic plants; 7) Overview of plant use (reference chart to the plants included in the lexicon); 8) Fourteen major hallucinogenic plants (detailed consideration of their cultural significance); 9) Mainstay of the heavens, amanita (fly agaric); 10) The hexing herbs (henbane, deadly nightshade, mandrake); 11) The nectar of delight, cannabis (hemp, marijuana, hashish); 12) St. Anthony's fire (ergot); 13) Holy flower of the north star, datura (thorn apple, toloache, torna loco); 14) Guide to the ancestors (iboga); 15) Beans of the Hekula Spirit (yopo); 16) Vine of the soul (ayahausca); 17) Trees of the evil eagle (floripondio); 18) The tracks of the little deer (peyote);

19) Little flowers of the gods, conocybe, panaeolus, psilocybe, stropharia (teonanacatl); 20) Cactus of the four winds, trichocereus (san pedro); 21) Vines of the serpent (morning glory) ololiuqui, badoh negro; 22) Semen of the sun, virola (epená); 23) Chemical structure of hallucinogens; and 24) Uses of hallucinogens in medicine.

502.   Shepard, Odell. **The Lore of the Unicorn.** Boston, MA: George Allen and Unwin Ltd., 1930 (third impression, 1978). 312p. illus. bibliog. index.

This work, first published in Great Britain in 1930, is a scholarly study of the unicorn legend. The book begins with a description of an ivory walking stick the author has in his possession, reported to be made from a unicorn horn, and several centuries old. It had been used to shield its former owners from perilous places, poisonous food and drink, epilepsy, many other ills, and as a weapon. Such horns sold for 20 times their weight in gold.

The author sets out to answer a number of questions concerning the unicorn. For instance, he asks: How did this horn acquire its great reputation? How was it supposed to act in detecting poison? How could it maintain its prestige while princes and dukes of Italy who owned it were dying suddenly from no apparent cause? Where did these horns come from, and what was the nature of the traffic that purveyed them? Was the belief in their powers only a vulgar superstition, or was it held by learned men and perhaps even by physicians? How old was this belief, and what was its origin?

The tale is well told. At the end of the book Shepard accounts for the ivory stick. It was the tusk of a narwhal, which is a little-known and elusive Arctic whale. The creature probably inspired the myth of the unicorn.

503.   Sperber, Perry A. **Drugs, Demons, Doctors and Disease.** St. Louis, MO: Warren H. Green, Inc., 1973. 294p. $15.50. LC 70-111808. ISBN 0-87527-127-8.

The author of this work wishes to give the non-professional an insight into the complex world of drugs. He traces the historical beginnings of medicine, but covers material up to our present state of knowledge. Drugs are emphasized, but other aspects of the medical field are examined.

The first few chapters are of most interest to the field under consideration in this bibliography. Chapter 1, "In the Beginning," takes up superstitions of primitive stone-age peoples regarding medicine. Plants used by them are discussed. Chapter 2, on ancient medicine, covers Babylonian, Egyptian, Greek, Jewish, Hindu, Roman, and Chinese medicine up until medieval times. Chapter 3 is on medieval medicine and discusses widespread charlatanism and quackery. At that time, world trade in drugs developed since demand was heavy and profits high. There was brisk traffic in materials like aloes, cloves, benzoin, camphor, cinnamon, cubebs, ginger, musk, mace, nard, nutmeg, opium, pepper, rhubarb, and sandalwood. Chapter 4, on seventeenth-and eighteenth-century medicine, presents biographic sketches on the great figures of the period and discusses medical procedures of the time. Pharmacopeias were developed. The chapter on the nineteenth century points out the remarkable advances in science and medicine of that time.

The remaining chapters (more than half the book) discuss modern medicine. There are separate chapters on drugs for various types of ailments, and also included are discussions of drug interations, the biological time clock, and pollution.

504.   Storms, G. **Anglo-Saxon Magic.** The Hague, Netherlands: Martinus Nijhoff, 1948; repr. Folcroft Library Editions, 1975. 336p. bibliog. index.

This scholarly work begins with a discussion of the characteristics of magic. The second chapter reviews the main sources of knowledge of magic in Anglo-Saxon times, the medieval manuscripts. Chapter 3 is on magical practices; chapter 4 on the structure and atmosphere of the ritual; and chapter 5 on how the manuscripts borrowed from the classics, Christian sources, and Germanic customs and practices.

The remainder of the book (over half) lists various physical conditions and diseases and tells what charms, herbs, treatments, or religious rituals can be used to combat them. An appendix provides prayers used as charm formulas. There is also a glossary listing plants by Anglo-Saxon names with modern English equivalents, Dutch names, and the internationally accepted Latin names. References are given to the charms in which the plants are used.

505. Thompson, C. J. S. **The Mystic Mandrake.** Introduction by Leslie Shepard. New Hyde Park, NY: University Books, 1968. 253p. illus. index. $5.00. LC 68-18751.

This book is evidently a reprint of a 1934 work, but with a new introduction.

The European mandrake plant has had a long history of fantasy and fiction and has played numerous witchcraft and magical roles, probably because its root bears a resemblance to the human figure. The plant does have medicinal properties, and it is poisonous. Powerful drugs can be prepared from the root (hyoscyamine, scopolamine, and mandragorine).

The book tells the story of the mandrake over a period of 3,000 years, covering myths, lore, and superstition. The author was a distinguished British physician-author and curator of the historical collection of the museum, Royal College of Surgeons of England. No formal bibliography is included, but numerous references are made in the text to classical works of yore.

The following chapters are presented: 1) Introduction. Mandragora–derivation of the name–description of the plant and its habitat; 2) The mandrake of the Hebrews–the mandrake of the Bible–Rachel and the mandrakes; 3) The mandrake in ancient Egypt, Assyria and Persia; 4) The mandrake in ancient Greece; 5) Demonology and plants; 6) Dioscorides on the mandrake; 7) Mandrake legends in China; 8) The mandrake of Josephus; 9) The Romans and the mandrake; 10) The mandrake in Britain–Anglo-Saxon times–traditions in England and Wales; 11) Mandrake in the Middle Ages–the demand for mannikins–how artifical mannikins were made; 12) The mandrake in Germany–strange stories of Alrauns–their occult powers–false mannikins; 13) The mandrake in France–Joan of Arc and the mandrake–the mandrake and mistletoe; 14) Ceremonies in gathering mandrake and other magical plants; 15) The mandrake and the gallows legend; 16) The mandrake in Italy–among southern Slavs and the Armenians; 17) The mandrake in the drama, poetry and story; 18) The mandrake in the herbals of the sixteenth and seventeenth centuries; 19) The medicinal and occult properties attributed to the mandrake; and 20) Mandragora in the light of modern science.

506. Wasson, R. Gordon. **Soma: Divine Mushroom of Immortality.** New York: Harcourt Brace Jovanovich, Inc., ca. 1971 (c1968). 381p. illus. (part col.). bibliog. index. (Ethno-Mycological Studies No.1). $15.00. LC 68-1197.

This scholarly work was written by a retired banker who is a noted specialist on the cultural role of mushrooms in history. He has travelled to many parts of the world, studying the use of hallucinogenic mushrooms and particularly their role in religious ritual. The exact identity of a plant called *Soma* in the ancient Aryan religion has never been known. It has sometimes been known as a plant, the juice of that plant, and sometimes a god. This book advances the theory and documents the thesis that

Soma was the fly-agaric (Amanita muscaria), a hallucinogenic mushroom. This book is an important contribution to the knowledge of hallucinogenic mushrooms.

507.   Wasson, R. Gordon. **The Wondrous Mushroom: Mycolatry in Mesoamerica.** New York: McGraw-Hill, 1980. 248p. illus. (part col.). bibliog. index. $525.00 deluxe ed. (Ethnomycological Studies No. 7). LC 79-26895. ISBN 0-07-068441-3; 0-07-068442-1 deluxe.

The deluxe edition of this work is a collector's item signed by the author and numbered. It is the report of several decades of research into the religious cult that has grown up around the hallucinogenic mushrooms of Mexico. The mushroom is said to be the only plant that has ever reached the status of a god. The author is a noted authority in this field.

The book is in two parts. The first two chapters describe the present, the other chapters the past. Chapter titles are: 1) A *Velada* in Huautla; 2) Traits of the Mesoamerican *Velada* and Kindred Topics; 3) Xochipilli, 'Prince of *Flowers*': A New Interpretation; 4) The *Flowers* in Pre-Conquest Nahuatl Poetry; 5) The Inebriating Drinks of the Nahua; 6) *Códices, Lienzos, Mapas*; 7) Piltzintli, Child God of the Nahua, and His Christian Progeny; 8) Teotihuacán and the Wondrous Mushrooms; 9) The Mushroom Stones of the Maya Highlands; 10) The Historical Record; and 11) The Shaman and the Mushroom: New Perspectives.

The first chapter tells the story of a *velada* (an all-night shamanic vigil where the divine mushrooms are 'consulted'), while the second presents the traits of the night time divination with hallucinogens. The purpose of the *velada* is to consult the mushrooms about a grave family worry.

The historical chapters explore literature, art, and various artifacts for folklore and information on rites and ceremonies involving the hallucinogens.

The book is handsome with fine illustrations that include photographs of present mushroom users and artistic works from the past.

Most works in this chapter are histories or exposés of the patent medicine era
or of other quackery. Much of the literature is nostalgic and entertaining, even though the
subject is serious. Several works express the view that quackery will always be with us
because of the psychology of the follower; he is eternally gullible.

It is obvious, and the point is made by some authors, that patent medicines
and quackery of yesterday are analogous to herbal remedies, cancer and arthritis cures,
and "health" and "natural" foods of today.

Some material in this chapter should be of interest to collectors, since patent
medicine advertisements, posters, bottles, proprietary medicine stamps, and the like
are popular collectibles. There are two good books on the stamps, those by
Griffenhagen and by Holcombe.

* * * * *

508.   Adams, Samuel Hopkins. **The Great American Fraud: Collier's Exposé of the
Patent Medicine Fraud, 1905-1906.** Denver, CO: Nostalgic American Research Foundation, 1978 (c1905). 146p. illus. index. $7.95. LC 78-104762.

This book is a reprint of the 1906 edition that was reprinted from a series of
articles published in *Collier's* weekly on the "nostrum evil and quacks." The introduction to that well-known series explained that patent medicine methods and their harm
to the public would be exposed. The series expressed the view that the patent medicine industry was founded "mainly on fraud and poison." The style of the work is
definitely one of exposé.

The articles reprinted here contain much interesting historical information,
illustrations and actual accounts of use and sale of many medicines available during
that era. Specific brand names are discussed throughout the book. One of the interesting themes found in the work is how reputable organizations (religious publications,
for example) were often "used" to advertise these products.

In addition to various patent medicines discussed, several articles evaluate non-
drug techniques such as vibration, magnetism, and the use of "mineral radium water"
for baths. The specific "doctors" associated with these cures are named in each case.

Contents of the work is as follows: Series I, The nostrum evil: introduction,
Peruna and the Bracers, Liquozone, the subtle poisons, preying on the incurables, and
the fundamental fakes. Series II, Quacks and quackery: the sure-cure school, the miracle workers, the specialist humbug, the scavengers. Early editions contained other articles: "The Patent Medicine Conspiracy against the Freedom of the Press," "Confidential" (the treatment accorded private letters by the nostrum manufacturers), and
"Patent Medicines under the Pure Food Law."

509.   Barrett, Stephen, and Gilda Knight, eds. **The Health Robbers: How to Protect Your Money and Your Life.** Philadelphia, PA: George F. Stickley Co., 1976. 340p. illus. $10.50. LC 76-22281. ISBN 0-89313-001-X.

Ann Landers wrote the foreword to this book. She begins by saying that Barnum was right: There's a sucker born every minute. And two to take him. The book is a special publication of the Lehigh Valley Committee Against Health Fraud, Inc. who sponsored the publication because quackery is thriving and they want to protect victims. They point out that some exploiters merely want money, while others, perhaps more confused than crooked, seek converts to their ignorance. The Committee hopes for stronger consumer protection laws and better health education.

Each chapter of the book is written by a respected authority in the particular field. The presentation is in two parts. The first is on health robbers and how to spot them, and the second is on the struggle to protect your money and your life. Following are some of the topics covered: exploiting cancer and arthritis victims, "tired blood," weight control, medical imposters, phoney sex clinics, food quacks, the "organic" rip-off, acupuncture, eye exercises, health gadgets, dubious dentistry, and faith healing.

510.   Carson, Gerald. **One for a Man, Two for a Horse: A Pictorical History, Grave and Comic, of Patent Medicines.** Garden City, NY: Doubleday and Co., 1961. 128p. illus. (part col.). bibliog. index. $6.50. LC 61-5590.

Hundreds of rare pictures, chosen from holdings of libraries, historical societies, archives, and private collections make up the largest part of this book. Captions and text, however, interpret and clarify the pictures in entertaining fashion. The book is called a "souvenir in words and pictures of the 'cures' and health devices of long ago." A great deal can be found in the book about the American heritage in medical history, advertising, publishing and mass distribution, public and private health, social legislation, taste and recreation, and the general level of culture.

Contents is as follows: 1) Materia *patent* medica; 2) "And her golden hair was hanging down her back"; 3) Weak women; 4) Indian cures; 5) She put it in her papa's coffee. . .; 6) Manhood: lost and found; 7) When it catches you *there*. . .; 8) It *looks* like whisky. . .; 9) The boys of '61; 10) The spice of life. . .; 11) Free show tonight; 12) The house that Jack($) built; 13) Some unforgettable characters; 14) It hung behind the kitchen stove; 15) The "medicine habit"; 16) Tapeworms; or, what have you?; 17) They work while you sleep; 18) "Gas pipe" therapy; 19) Right off the cob; 20) In the wake of the news; 21) Follow the leader; 22) It pays to advertise; and 23) Louisiana hayride.

The book is amusing. All manner of odd panaceas are presented including Pasture Weed, Kickapoo Indian Cough Cure, Hostetter's Bitters (Generously spiked with whisky), Barker's liniment, Salvation Oil, Dr. King's New Discovery for Consumption, Pluto Water, Hamlin's Wizard Oil, Dalley's Magical Pain Extractor, and many more.

511.   Clark, Thomas D. **Pills, Petticoats, and Plows: The Southern Country Store.** Indianapolis, IN: Bobbs-Merrill Co., 1944; repr. Norman, OK: University of Oklahoma Press, 1964. 306p. illus. bibliog. LC 64-11333. ISBN 0-8061-0593-3.

In post-Civil War times, in the rural areas of the South particularly, the country store was an important part of the lives of its customers. It was the gathering place for the community, a credit source, a public forum, a news exchange, and much more. Nearly everything was sold there, including many patent medicines.

This book covers all features of the country store, but chapters of most interest here are those called "The Halt, the Lame, and the Bilious," "The Farmer and His Almanac," and "Death Always Came at Night."

Stores sold vast quantities of tonics, pills, ointments, liniments, and dry-herb mixtures which were manufactured in larger cities. Alcohol-laden bitters was another popular product. A number of products and companies that produced them are discussed. It is said that country stores were the most important source of income for patent medicine manufacturers. The book also points out that almanacs and calendars were turned out in astronomical numbers by the Chattanooga Medicine Company, and that they were more widely read than most volumes of southern history.

The book is a humorous, fascinating, and touching account of an institution now gone from the American scene.

512.   Cook, James. **Remedies and Rackets: The Truth about Patent Medicines Today.** Introduction by Oliver Field. New York: W. W. Norton and Co., 1958. 252p. bibliog. index. LC 58-10477.

Although this is an older book, it is still pertinent. It grew out of a series of articles originally published in *The New York Post.* About a billion dollars are spent for patent medicines each year, which is money down the drain, the author states. Some of the purchased "cures," "remedies," and "aids" may help slightly; some may do harm; and most are probably worthless against the ailments they are supposed to treat. Although Cook was talking about what has been called "patent medicines" and, to some extent, all non-prescription drugs, the same situation exists with herbal medicines and "natural" remedies and foods that are so popular now. They are the "patent medicines" of today.

Following are chapter headings: 1) Our Billion-Dollar Medicine Show; 2) The Chamber of Horrors: A Brief History; 3) Tired Blood; 4) Aspirin: Plain and Fancy; 5) Teasing the Arthritics; 6) Vitamins and Voodoo; 7) Tonics and Salesmanship; 8) Cold Cures and Rocket Techniques; 9) Reducing Pill Razzle-Dazzle; 10) The Imitation Tranquilizers; 11) Laxatives, Antacids, and Myths; 12) The Truth about Drug Prices; 13) Adventures in the Skin Game; 14) How to Grow Old Gracelessly; 15) The Triumph of Liver Pills; 16) Cancer and Quackery; 17) Nostrums in New York; and 18) 170,000,000 Guinea Pigs.

In the final chapter, Cook remarks that "it is impossible to escape the conclusion that flimflam—embodied in phoney arthritis remedies, overpriced and overadvertised vitamins, worthless tonics, ineffective cold medicines, fake reducing pills, pseudo-tranquilizers, deceptively-promoted and hazardous laxatives, bogus skin treatments, and deadly cancer cures—can be found in almost every area of the country's patent medicine trade." He advocates educating the public about the nature of the human body and the effects of substances on it so as not to be deceived by exaggerated claims of advertisers. The government gives some protection, he says, "but generally speaking, in the patent medicine jungle it's every man for himself."

513.   Dukes, M. N. G. **Patent Medicines and Autotherapy in Society.** Patent-geneesmiddelen en Zelfbehandeling in de Samenleving (met Nederlandse samenvatting). 2d rev. ed. Den Haag, Holland: Drukkerij Pasmans, 1963. 191p. bibliog.

This work was first printed as an academic thesis in the Faculty of Medicine, University of Leyden. It is the study of the drugs and traditional empiric treatments used (or misused) by patients who treat their own ailments without professional medical assistance. The use of patent medicines and other kinds of self-treatment by the public is much greater than is commonly realized, according to the author. The study is in two parts. The first part discusses self-treatment of illness—its history, its current volume, reasons for it, and to what extent it should be incorporated into an ideal system of health care. The second section takes up specific problems in detail. Included are discussions on the proper scope of self-medication, the retail sale of patent medicines, formulation of patent medicines, public advertising and promotion of medicaments, and the proprietary borderland.

Dukes believes that in the Middle Ages the basis of autotherapy was the traditional folk remedy, which was in general synonymous with herbal medicine. Since the latter was based on lore handed down from one generation to another, it was bound up with the relatively stable medieval village community and receded rapidly with the rise of industrialism from the eighteenth century onward. The rise of the vendor of secret remedies came next, followed by the growth of the so-called "patent" medicine industry in recent times.

The author looks at repressive legislation in a number of countries. The role of the druggist and advertising are discussed. Dukes points out that substances closely allied to drugs, such as "health" foods, therapeutic apparatus, contraceptives, and cosmetics should be given the same attention as drugs.

The author says repressive legislation will not bring about a retreat of medical quackery. As is the case with prostitution, alcoholism, and other similar social-physical problems, the roots of these things lie in demand as well as supply. The charlatan will not vanish until the patient ceases to ask for him.

514.   Fishbein, Morris. **The New Medical Follies.** New York: Boni and Liveright, 1927; repr. New York: AMS Press, 1977. 235p. LC 75-23711. ISBN 0-404-13262-6.

The late author of this work was for many years editor of the *Journal of the American Medical Association* and of *Hygeia*, contributed to other periodicals, and was the author of many medical reference books for the lay public. This book was reprinted with no new introductory material; presumably the reprint publisher felt that what was said about medical follies and quackery 50 years ago is still apropos today.

Most of the essays and/or chapters appeared previously as journal articles. Titles are as follows: 1) An Encyclopedia of Cults and Quackeries; 2) The Cult of Beauty; 3) The Craze for Reduction; 4) Rejuvenation; 5) Rejuvenation: The Mechanical and Glandular Methods; 6) Bread and Some Dietary Fads; 7) The End of Eclecticism; 8) Physical and Electric Therapy; 9) Psychoanalysis– A Cultist Movement?; 10) Ethics—Medical and Otherwise; and 11) The Physician of the Future.

The book handles cults and fads in exposé fashion. Some of the author's remarks seem dated, but much material is still relevant, and all is interesting if only for the history.

The last two paragraphs seem prophetic: "The general extension of human existence will undoubtedly bring new problems of overpopulation and of economic adjustment in daily life. It is unreasonable to believe that medicine will play any great part in solving this question, unless it develops, as it may, some system of immunization against conception. But even this will be used by the intelligent and avoided or misused by the unintelligent."

"Quackery, cultism and frauds of all types will continue to take their toll among the ignorant who are uninformed, and among the educated who know enough to be easily misled. The fertile mind of the quack avails itself of new plans as rapidly as scientific medicine develops new ideas for human benefit. It is inconceivable that the time will ever come when the percentage of persons misled by quackery will be greatly reduced, except to the extent that the coming generations are educated in the fundamental facts concerning the human body."

515.   Francesco, Grete de. **The Power of the Charlatan.** Translated from the German by Miriam Beard. New Haven, CT: Yale University Press, 1939; repr. New York: AMS Press, 1979. 285p. illus. bibliog. index. $31.50. LC 79-8609. ISBN 0-404-18471-5.

Because the charlatan is always with us, this older work is still of interest. It presents in scholarly fashion an account of charlatans of early times, particularly during the eighteenth century, with many comments about how they operated and why they were successful. The psychology of both offender and follower is explored. Many illustrations from early books are included.

Chapter 1, "The Charlatan: The Man and His Power," traces the origin of the word "charlatan" and how it has been used. Dupes are also discussed. Chapter 2, on "Alchemy and Its Charlatans," points out that alchemy was the scientific handmaid of the charlatan. There is a section on the gold maker Bragadino, and one on Leohnhard Thurneisser, a scientific charlatan. Chapter 3, "Power through Propaganda" takes up the evolution of the medicine show. American medicine shows are not covered, only European. Also presented is a discussion on Buonafede Vitali (1686-1745), a physician esteemed in his time who voluntarily turned from university professor to a mountebank. Chapter 4, "The Higher Charlatantry," discusses courtier charlatans. There is a section on "The Charlatan as Dramaturge and Child of Nature." In the eighteenth century, the taste for nature and natural scenery was popular. "Mountain doctors" worked cures against a fashionably rugged background. The "quack of quacks" Cagliostro is discussed at some length. The last chapter is on "The Marvels of Technology, A New Form of Magic." There is a section on the Enlightenment and its automata and one on Gottfriend Christoph Beireis (1730-1809), a court councillor, charlatan, and professor at the University of Helmstedt.

In conclusion, the author points out that the power of the charlatan is based not upon direct lies but upon falsification. His power will not wane as long as he can find so many overcredulous persons who shrink from experiencing the whole truth. Francesco believes that in the past effective confrontation of charlantanism usually came from a small minority of solitary men, not from scholars or political leaders.

516.   Gillespie, L. Kay. **Cancer Quackery: The Label of Quack and Its Relationship to Deviant Behavior.** Palo Alto, CA: R & E Research Associates, 1979. 130p. illus. bibliog. LC 78-68453. ISBN 0-88247-563-0.

This study was undertaken to increase available knowledge about treatment of physical ailments by unconventional methods—methods that licensing agencies and physicians call "quackery." The author attempts to enter the subjective world of the quacks in order to present that world to others. The study was primarily conducted within Utah, where the culture reflects the values of the predominant religious denomination, the Church of Jesus Christ of Latter-Day Saints.

Chapter headings are: 1) Quackery: The Sociological Task—Definition and Differentiation; 2) Review of the Literature; 3) Theory and Methods; 4) Quackery as a System; 5) The Quackery Process; and 6) Conclusion.

The author concludes that quackery is hard to prove unless it is officially and clearly defined. In Utah, the courts have been unsuccessful in controlling unconventional practitioners, and attempts at public education have met with opposition and skepticism. It was found that the label "quack" applied to unconventional practitioners did not match the stereotypes held by the general population. Gillespie concedes that the study has raised unanswered questions that point to further research. Areas suitable for inquiry include: 1) Cross cultural comparisons of conventional and unconventional practice; 2) Historical development of quackery and the process by which it came to be defined as deviant; 3) Subjective world of those who patronize quacks and their rationale for doing so; and 4) Relationship between the social control agencies and the criminal justice process in defining and labeling quackery.

517.   Griffenhagen, George B. **Private Die Proprietary Medicine Stamps.** Milwaukee, WI: American Topical Association, 1969. 78p. illus. bibliog. index. (Medical Series V.4; Handbook No. 66). $4.00pa.

The early patent medicine business was so lucrative in the United States that it was one of the first to be taxed to gain revenue for the Civil War. This handbook is the story of this revenue tax, the firms involved, and the products that were taxed Imprinted seals and stamps were used as a means of securing this revenue. Certain manufacturers wished to print their own distinctive stamps for advertising, which was allowed. The stamps were called private die stamps, and *Scott's Specialized Catalogue of the United States* provides descriptions and current values of them.

The introduction of this pamphlet provides background information. The main section is a list of company names with historical information about the firm, its products, and its stamps. Also provided is an index of the proprietary medicines mentioned in the various monographs. After the stamp tax law was repealed in 1883, many companies printed and used labels similar to the stamps. An appendix provides a list and description of such labels.

Both the stamps and the labels are prized by collectors.

518.   Hechtlinger, Adelaide. **The Great Patent Medicine Era: or Without Benefit of Doctor.** New York: Madison Square Press, Grosset and Dunlap, Inc., 1970. 248p. illus. (part col.). $14.95. LC 70-122554.

This profusely illustrated, quarto-sized book relates the story of American folk medicine from the end of the Civil War until about 1906, when the Pure Food and Drug Act was passed by Congress. The introduction points out that physicians' services were scarce and expensive before 1900, and much treatment was domestic and primitive. Herb recipes were passed along from person to person as well as being available in herbals. If home remedies did not help, the frontiersman called upon patent medicines. Doctors were consulted only in emergencies. It was a time of such remedies as Indian Snake Root Oil, electric belts, tonics, hair restorers, Lydia E. Pinkham's Vegetable Compound, liniments, wizard oil, elixirs, and mustard plasters.

The book presents a large number of illustrations of advertisements, almanacs, catalogs of drugs, and descriptions of medical books and superstitions. It is a delightful collection of material.

Following are section headings: 1) Introduction; 2) Books to aid afflicted; 3) Parts of the body; 4) Home remedy books; 5) Indian doctor's dispensatory; 6) The Indian doctor; 7) Passions and sex; 8) The guide board; 9) Health and disease; 10) Book advertisements; 11) Almanacs of patent medicines; 12) Labels of old patent medicines; 13) Sears & Roebuck; 14) Aphrodisiacs; 15) Electricity; 16) Dr. Pierce; 17) The Indian vegetable family instructor; 18) Dr. Chase's recipes; 19) Medicology; 20) Advertisements; 21) Trading cards; 22) Medicinal plants; and 23) Medical folklore.

An index would have added value to the book.

519.   Helfand, William H. **James Morison and His Pills: A Study of the Nineteenth Century Pharmaceutical Market,** and Crellin, J. K. **A Note on Dr. James's Fever Powder.** London: British Society for the History of Pharmacy, 1974. 101-143p. illus. bibliog. (Transactions of the British Society for the History of Pharmacy. Vol.1, no.3, 1974). £1.50.

This publication contains two monographs that give accounts of the use of two widely used patent medicines of the eighteenth and nineteenth century in Great Britain. Both were ineffective, contained harmful ingredients, and evidently caused a number of deaths. However, they were promoted and sold for some years in spite of exposure and criticism from reliable sources.

520.   Holcombe, Henry W. **Patent Medicine Tax Stamps: A History of the Firms Using United States Private Die Proprietary Medicine Tax Stamps.** Lawrence, MS: Quarterman Publications, Inc., 1979. 604p. illus. bibliog. index. $50.00. LC 76-51546. ISBN 0-88000-098-8.

The author of the 137 reprinted articles collected in this volume died in 1973. George B. Griffenhagen, a distinguished pharmacist, philatelist, and pharmacy historian completed the book for publication. Holcome wrote the articles for six philatelic magazines between 1936 and 1957. They deal with the proprietary medicine companies that, during the Civil War and until 1883, designed stamps to be affixed to their packages signifying the payment of excise tax levied to meet wartime needs. Also included here in this book are a series of Holcombe's articles dealing with companies using similar tax stamps during the Spanish-American War. The stamps are now collector's items and are scarce because they were usually torn when packages were opened. Along with material about the companies, the stamps are described and often pictured. An index of *Scott United States Stamps Catalogue Specialized* listings for the stamps is included.

Material presented in the book is significant because not a great deal is known about medicine proprietors before the federal food and drug laws. They advertised spectacularly and boastfully, but kept secret business practices and ingredients in pills and potions. The book contains vignettes of about 140 companies and many products with such trade names as Williams's Pink Pills for Pale People, Hostetter's Celebrated Stomach Bitters, Dalley's Magical Pain Extractor, Mrs. Winslow's Soothing Syrup, Clark's Anti-Bilious Compound, and Peruna. The largest single class of medicinals promoted by the firms was bitters, with cathartics and plasters tying for second place. Other popular remedies were liniments, eyewashes, liver and kidney remedies, vermifuges, blood purifiers, analgesics, catarrh remedies, tonics, cough syrups, carminatives, medicinal foods, hair preparations, and other cosmetics. There are indexes by persons, firms, and products.

This is a fascinating book of interest to many groups, including stamp collectors; pharmacists; pharmaceutical, medical, and social science historians; and medicine bottle and proprietary medicine ephemera collectors.

521.   McNamara, Brooks. **Step Right Up.** Garden City, NY: Doubleday and Co., 1976. 233p. illus. (part col.). bibliog. index. $12.95. LC 73-20522. ISBN 0-385-02959-4.

This book is a history of the patent medicine show. The author of the well-documented account is a professor of drama, and the emphasis is on the show rather than the medicines. Many patent medicines are mentioned, however, and it can be seen how such preparations as Pink Pills for Pale People and Kickapoo Indian Sagwa were sold to the public by quacks of all kinds, sometimes exotically garbed as Indians, Turks, or sorcerers. The last of the shows described are those of the Hadacol Caravans in the 1950s. They covered several southern states and featured well-known Hollywood stars.

Chapter titles are: 1) Step Right Up; 2) Pitchmen, High and Low; 3) The Medicine Show; 4) Wizard Oil; 5) The Kickapoo Idea; 6) The Kickapoo Shows; 7) Indian

Shows and Showmen; 8) Oregon; 9) Up in All the Acts and Bits; and 10) For a Better Tomorrow. Appended are sample dialogues from shows and a glossary of pitchmen's terms.

The author's view is that the medicine show was extremely influential, expecially in rural areas. In later years the showman began to assume the stature of an American folk hero (or, more accurately, anti-hero).

To set the stage, the book begins with the following quotation: "Step right up—here you are!—...This little box will save your life one dose alone irrevocably guaranteed to instantaneously eliminate permanently prevent and otherwise completely cure toothache sleeplessness clubfeet mumps stuttering varicoseveins youthful errors tonsilities...and falling down stairs or your money back."

522.   **The Medicine Show: Consumers Union's Practical Guide to Some Everyday Health Problems and Health Products.** By the editors of Consumer Reports Books. 5th ed. New York: Pantheon Books, 1980. 383p. illus. index. $10.00; $5.95pa. LC 78-20413. ISBN 0-394-51106-9; 0-394-73887-Xpa.

This fifth edition, like earlier ones, is based on articles originally appearing in *Consumer Reports*. The work first appeared over 25 years ago. Material presented has been developed with the assistance of medical advisers, and standard sources of information have been consulted.

The emphasis of the book is on over-the-counter drugs and health products, but also included are chapters on estrogens, generic drugs, and antibiotics. In addition, a great deal of information has been provided on the disease or condition for which the various products are used. There is also a chapter on poison emergencies and one on evaluating news about miracles. A glossary of medical and technical terms is appended.

In general, material in the book is accurate and valuable as well as expertly written. Some commonly used products and drugs are reported to be of little value; at least their limitations are noted. Other products are recommended. Cautions about possible undesirable effects have been included. The pros and cons about the use of a great many commercial health products and remedies are placed in proper perspective.

The authors of this work evidently think today's advertising of nonprescription drugs and health products is analogous to the pitch of the patent medicine salesman of yesteryear. However, nothing is said about the current craze for herbal remedies and "health" foods that are even more potentially dangerous because they are under no control by pharmacists or physicians.

523.   **Patent Medicines and Proprietary Articles: A Reproduction of a Section of the Meyer Bros. and Co. Wholesale Drug Catalog of 1887.** With an Introduction by Jack K. Rimalover. Princeton Junction, NJ: Stonybrook Associated, 1970. 45p. illus.

Meyer Brothers and Co., established in 1852, were importers and wholesale druggists who supplied drug stores with products listed in this wholesale catalog of 1887. This reprint was made available primarily so collectors of patent medicine bottles found in attics, old trash dumps, or antique shops could identify them.

The introduction of the reprint provides information on the patent medicine era of the late 1800s. The listing of patent medicines and proprietary articles is arranged alphabetically by name or type of product with the price. The manufacturer's name is usually given. Representative advertisements of the time are reproduced on the last few pages.

524.   Schaller, Warren E., and Charles R. Carroll. **Health, Quackery and the Consumer.** Philadelphia, PA: W. B. Saunders Co., 1976. 426p. illus. bibliog. index. $12.75. LC 75-5058. ISBN 0-7216-7949-8.

The authors of this textbook think there are at least two reasons for examining the health care system in the U.S. today. The first is to identify, understand, and utilize components of the system that are legitimate and productive in promoting health; the other reason is to recognize health quackery that results in reduced chances of recovery from illnesses.

Material is divided into three general areas. Discussed first are parameters of health and disease, consumer behavior, prevention of illness, and utilization of health services. The second section deals with questionable health practices, and the third focuses on changes that may be forthcoming in our health care delivery system and provides assistance to those who are involved with consumer health education. Selected methods and learning activities for students grades K through 12 and for college students and adults are outlined. Each chapter concludes with discussion questions and activities for students.

The questionable health practices discussed include osteopathy, chiropractic, naturopathy and naprapathy, homeopathy, spiritualism, and psychic healing (such as faith healing, Christian Science, and laying on of hands), acupuncture, zone therapy (reflexology), folk medicine, and hot-cold therapy. Also discussed are the use and abuse of health products, device quackery, and nutritional quackery. There are separate chapters on arthritis and cancer quackery.

The book covers a great many topics, but does not delve into each very deeply, probably because of space limitations.

525.   Smith, Ralph Lee. **The Health Hucksters.** New York: Thomas Y. Crowell Co., 1960. 248p. index. LC 60-15098.

"Health huckstering" is described by the author of this book as the falsifying or distortion of medical truth for commercial profit. He says it is a billion-dollar industry that is carried out, with the assistance of advertising agencies, by certain manufacturers and distributors of drugs, foods, and cosmetics. One of its powerful underlying currents is to keep you away from your doctor, at least until you have made a self-diagnosis and bought the advertiser's remedy. The book specifies common abuses, examining why they are thriving and what can be done about the problem.

Chapter headings are: 1) The Health Husksters; 2) The Gold Rush in Vitamins and Minerals; 3) Big Firms Lead the Way—Dentifices and Cold Remedies; 4) Fact and Fiction about Your Weight; 5) Advertising and Your Heart; 6) Putting the Heat on Your Doctor—Ethical Drugs; 7) The Arthritis Business; 8) Hucksters in the Saddle—The Cigarette Ads; 9) The Booming Food Fads; 10) Are Cosmetics Medicine?; 11) The Promoters at Work—An Inside View; 12) Modern Advertising vs. Horse-and-Buggy Law; and 13) Needed: A Consumer's Bill of Rights.

The chapter on food fads is of special interest. It puts "health foods" in proper perspective. The question is asked how an enlightened society can believe the statements of many publications on "health foods"; the answer is that food has an emotional as well as biological value. The emotional basis of many food fads can be seen in statements such as those on white bread. What is involved is the rejection of modern, "machine age" methods and preference for the old, simple and allegedly "natural" way of eating. Food faddism comes close to being a way of life, a dislike for the changes and revolutions through which our society is going. The belief in food fads is often accompanied by denunciation of "Big Business," "The Chemical Interests," and "Fragmentary Scientists" who are alleged to be joined in a "Giant Unholy Alliance" to separate people from the natural soil and its fruits. Common sense rejects this view, but emotions understand it. The chapter on food fads criticizes works by Adele Davis (see entry 543), D. C. Jarvis (see entries 343,384), and those of J. I. Rodale (see entry 306), and Rodale Press.

Most of the book, however, is concerned with the advertising of large firms. The drug industry and the advertising profession are asked to face up to their breach of faith with the people.

526.   Stage, Sarah. **Female Complaints: Lydia Pinkham and the Business of Women's Medicine.** New York: W. W. Norton Co., 1979. 304p. illus. bibliog. index. $10.95. LC 78-14414. ISBN 0-393-01178-X.

The author relates in the foreword that Lydia Pinkham had gone respectable by the time she had an opportunity to meet her. Her oil painting hung on the wall of Radcliffe's Schlesinger Library, next to portraits of the library's donors in a room dedicated to the country's outstanding women. It was not always so. The Lydia E. Pinkham Medicine Company began as a kitchen concern in 1875, manufacturing Pinkham's Vegetable Compound for "female complaints." The product was destined to become famous; the company grew into a multi-million-dollar business. However, jokes about the medicine were common for many decades.

An early label for the compound enumerated various female complaints for which the product was to be used; a later bottle listed only the ingredients which were said to be crystalline vitamin B_1, gentian, black cohosh, true and false unicorn, life and pleurisy roots, dandelion, chamomile, and alcohol (15%) as a solvent and preservative.

The book skillfully weaves together the biography of Mrs. Pinkham and her associates, history, business, advertising, and medicine. The author shrewdly analyzes why the business was so successful. Women were distrustful of treatment offered them by conventional medicine. Pinkham advertising exploited dissatisfaction with the medical profession and provided a criticism of gynecology in what was called The Age of the Womb. Quite possibly the vegetable compound treated many imaginary illnesses, but it did no harm, and provided what seemed to be an option to the unsatisfactory treatment physicians provided. The advertising also reproduced and reinforced conceptions about women and their health that were current in the culture of the time.

The history of the company is well told. After long-standing family feuds, the company was sold in 1968 and moved to Puerto Rico. Cooper Laboratories, a large diversified pharmaceutical company, continues to make the medicine and sell it to an ever-shrinking clientele.

Stage comes to some interesting conclusions. She thinks the history of the Pinkham Company speaks to changes in the lives of American Women, to changing cultural attitudes toward female sexuality, and to the prolonged failures of the medical profession to provide adequate treatment for women's health problems. Stage prophesies that while it is unlikely that Lydia Pinkham's Vegetable Compound will share in the new popularity of "natural" medicines, it would not be surprising to see new similar products appear on the market, claiming to relieve gynecological symptoms through some combination of "natural ingredients."

527.   Young, James Harvey. **American Self-Dosage Medicines: An Historical Perspective.** Lawrence, KS: Coronado Press (Box 3232, Lawrence, KS 66044). 1974. 75p. bibliog. (Logan Clendening Lectures on the History and Philosophy of Medicine, New Series, No.1). SBN 87291-068-7.

The author of this brief work has written other books on health quackery in the United States. This publication is a scholarly lecture that focuses on the "emergence from quackery of American proprietary medicines and their ascent under pressure to successive levels of greater respectability, suggesting at the end that we are today writing the latest chapter of this ancient and continuing tale."

The work is primarily concerned with the history of laws and regulations regarding drugs used for self-medication.

528. Young, James Harvey. **The Medical Messiahs: A Social History of Health Quackery in Twentieth-Century America.** Princeton, NJ: Princeton University Press, 1967. 460p. illus. bibliog. index. $9.00. LC 67-21031.

This well-documented work is a sequel to the author's *The Toadstool Millionaires* (see below), in which he described the origin of patent medicines in America from colonial days up to 1906. This later work covers the twentieth century up until the mid-1960s. It is paradoxical that the present irrational approach to the pursuit of health comes at a time when medical science has developed effective therapeutic procedures, the educational level of the public is higher than ever before, and more stringent laws are in effect. Young thinks medical quackery is more prevalent now than ever before, and the book is concerned with this paradox.

The book also attempts to interpret quackery and self-medication in relation to trends in science, marketing, and government. Modern advertising, laws to curb quackery, and educational efforts of such groups as the American Medical Association are discussed. Primary concerns of the author include promotion of drugs, food supplements, and devices. Case examples cited include tuberculosis-curing liniment, mail-order health, radio therapeutic instruments, weight-reducers, vitamin and iron promotion, nutritional products vended by an itinerant "lecturer," and diabetes and cancer "clinics."

Young concludes that although knaves and fools will always be with us, there is room for guarded optimism that the high tide of medical quackery at the middle of the twentieth century might be pushed back. He was writing in the mid-1960s, before the recent rise of the herb and "natural" food fads. He was overly optimistic.

529. Young, James Harvey. **The Toadstool Millionaires: A Social History of Patent Medicines in America before Federal Regulation.** Princeton, NJ: Princeton University Press, 1961. 282p. illus. bibliog. index. LC 61-7428.

This is a significant history of proprietary medicines in America, from the early eighteenth to the early twentieth century. The title was suggested by a quotation from Oliver Wendell Holmes, "Somebody buys all the quack medicines that build palaces for the mushroom, say rather, the toadstool millionaires." Various stages in the origin and development of patent medicines, their promotion, and criticism are covered. The subject is related to broad trends in health, education, journalism, marketing, and government. A number of case histories are provided throughout.

Chapter coverage is as follows: 1) English patent medicines in colonial America; 2) American independence in the realm of pseudo-medicine; 3) The expansion of American nostrums during the early nineteenth century; 4) Thomsonianism, a democratic system of patented medication; 5) The first significant critique of patent medicines; 6) Patent medicines and the press; 7) The Civil War, its aftermath, and the great boom; 8) Patent medicine advertising by paint and poster; 9) The patent medicine almanac; 10) Quackery and the germ theory; 11) An analysis of the psychology of patent medicine advertising; 12) The linking of entertainment to nostrum promotion;

13) Acceleration of the patent medicine critique; 14) The passage of the Pure Food and Drugs Act of 1906; and 15) Sobering continuities in the realm of patent medicines.

Young makes it clear that quackery is not dead today in spite of regulatory legislation.

15

"NATURAL,"
"HEALTH," AND "ORGANIC"
FOODS; NUTRITION; AND DIETS

Several types of materials are included in this section. Some books promote the use of "natural," "health," and "organic" foods; other works debunk the concept and point out fallacies in proponents' views.

It is important to realize that scientists do not use the terms "natural" or "organic" in the same way "health" food proponents do. When a scientist speaks of a natural product he means one that is not synthetic in origin. All foods are natural products. Popular writers use the term "natural" to mean a food that contains no additives and has not undergone any kind of processing. "Organic" materials to the scientist are those that have been derived from an organism, and organic chemistry is the study of carbon compounds as compared to inorganic chemistry which is the study of materials that do not contain carbon. All foods are organic because they contain carbon. Laypersons have been using the term "organic" to mean plant foods that have been grown without the use of chemical fertilizers or insecticides. Those accustomed to scientific terminology find the layperson's usage of these term imprecise and confusing, although a few popular books have defined the terms in the way they use them.

A number of the books imply that "natural" food plants are healing plants, and advocates seem to aspire to superhealth through nutrition. Scientific evidence is not available to back up most of these claims. Personal testimonials are not good evidence. However, many individuals are being brainwashed by the multi-billion dollar nutrition cultism industry and by popular books on the subject. Furthermore, a number of "doctors" who write these books and special diet books are Doctors of Naturopathy or Ph.D.s in unrelated fields, although a few are M.D.s who should know better. The special (fad) diet book has become very popular, and several are reviewed in this section.

Several books on vegetarianism are listed. Vegetarians seem to believe that meat eating is immoral, and the books allege that "natural" foods from plants are superior to other foods. Some even claim meat is poisonous.

A few cookbooks are included in this chapter (although those dealing more specifically with herbs are listed in chapter 7). The books discuss cooking with honey and fructose, low fat, salt and sugar-free cookery, vegetarian recipes, and the like.

In all fairness to "health" food advocates, it should be said that the movement grew out of the bad publicity given food additives of recent years. The government does not entirely protect against the use of some additives that may be harmful. Also, the public became disillusioned with conflicting reports in the news media about such matters. However, it should be understood that food labeled "health" food isn't always healthy; some foods naturally contain small amounts of poisonous materials, a fact seldom recognized.

The books on the subjects treated in this chapter tend to be repetitive, and an attempt has been made to add some related materials. The title by R. J. Taylor on *Food Additives* presents the case for the use of additives; the title by Wertheim discusses natural poisons in foods.

* * * * *

530.   Adams, Rex. **Miracle Medicine Foods**. West Nyack, NY: Parker Publishing Co., Inc., 1977. 230p. $9.95. LC 77 6245. ISBN 0-13-585463-6.

This book is made up of 16 chapters, covering topics that range from foods for "Instant pain relief" to foods for "new youth." A large number of ailments and diseases are mentioned throughout these chapters, and all kinds of treatments (not necessarily limited to foods and diet) are reported.

The basic approach of the book is to report cases in which a specific food or treatment was used and "miracle" healing was accomplished. Few cases are documented, but occasionally reference is made to a medical journal article.

The book has an aura of sensationalism about it, presenting material in a style similar to popular tabloids. Paragraphs often begin with an exclamation such as "Breast cysts relieved!"or "Praised the world over!" or "Bleeding gums healed!" or "Instant relief for kidney, bladder, and urinary problems!"

Specific dosages, formulas, or recipes are *not* given. There seems to be a preponderance of cases using garlic as the miracle treatment.

The lack of an index makes this book difficult to use for reference, but it is unlikely that it could serve that purpose anyway.

531.   Adams, Ruth, and Frank Murray. **Health Foods**. New York: Larchmont Books (25 West 45th St., New York, NY 10036), 1975. 351p. index. $2.25pa.

This work describes 49 different foods or classes of foods that the authors consider health foods. Arrangement is alphabetical by name of the product. Each monograph is several pages, and sample recipes have been included in many instances. In addition to foods that the authors say were introduced to the nation by health food stores, some ordinary foods have been included such as bread, eggs, peanuts, brown and wild rice, margarine, and gelatin. Some foods in the former category include wheat germ, kefir, many seeds, and brewers yeast. Several monographs are on classes of substances such as enzymes, herbs, juices, meat substitutes, and protein and protein supplements.

532.   Airola, Paavo. **How to Get Well: Dr. Airola's Handbook of Natural Healing**. Phoenix, AZ: Health Plus Publishers, 1974. $12.95. 303p. bibliog. index. ISBN 0-932090-03-6.

This popular best seller has been sub-titled "therapeutic uses of foods, vitamins, food supplements, juices, herbs, fasting, baths, and other ancient and modern nutritional and biological modalities in the treatment of common ailments." It presents therapeutic approaches called "biological medicine," said to be based on harmless nutritional and naturopathic methods of correcting disease and restoring health.

The book is in five parts: 1) How to get well; 2) How to protect yourself against common poisons in food, water, air and environment; 3) Directions (descriptions and instructions regarding nutritional, herbal and other therapies recommended in part 1 of the book); 4) Recipes for special foods and dietary supplements recommended in this book; and 5) Charts and tables.

Part 1 makes up about half the book. It lists common diseases and disorders alphabetically and tells how each condition can be treated, by diet, fasting, herbs, or other means.

533.   Atkins, Robert C. **Dr. Atkins' Diet Revolution: The High Calorie Way to Stay Thin Forever.** Recipes and menus by Fran Gare and Helen Monica. New York: David McKay Co., 1972. 310p. index. $6.95. LC 72-75458.

Dr. Atkins believes that overweight is not caused by overeating but is the result of metabolic imbalance, a view not held by most experts. Balanced diets are usually about 50 percent carbohydrate, 30 percent protein, and 20 percent fat. Dr. Atkins' diet initially cuts out carbohydrates entirely, and then limits them permanently. Atkins says the diet isn't just a reducing diet. It is also recommended for those with adult-onset diabetes, cholesterol problems, ulcer problems, migraine, heart and arterial diseases, and fatigue and emotional disturbances that accompany hypoglycemia.

Contents is as follows: 1) What this book will reveal to you; 2) The diet revolution: it will change your life; 3) How I arrived at this diet revolution; 4) I promise you that you will never feel a hunger pang; 5) If you're always fighting fat, chances are you're "allergic" to carbohydrates; 6) What causes this twentieth-century plague; 7) It's a new energy diet—both psychological and physical; 8) To stay fat—keep on counting calories; 9) To stay flat—start counting carbohydrate!; 10) How to take your own dieting case history; 11) Before you start on this diet; 12) The revolutionary never-hungry no-limit steak-and-salad-plus diet; 13) How to follow the diet—level by level; 14) Why one dieter in ten gets stuck temporarily; 15) Meal plans and recipes; 16) Maintenance: staying at your best; 17) Answers to the questions patients most often ask; and 18) Why we need a revolution, not just a diet.

The chapter on meal plans and recipes is about 50 pages. Recipes do indeed appear appetizing, mainly because most call for large amounts of heavy cream and butter.

534.   Atkins, Robert C. **Dr. Atkins' Nutrition Breakthrough: How to Treat Your Medical Condition Without Drugs.** New York: W. Morrow, 1981. 367p. bibliog. index. $12.95. LC 80-39910. ISBN 0-688-03644-9.

This is Dr. Atkins' third book on nutrition therapy. His "breakthrough" therapy involves maintenance of health and treatment of illness by use of doses of vitamins and minerals in conjunction with certain dietary practices. He believes in "health" foods.

535.   Bäiracli-Levy, Juliette de. **Nature's Children: A Guide to Organic Foods and Remedies for Children.** New York: Schocken Books, 1978. 146p. illus. index. $2.95pa. LC 78-163326. ISBN 0-8052-0580-2.

About half of this book is devoted to general discussions of the dietary needs and problems of mothers, fathers, infants, and children. Birth and lactation are also discussed. Various foods and food groups are recommended with emphasis on "organic" foods and herbs. Warnings against certain eating habits and types of food are given throughout.

The last half of the book is concerned with "natural" medicines and recipes for them. The chapter on "natural" medicines is an alphabetical listing of various maladies. Each entry includes various herbal and dietary treatments with the emphasis again on what is considered "natural" or "organic." A short section on first aid is an interesting feature of this section.

The chapter with recipes is similar to a cookbook, but most recipes contain uncooked, "natural" foods. Many call for cooling and refrigeration, however. Also included is a short section on "natural" cosmetics.

The book is apparently based on the author's first-hand knowledge and experience.

536.   Berto, Hazel. **Cooking with Honey.** New York: Gramercy Publishing Co., 1972. 234p. index. $4.98. LC 72-185094. ISBN 0-517-50115-5.

The recent emphasis on "natural" foods has brought about increased interest in the use of honey, an age-old sweetening agent.

The introduction to this cookbook discusses the history of the use of honey. The rest of the book is made up of over 300 recipes, except for the last chapter which is on varieties and flavors of honey. The flavor and color of honey varies from area to area; the flavor especially depends on the floral source. A list of a few kinds of honey available commercially is provided with comments about color and flavor.

The recipes are arranged under the following chapter headings: 1) Main Dishes to Treasure; 2) Vegetables with a Difference; 3) Salads for Every Occasion; 4) Breads, Today's and Yesterday's; 5) Cakes and Cookies; 6) Pastries, Desserts, and Candies; and 7) Beverages Past and Present. Interspersed among the recipes are many comments by the author, particularly emphasizing history and tradition. Some material is peculiarly placed; for instance, a few paragraphs on great-grandma's household hints on cleaning are in the salad chapter, and a section on honey in great-grandma's medications is in the vegetable chapter.

537.   Calella, John R. **Cooking Naturally: An Evolutionary Gourmet Cuisine of Natural Foods.** Berkeley, CA: And/Or Press, 1978. 112p. illus. bibliog. index. $4.95pa. LC 78-54342. ISBN 0-915904-35-7.

The author, who has had a television show on "natural" cookery, provides information on how to combine "natural" vegetable foods for the best flavor and attempts to show that good nutrition need not be sacrificed for good taste. Also included are the author's views on how diet can be enhanced by attention to pure water and air, exercise, weight control, relaxation, and inner tranquility. There is a section on fasting, and food charts and menus are provided.

538.   Cannon, Minuha. **The Fructose Cookbook.** Charlotte, NC: East Woods Press, Fast and McMillan Publishers, Inc. (820 East Boulevard, Charlotte, NC 28203), 1979. 128p. illus. index. $5.95pa. LC 79-4902. ISBN 0-914788-18-3.

This book presents over 120 recipes for dishes prepared without regular table sugar (sucrose) by substituting fructose (often called fruit sugar or levulose and found naturally in sweet fruit, berries, honey, and vegetables). In addition, many recipes make use of the popular so-called "natural" foods such as seeds, whole grain flours, bran, yogurt, and carob powder (in place of chocolate).

The viewpoint of the author is that fructose is superior to sucrose. Since fructose may not be readily available in groceries or health food stores, a few suppliers are listed at the end of the book. Although the book does not mention it, crystalline frutose if much more expensive than sucrose, even when its greater sweetening power is taken into account.

539.   Ceres. **Herbs and Fruits for Vitamins.** Drawings by Alison Ross. Wellingborough, Northamptonshire, England: Thorsons Publishers, Ltd., 1978. 63p. illus. ISBN 0-7225-0301-6.

In the introduction to this work, the author expresses the view that present-day diets should be changed by adding more "natural" whole foods that contain "natural" vitamins. The primary foods in this natural diet should be "organically" grown wholewheat bread, other whole grains like brown rice; ripe uncooked fruit (without sugar); and fresh salad and green vegetables. Also, unprocessed milk and cheese and fresh butchers' meat are better than products that have been 'treated' to keep, it is said. The introduction also lists the vitamins with a little information about each.

The main section of the book is a list of 20 plants, many of them wild, presumed to be especially nutritious. Information is given on cultivation; production; nutritional and medical value; use; and a little historical background. Each plant is illustrated with a line drawing.

The book has popular appeal, but provides only limited and perhaps misleading scientific information. The most interesting aspect of it is the historical material.

540.   Cheraskin, E., and W. M. Ringsdorf, Jr., with Arline Brecher. **Psychodietetics: Food as the Key to Emotional Health.** Toronto, New York, London: Bantam Books, 1974. 239p. bibliog. index. $1.95pa. ISBN 0-553-02125-7.

The author of this work believes that emotional problems may be rooted in improper diet and nutrition. The book offers step-by-step programs to treat such illnesses through diet.

Following are chapter titles: 1) From Food to Mood: What Psychodietetics Is All About; 2) What Causes Emotional Illness: Is Something Eating You? Or Can It Be Something You're Eating?; 3) The Dieting Craze: It Can Drive You Crazy!; 4) Alchololism Is a "Social" Disease: Fact or Fancy?; 5) Schizophrenia Is a Mental Disease: Fact or Fancy?; 6) Hypoglycemia, the Nondisease: Can a Sweet Tooth Lead to a Sour Disposition?; 7) "Mental" Illness: The Twilight Zone; 8) Drug-Induced Mental Illness: Psychodietetic Help for the Addicted; 9) Problem-Solving: The Psychodietetic Approach to Sexual Inadequacy, Hyperactivity Senility, Allergy; 10) Hidden Nondietary Factors that Influence Emotions; 11) Are You Going to Crack Up?; 12) The Balanced Diet Myth; and 13) The Optimal Diet.

The authors of the book are qualified physicians, and the optimal diet they suggest is good, indeed it seems to be a "balanced" diet. In addition, there seems to be some basis for their belief in a close relationship between diet and mental health. However, the documentation provided is open to question. Many sources listed are to non-scientific materials of questionable quality.

541.   Dalrymple, Fay Lavan, and Jean Dalrymple. **The Folklore and Facts of Natural Nutrition: A Guide and Reference Book with 100 "Miracle" Case Histories (in Letter Form), Diet, and Menus Showing How Nutrition and Vitamins Can Help You.** New York: Exposition Press, 1973. 192p. bibliog. index. $6.50. LC 72-86587. ISBN 0-682-47536-X.

The subtitle of this work provides a resumé of it. Like many recent popular books on nutrition and "natural" foods, this one contains many controversial statements, along with some accepted views.

The work is presented in three sections. The first section is made up of testimonials from people who say their condition has improved because of some change in diet. The material is grouped by disease or condition. The second part, called "Cooking for Health," discusses nutrition and proper diet and includes menus and recipes. Part three, on nutritional supplements, deals with vitamins and minerals. There are lists of recommended foods, vitamins and minerals for specific conditions, and food values. A section on folklore in foods and nutrition has also been provided.

542.   Das, Swami Harihar. **The Healthy Body Handbook: A Basic Guide to Diet and Nutrition, Yoga for Health, and Natural Cures.** New York: Harper and Row, 1980. 113p. illus. bibliog. $5.95pa. (Harper Colophon Books). LC 79-2802. ISBN 0-06-090730-4.

The author of this handbook is said to be a native Indian herbal doctor and yogi. He has developed a health program inspired by yogi tradition and adapted to Western use. The object is to help people maintain their health, and perhaps even increase energy and vitality.

Material is presented in three sections: the diet, yoga for health, and natural cures. In regard to diet, Das suggests avoidance of prepared foods, especially those chemically treated or artificially flavored. Few meats are allowed; use of vegetable and fruit juices is encouraged. It is hoped that few would agree with the author's statement that "pasteurized milk is almost devoid of nutritive value." International vegetarian menus and recipes have been included.

In the section on yoga, a number of exercises are described and illustrated. The section on natural cures presents folk remedies for a range of ailments. These are given under such headings as skin, eyes, stomach, head, and women's problems.

Swami Das believes that maintaining physical health is the way to an enlightened mind and spirit.

543.   Davis, Adelle. **Let's Have Healthy Children.** New and expanded ed. New York: Harcourt Brace Jovanovich, 1972. 486p. illus. index. $6.95. LC 77-160400. ISBN 0-15-150440-7.

This book is a nutrition guide, primarily for mothers and expectant mothers. There are chapters dealing with prenatal care, the feeding of children, and good nutrition in preventing disease. In general, the advice given is probably good, but many claims made for vitamins and "proper" diets seem to be exaggerated, or at least over-emphasized. There is a growing awareness among experts that many Americans are over-dosing themselves with vitamins and minerals, and that this is harmful (as well as expensive) as toxic symptoms develop. It is felt that a doctor's advice should be sought before using vitamins. The author puts a great deal of emphasis on the value of Vitamin E. However, many reputable nutritions question its role at all in ordinary nutrition. The author has a reasonably sound scientific background, but many other scientists do not agree with her views on several matters, for instance, the importance placed on "organically" grown food and her criticism of the use of pesticides in agriculture.

The book contains useful tables of recommended daily dietary allowances and of food composition.

Numerous references are made in the text to scientific studies, but no literature references are included. However, the author has written other books on nutrition where much scientific documentation was included. This book was obviously intended for lower-level lay audiences, and perhaps this is where the fault lies. The material is oversimplified.

544.   Gare, Fran, and Helen Monica. **Dr. Atkins' Diet Cook Book.** Under the supervision and with an introduction by Robert C. Atkins. New York: Crown Publishers, 1974; repr. Bantam Books, 1975. 291p. illus. index. $1.95pa.

Recipes presented in this cookbook are based on principles set forth in the book *Dr. Atkins' Diet Revolution* (see entry 533). Atkins' view is that most obesity results from the body's inability to deal with carbohydrates in the diet. Consequently, his book and this cookbook stress low-carbohydrate foods and recipes. Indeed, practically no carbohydrates are used. The cookbook contains recipes for a wide variety of dishes. Sugar substitutes are called for, but many recipes include large amounts of fats. Menus are provided, including suggestions for foods to choose from restaurant menus.

The prescribed diet can be considered a "fad" type because most nutritionists believe the correct diet should be balanced to include proteins, carbohydrates, and fats.

545.   Gibbons, Euell, and Joe Gibbons. **Feast on a Diabetic Diet.** Rev. ed. Greenwich, CT: Fawcett Books, 1973. 314p. (A Fawcett Crest Book). bibliog. $3.95pa. LC 49954.

Because Joe Gibbons was a diabetic, he asked his author-brother, Euell, to help him write a book about better eating for the diabetic. Although Euell Gibbons had written several books that were best sellers about herbs and wild foods, this one is not entirely herbal in its concepts. It is a special cookbook with information on planning and preparing meals for the diabetic. It deals with values, exchange systems, and encourages the reader to convert and create recipes. A variety of recipes are included.

Three other books by Euell Gibbons are reviewed in chapter 17 (see entries 602, 603, 604).

546.   Goldbeck, Nikki, and David Goldbeck. **The Supermarket Handbook: Access to Whole Foods.** Drawings by Ellen Weiss. New York: Harper and Row, 1973. 413p. illus. index. $8.95. LC 73-4084. ISBN 0-06-011581-5.

An attempt is made in this book to educate people about selecting and preparing foods in a manner that allows the least possible use of additives or processed foods that the authors consider unsafe or inferior. Much money, they say, is spent on promoting concocted foods when real basic foods exist. The book is designed to guide consumers "past the nonnutritive, chemically laden nonfoods in the supermarket to the whole, healthy items that are still available."

The presentation is in two parts. The first part is on shopping and selecting foods, the second on preparing food in the home kitchen. Best brands of foods are named (a great many unfamiliar, at least in the Midwest), recipes provided, and tips for selection and preparation given. A glossary is included that explains the way certain terms are used throughout the book. Following are extracts that give some indication of the tone of the book: Additives (materials used to enhance final product, either natural or chemical in origin); Natural foods (those free of chemicals in their production); Organic foods (those grown without pesticides, in soil untreated with artificial fertilizers and not treated with any preservatives or synthetics); Processed foods (those manufactured in some way; refined, cooked, or combined with other food ingredients); Whole foods (the focal point of the book; foods offered for sale free of chemical additives, colorants, or artificial flavoring, left in the whole, unrefined state, or processed as little as possible).

Most material is correct, and good advice is often given, although there are some statements open to question. For instance, many will not agree that pork is a "questionable buy." In addition, repeated remarks in books such as this one about the undesirability of salt, white sugar, white flour, refined foods, processed foods, artificial flavors, artificial fertilizers, pesticides, food additives and "chemicals," sound like a broken record. Many of these materials serve a useful purpose and probably cause little or no harm. Sugar, salt, and some additives are preservatives, for instance. In all fairness, though, this book is better balanced than most of its kind.

547.   Hall, Dorothy. **The Natural Health Book.** Illustrated by Richard Gregory. New York: Scribner's, 1976. 322p. illus. index. $6.95pa. LC 77-74715. ISBN 0-684-15228-2.

The author of this guide to health has had a commercial herb nursery and is a professional naturopath, treating and advising patients on the use of "natural" remedies and foods.

The chapter headings are: 1) Vitamins; 2) Mighty Minerals; 3) Instinctive Eating; 4) Good, Bad, and Indifferent Food; 5) Organic Growing; 6) Wild Plants and Weeds; 7) Simple Home Remedies for Everyday Ills; and 8) What Is Health?

The chapter on wild plants and weeds lists some common weeds that are of benefit to mankind. The chapter on home remedies lists a few common ailments and suggests such remedies as garlic, honey, eucalyptus oil, castor oil, mustard plaster, boiled onions, wintergreen oil, and rosemary oil. The main thrust of the book is on prevention of health problems through "natural" nutrition and a feeling of well-being.

548.   Herbert, Victor. **Nutrition Cultism: Facts and Fiction.** Philadelphia, PA: George F. Stickley Co., 1980. 234p. bibliog. index. $12.95. LC 80-51835. ISBN 0-89313-020-6.

The author of this hard-hitting work is a distinguished attorney, physician, and nutrition scientist who has impressive credentials, unlike many who write nutrition books for the lay public. He has produced a book that is needed as an antidote to many popular works.

The introduction to the book is a kind of who's who in the field of nutrition quackery and includes such figures as Adelle Davis, the Shute brothers, J. I. Rodale, and Linus Pauling. Specific details are provided about their questionable activities and views. In addition, the text throughout makes references to others who are said to be frauds and quacks. Suitable documentation is provided. The author has especially focused on the use of laetrile, vitamin A megadoses, and pangamic acid (called vitamin B_{15} by proponents).

The main presentation is in three parts. The first, "Nutrition Cultism—Laetrile: the Cult of Cyanide—Promoting Poison for Profit," presents a complete picture of the substance, including its chemistry, promotion, dangers, fallacious legal defense, and the actions of its proponents. Also considered in this section is the pseudovitamin B_{15} that is said to have been promoted by the creator of laetrile. Megavitamin therapy is also shown to be without value and harmful.

The second section of the book, on "Ethical Medicine," considers acquiring new information while retaining old ethics; medical, legal and ethical considerations in the use of drugs having undesirable side effects; and the matter of fat, cholesterol, and free scientific inquiry.

Part 3, "Nutrition Facts," deals with basic matters of nutrition and includes the American Medical Association's concepts of nutrition and health, and guidelines for healthful diets of the National Academy of Sciences.

The author appropriately dedicates his book "To those I cherish; that they may not fall victim to the gurus, the hucksters, or the arrogance of ignorance."

549.   Hess, John L., and Karen Hess. **The Taste of America.** New York: Penguin Books, 1977. 384p. bibliog. index. $2.95pa. LC 77-23938. ISBN 0-14-004535-X.

The authors of this book present a diatribe concerning the diet of Americans. They say our food has been drained of flavor and nourishment, loaded with additives, and disguised by fancy packaging. In addition, they remark that cookbooks are full of nonsense and that fine restaurants serve frozen food with French names at intolerable

prices. Worse yet, so-called food experts encourage food-snobbery and promote ignorance. The book takes up most facets of food. The authors plead a case for simple,
fresh food, prepared with loving care.

The authors conclude that there is a gleam of hope for us through the "health"
food and "organic" food movements, and that the counter culture has made promising
steps toward reviving the taste of our food. It has encouraged the use of unbleached
flour, for instance, and a resurgence of home baking and gardening is taking place.

This is a difficult book to judge. There is truth in what is said, although many
questions are not adequately answered. For instance, how does an urban family get
fresh-from-the-garden food? How can food be preserved "naturally" without additives
or freezing? And more important still, how does the average working wife and mother
find time to bake the family's bread? The back-to-nature movement has appeal, but
how realistic is it?

550.   Hodges, Robert E., ed. **Nutrition: Metabolic and Clinical Applications.** New
York: Plenum Press, 1979. 478p. bibliog. index. (Human Nutrition: A Comprehensive Treatise, v.4). $37.50. LC 78-27208. ISBN 0-306-40203-3.

The science of nutrition has advanced quite rapidly the past two centuries.
Although early books on herbal foods are being made abundantly available in reprinted
editions, it is well to bear in mind that modern scientific works such as the one under
review exist. Designed primarily for the researcher or advanced student of nutritional
science, each chapter has been written by an expert. The topics covered, however, are
of interest to laypersons and scientists and physicians alike.

People in all walks of life are interested in nutrition and are seeking satisfactory
answers to questions regarding it. Until recently, according to the editor, medical
schools have taught little about the subject, and doctors often cannot help. Consequently, the public turns to self-professed nutrition or "natural" food experts who make
extravagant claims and exhibit their paper-back books in supermarkets and "health-
food" stores. There is a need for accuracy, up-to-date information, and factual interpretation of the subject. It is intended that this book will fill such a need, and it does so
very well.

The following chapters are presented: 1) The Hemotopoietic System; 2) Nutritional Disorders of the Nervous System; 3) Nutrition and the Musculo-skeletal System;
4) The Interaction between the Gastrointestinal Tract and Nutrient Intake; 5) Nutritional Effects of Hepatic Failure; 6) Cardiac Failure; 7) The Relationship of Diet and
Nutritional Status to Cancer; 8) Mutual Relationships among Aging, Nutrition, and
Health; 9) Effects of Organ Failure on Nutrient Absorption, Transportation, and Utilization: Endocrine System; 10) Megavitamins and Food Fads; 11) Effects of Ethanol on
Nutritional Status; 12) Infectious Diseases: Effects of Food Intake and Nutrient Require-
ments; 13) Obesity: Its Assessment, Risks, and Treatments; and 14) Nutrition and the
Kidney.

551.   Hoffer, Abram, and Morton Walker. **Orthomolecular Nutrition: New Lifestyle
for Super Good Health.** New Canaan, CT: Keats Publishing Co., 1978. 209p. bibliog.
index. $8.95; $2.25pa. LC 77-91335. ISBN 0-87983-153-7; 0-87983-154-5pa.

Linus Pauling, known as an advocate of vitamin therapy, has provided an introduction to this work. His views are somewhat controversial. The senior author, Dr.
Hoffer, says he discovered through his psychiatric practice that food allergies were
responsible for certain behavioral disorders. This led him to advocate the practice of
orthomolecular medicine, a system that depends on nutrition therapy, particularly the

use of vitamins. Emphasis is given, however, to the differing nutritional needs of each patient. Case histories of cures for both mental and physical illnesses by the use of mega-vitamin therapy are cited.

The book includes a compilation of vitamins and minerals and their functions.

552.   Jencks, Tina. **In Good Taste: A Creative Collection of Delicious Easy to Prepare, Low-Fat Recipes, Free of Sugar and Salt.** Illustrated by Paula Morrison; introduction by Eileen Poole. Berkeley, CA; Lancaster-Miller, 1980. 142p. illus. $4.95pa. LC 80-82395. ISBN 0-89581-020-4.

The author of this book takes the view that nutritious food should be low in fat and free of salt and sugar. She attempts to provide recipes for a range of dishes that are enticing and still free of salt, sugar, and fat. More than 100 recipes are presented with rather handsome illustrations complementing the text.

553.   Jordan, Julie. **Wings of Life: Vegetarian Cookery.** Trumansburg, NY: The Crossing Press, 1976. illus. index. (A Crossing cookbook). $5.95pa. LC 76-43075. ISBN 0-912278-82-X; 0-912278-77-3.

The author of this cookbook, a vegetarian, presents here recipes she has developed using no meat. She does, however, cook with eggs and dairy products. The recipes make heavy use of the usual "health" foods such as whole grain cereals, honey, yogurt, nuts, seeds, herbs, and spices. Old-fashioned methods are suggested for preparing the foods, for instance, grinding one's own grain in a hand grain mill and using a mortar and pestle for grinding herbs and spices. Instructions are included for making homemade yogurt, buttermilk, sauerkraut, and for sprouting beans. It is only fair to say, though, that the buttermilk recipe is for making cultured buttermilk rather than the "real" product which is a by-product of butter making.

For the most part, the recipes are appealing, and exaggerated claims are not made for benefits from eating the foods.

554.   Kilham, Christopher. **The Complete Shopper's Guide to Natural Foods: Vitamins, Supplements, Cosmetics, Kitchenware, and Bodycare Tools.** Illustrated by Mary Schweninger. Brookline, MA: Autumn Press; distr. Random House, 1980. 176p. illus. bibliog. index. $2.95pa. LC 80-66696. ISBN 0-394-73983-3.

Easy to read and concise, the aim of this guide is to assist the shopper in selecting "natural" foods and other "natural" products. Products covered include: beverages, vitamins, food supplements, medicinal herbs, spices, "natural" cosmetics, body care tools, household cleaners, pet foods, grooming products, and staple and prepared "natural" foods. Recipes, cooking suggestions, and comments about nutrition are included.

555.   Lappé, Frances Moore. **Diet for a Small Planet.** Rev. ed. Illustrated by Kathleen Zimmerman and Ralph Iwamoto. New York: Ballantine Books, 1975. 410p. illus. bibliog. index. $2.50pa. ISBN 0-345-27429-6.

The view taken by the author of this book is that people of the United States are wasteful in their food habits. They eat and waste millions of tons of high-grade protein. Lappé believes this is reducing the capacity of the earth to provide; the earth is only a small planet, she says. She has a plan to help make the most of the protein the earth makes available.

The book provides food preparation hints and recipes, using mostly vegetable products, that will produce high-grade protein nutrition said to be equivalent to or better than meat protein. Matters such as "natural" foods and food polluted with pesticides are referred to throughout.

The book is presented in these sections: 1) Earth's labor lost; 2) Bringing protein theory down to earth; 3) Eating from the earth: *where* to get protein without meat; and 4) Eating from the earth: *how* to get protein without meat. Appendices include the following: 1) Definitions and basic cooking instructions for beans, grains, nuts, and seeds; 2) Calorie/protein comparisons; 3) Protein cost comparisons; 4) Meat equivalency.comparisons and sample calculations; 5) Pesticide residues in the American diet, 1964-1970; 6) Whole wheat flour compared to white flour; 7) Brown rice compared to other types of rice; and 8) Sugars, honey, and molasses compared to each other.

Nutritionists generally believe that it is virtually impossible to get complete proteins necessary for a proper diet using vegetable products alone. However, if animal products such as eggs, cheese, and milk are added it is possible. Some recipes given in the book make use of these animal products.

556.   Levy, Robert I., and others, eds. **Nutrition, Lipids, and Coronary Heart Disease, A Global View.** New York: Raven Press, 1979. 566p. bibliog. index. (Nutrition in Health and Disease: v.1). $52.00. ISBN 0-89004-181-4.

Important information about diet is given in this work, uninfluenced by fads. Sources for reliable material in this area are somewhat scarce, and a well-integrated, well-documented account of the relation between diet and coronary artery disease is presented. Many issues of current concern are covered, such as fiber in the diet, megavitamins, minerals, diet for children, and the question of whether there is an optimum diet for everyone.

Following are section headings: 1) Epidemiology of diet, lipids, and heart disease; 2) Role of dietary components in lipid metabolism; 3) Use of diet in preserving health and treating disease; 4) Methods for changing dietary habits; 5) The changing food supply and consumption patterns; 6) Nutrition in relation to other aspects of cardiovascular disease.

The book is especially recommended for physicians who must give diet information to patients.

557.   Linn, Robert, with Sandra Lee Stuart. **The Last Chance Diet—When Everything Else Has Failed.** New York: Bantam Books, 1977. 206p. bibliog. $1.95pa. ISBN 0-553-10490-X.

Here is another popular diet book, this one calling for a "protein-sparing fast program" to be undertaken only under a doctor's supervision. The author, evidently an osteopath, presents discussions of why a person gets fat, diet fads and their fallacies, the history and psychology of fasting, and the dangers of total fasting. Also included is a maintenance diet to be followed after the desired weight is obtained.

The substance used in Dr. Linn's "protein-sparing fast program" is a liquid protein called "Prolinn." Diets exclusively made up of liquid protein (as this book suggests) have received adverse publicity recently as being dangerous.

558.   Margolius, Sidney. **Health Foods: Facts and Fakes.** New York: Walker and Co., 1973. 293p. bibliog. index. $6.95. LC 75-186187. ISBN 0-8027-0375-5.

Written by an expert on consumer problems and money management, this is one of the best books on the subject of "organic" and "natural" foods. Margolius has attempted to evaluate many controversial concerns that have led to the growing health food movement and to evaluate claims made by health food faddists. He says it was a formidable task, partly because of the unsettled nature of some issues and emotions involved on both sides. However, he has taken a look at the cult, the facts, myths, and psychological impulses behind it, and the exploitation of understandable fears by commercial interests. He found that food faddists tread on dangerous grounds in their claims, some merely foolish (such as health foods to increase sexual powers) and some dangerous (such as massive doses of vitamins.).

Margolius lays some of the responsibility for food faddism on the U.S. government departments, Congress, and industries. The public may think it is adequately protected against additives and pesticides in the food supply, and then finds this is perhaps not so when new research results are made public indicating harmful effects of some of them.

Chapter headings are: 1) Panic in Healthfoodland; 2) Cashing in on Mother Nature; 3) Deceptions and Self-Delusions; 4) Evaluating the Foods of the Revolutions; 5) Vegans and Protein-Eaters from Sense to Zens; 6) Fats, Oils, and Lecithin; 7) Natural Vitamins and Unnatural Kidding; 8) Bread vs. the Stuff You Eat; 9) Milk vs. the Stuff They Drink; 10) The War over Additives; 11) Organic Fertilizer Claims and Facts; 12) Pesticides and Problems; 13) The Natural Skin Game; 14) How to Live to the Last Minute; 15) Nutritional Exaggeration on Both Sides of the Compost Heap. There are several appendices and tables included. Some interesting ones include: a list of government food and environmental offices, a glossary of nutrition and health food terms, and nutrients in "health" and various common foods. The appendices on additives are especially enlightening. Representative ones are listed with the use or function and source. About half are natural, the others synthetic. Also types are named with explanations of their purposes. These include: nutritive additives, flavor additives, antioxidants, microorganism spoilage controls, emulsifiers (enable oil and water to mix and stay mixed), stabilizers and thickeners, acidity or alkalinity controls, leavening agents, color additives, bleaching and maturing agents (used especially in flour milling and bread baking), sequestrants (used in food processing to set apart or separate traces of substances that otherwise interfere in the processing), humectants (keep moisture in foods), anticaking agents (keep salts and powders free-flowing), clarifying agents (settle out traces or small particles), curing agents (used to preserve meat), foaming agents and inhibitors, and solvents (carriers for flavors, colors, etc.). Some of these are more useful than other, obviously; a few are used for cosmetic purposes only.

559.   Miller, Marjorie. **Introduction to Health Foods.** New York: Dell Publishing Co., 1972. 196p. $ .95pa. ISBN 0-440-14087-0.

Here is a good example of a "health food" book with the usual views held by those promoting the movement. Frequent references are made to the simpler, earlier times and foods direct from the soil without preservatives or processing of any kind. Insecticides and chemical fertilizers are considered bad. Honey is to be used in place of sugar or, if sugar must be used, it should be brown sugar. Whole grains are highly regarded for the diet. There are other foods considered of particular value, as can be seen by the list of foods covered.

The first chapters provide basic information on nutrition. "Naturalness" is emphasized. The next section, called "Handbook of Health Foods," takes up the following foods: cheese, nuts, raw certified milk, vegetables, fruits, seeds, sprouts, honey, blackstrap molasses, wheat germ, alfalfa, bone meal, desiccated liver, brewer's yeast, fish liver oils, rose hips, kelp, meat, poultry, fish, natural vegetable oils, herb teas, wines, pop wines, yogurt, cereals and bread, vitamin supplements, soybeans, and raw juices. The last section, "Far-In Recipes," provides a few examples of dishes made with "health foods."

As with most books on this subject, some material presented is scientifically sound and some is not; there's a strange mixture of good advice and nonsense.

560.   Poulos, C. Jean, Donald Stoddard, and Kay Carron. **Alcoholism, Stress, Hypoglycemia, with Diets.** Santa Cruz, CA: Davis Publishing Co., 1976. 131p. illus. bibliog. $6.95pa. LC 76-24383. ISBN 0-89368-600-X.

    This work summarizes a two-year research project conducted to determine the relationship of hypoglycemia and stress to alcoholism. It is not a typical research report in that it is written for the average reader in oversimplified fashion rather than for researchers in their language. In addition, the authors frequently take positions contrary to those held by most authorities.

    The hypothesis is that hypoglycemia plays an important role in the causes of alcoholism, a resultant symptom that occurs from an unknown cause or causes. This interrelationship is examined in detail and is supported with references to selected research findings and research carried out by the authors. Included at the end is a section on miscellaneous substances: protein, carbohydreates, fats, vitamins, minerals, sugar, tobacco, and caffeine. Diet suggestions are included. There is a list of suggested readings, mostly popular "health food" and nutrition books. References to scientific literature have been included in the text, however.

    Presumably, material on nutrition has been included to give suggestions on how to improve the diet and avoid various undesirable conditions such as alcoholism, stress, and hypoglycemia.

    The publication is a curious mixture of the scientific and the popular. It suffers from poor organization and format; there is no table of contents or index, and no chapter titles have been used.

561.   Reuben, David. **The Save Your Life Diet: High-Fiber Protection from Six of the Most Serious Diseases of Civilization.** New York: Ballantine Books, 1975. 172p. bibliog. $1.95pa. LC 75-6643. ISBN 0-345-25350-7-195.

    Dr. Reuben, the author of several best-selling works on sex, says he wrote this book because he was convinced that a high-fiber diet has great potential as a tool of preventive medicine. He thinks there is compelling evidence in medical literature to show that added roughage to our daily diet provides protection from cancer of the colon and rectum, ischemic heart disease, diverticular disease of the colon, appendicitis, phlebitis and resulting blood clots to the lungs, and obesity.

    The book discusses each of these conditions and the high-roughage diet that is presumed to prevent them. The last chapter presents high-roughage recipes and menu hints. Bran or high-roughage cereals are added to standard recipes in most instances. Other diet modifications suggested are the use of honey instead of white sugar, whole grain flour instead of refined flour, and fresh fruits and vegetables with little peeling. Herbal seasonings are often included.

    An appendix points out that there is scientific evidence against use of roughage in the diet, but Reuben concludes that the adverse findings are not strong.

562.   Schwartz, George. **Food Power: How Foods Can Change Your Mind, Your Personality, and Your Life.** New York: McGraw-Hill, 1979. 189p. bibliog. index. $10.95. LC 78-32115. ISBN 0-07-055673.

    The author of this work is a physician and professor. He primarily examines the beneficial effects of food on behavior. Areas touched upon include effects of certain foods on sleep, creativity, sexuality, and depression. Also included are discussions on fasting and misconceptions about certain foods.

563.　Shulman, Martha Rose. **The Vegetarian Feast**. Illustrated by Beverly Leathers. New York: Harper and Row, 1979. 319p. illus. index. $12.95. LC 78-2166. ISBN 0-06-013997-8.

The author of this vegetarian cookbook is a professional cook and caterer. She presents a variety of recipes, including some for international dishes. Menus are suggested, and advice is given for large and small scale entertaining, as are ideas for everyday family dining and holiday meals.

Adequate protein is a tricky problem for vegetarians and, in this case, the author makes use of dairy products and eggs. She also stresses the use of high-protein vegetables.

564.　Speer, Frederic. **Food Allergy**. Littleton, MA: PSG Publishing Co., 1978. 165p. bibliog. index. $16.00. LC 76-45950. ISBN 0-88416-184-6.

This is a book on food allergy for the physician and the patient, written by a physician. Many of the individual plant foods mentioned in the book are common herbs or wild foods.

The first chapter includes the history of food allergy, the mechanism, inherited factors, and incidence. Chapter 2 covers nonallergic reactions to foods such as toxins naturally occurring in foods and bacterial food poisoning. Chapter 3 covers manifestations of food allergy. The next chapter, on the biological classification of foods, points out that this classification is important in dealing with plant food allergy. There is usually little correspondence between conventional and biological classifications. For example: peanut is related to soybean, not pecan; cinnamon is related to avacado, not ginger; red pepper is related to potato, not black pepper; and potato is related to eggplant, not sweet potato. The chapter contains tables that place foods in the proper plant family. Chapter 5 is a discussion of individual foods. Common offenders are covered as are food additives. The remaining chapters cover the detection of food allergens, treatment, allergic cookery, and food allergy in infancy.

The book serves as a reminder that "natural" foods may cause as much trouble as any other food.

565.　Switzer, Larry. **Spirulina: The Whole Food Revolution**. Berkeley, CA: Proteus Corp. (2000 Center St., Suite 1221, Berkeley, CA 94704), 1980. 75p. illus. bibliog. (An Earthrise Book). $4.95. LC 80-133429.

The Proteus Corporation, who published this small book, manufactures Earthrise Spirulina, which is said to be becoming well-known in the "natural" food market. The book provides information about the food with recipes on preparation. Also included are details about how Spirulina is grown, harvested, and produced. It is said to be high in protein and of relatively mild flavor.

The book predicts that Spirulina will become a world food commodity suitable for alleviating the scarcity of food in the future. It has evidently had a history of use for human consumption in Mexico and East Africa, and it grows in freshwater lakes in these areas. It is a type of vegetable plankton, a blue-green algae.

566.　Tarnower, Herman, and Samm Sinclair Baker. **The Complete Scarsdale Medical Diet Plus Dr. Tarnower's Lifetime Keep-Slim Program**. New York: Bantam Books, 1978. 225p. index. $3.25pa. ISBN 0-553-20228-6.

The late author of this book was a cardiologist and internist who became well-known for his "Scarsdale Medical Diet." He became even more widely known after he was shot to death by a woman friend.

Contents of the book is as follows: 1) A private diet goes public...Why the phenomenal success of the Scarsdale Medical Diet; 2) The ingredients of the successful Scarsdale Medical Diet; 3) The mystery of diet chemistry; 4) The complete Scarsdale Medical Diet; 5) Answers to your questions on beginning the Scarsdale Medical Diet; 6)..."What do I do now?" Scarsdale keep-trim diet to stabilize weight loss; 7) Scarsdale two-on—two-off program: keep trim for your lifetime; 8) Scarsdale gourmet diet for epicurean tastes; 9) Scarsdale money-saver diet to save pennies and lose pounds; 10) Scarsdale vegetarian diet; 11) Scarsdale international diet; 12) Be a Scarsdale loser and a lifetime winner; 13) Answers no more; questions you may have after being on the Scarsdale Diet; 14) Special information that will help you; and 15) Shape up and count your blessings. Also included is a medical appendix called "You and your physician—some medical problems that are affected by diet."

The chapter on special information provides a useful table of composition of foods, and menus are included in several chapters.

Tarnower's approach is not entirely unconventional, but he suggests relatively higher protein and lower carbohydrate intake than is standard. Also, he suggests a very low calorie diet, only 1,000 per day. Most authorities believe 1,200 calories per day is a more realistic and safe, although, of course, weight is not lost as quickly. Tarnower does not make exaggerated claims or attempt to sell any products through his book.

The book is popularly written and has been a best seller.

567.   Taylor, R. J. **Food Additives.** New York: John Wiley and Sons, 1980. 126p. bibliog. index. $30.00. (The Institution of Environmental Sciences Series). LC 79-42729. ISBN 0-471-27684-7; 0-471-27683-9pa.

The intent of the late author of this work was to present the case for the use of food additives to lay people and science students. There has been much criticism of food additives recently, particularly by proponents of "natural" foods.

Chapter 1 takes up the origins and development of food sources and points out that many foods commonly used naturally contain toxic materials. The next chapter is called "The Case for Food Additives." Another chapter discusses the character of additives, including antioxidants, preservatives, emulsifiers and stabilizers, food colors, flavors, sequestrants, anticaking agents, acids, buffers and bases, humectants, firming and crisping agents, sweeteners, enzymes, nutritive additives, and flour and bread additives. The chemistry of the substances, including structures, is often given. The next chapters are devoted to legislative processes, safety testing, and like matters. Appended materials include lists of food additives and toxic materials found naturally in foods.

568.   Thomas, Anna. **The Vegetarian Epicure.** Illustrated by Julie Maas. New York: Vintage Books, 1972. 305p. illus. LC 73-39176. ISBN 0-394-71784-8pa.

The author of this work on vegetarian cooking does not approve of eating meat, but she uses milk products and eggs in her recipes. She attempts to show that vegetarian meals are interesting rather than dull and tasteless as is often believed.

There are sections on entertaining, menus, and on holidays and traditions. Recipes given include breads, soups, sauces, salads, vegetables, souffles, omelettes, cheeses, rice, pasta, curries, and sweets. The author does not always use "health" or "natural" foods in her recipes; she occasionally uses sugar and white flour.

569.   Thomas, Anna. **The Vegetarian Epicure, Book Two.** Illustrated by Julie Maas. New York: Knopf; distr. Random House, 1978. 401p. illus. index. $10.00; $6.95pa. LC 77-16685. ISBN 0-394-41363-6; 0-394-73415-7pa.

A sequel to the title reviewed above, this book was inspired by the author's travels over a four-year period in Europe, the Middle East, and Mexico where she sought new ways of preparing vegetarian dishes. Recipes provided are typical dishes of the different countries visited.

570.   Vander, Arthur J. **Nutrition, Stress, and Toxic Chemicals: An Approach to Environment-Health Controversies.** Ann Arbor, MI: University of Michigan Press, 1981. 370p. bibliog. index. $18.00; $9.95pa. LC 80-28078. ISBN 0-472-093290; 0-472-06329-4pa.

The author of this admirable work is a physician and a professor of physiology at the University of Michigan. The book deals with the influence of certain environmental factors, broadly defined, on human health. It treats questions of recent controversy such as: Do high-fat foods increase the risk of heart attacks? Does saccharin in moderate amounts cause cancer? Is stress a major cause of physical disease? Can vitamin C prevent colds? An attempt is made to present the current state of knowledge in these and other areas. The author warns, however, that conclusive answers cannot be given to many questions of this kind. Research into them is hard to perform.

The presentation is in four parts: First principles, Nutrition, Stress, and Toxic chemicals. Chapter headings are: 1) Methods for Detecting Environmental Factors in Disease; 2) Biological Responses to Environmental Challenges; 3) The Task of Nutritional Science; 4) Protein Nutrition: The Problems of Setting Minimal Dietary Requirements; 5) The Iron-Enrichment Controversy; 6) Cholesterol, Fats, and Heart Disease; 8) The Body's Responses to Environmental Chemicals; and 9) Saccharin, Cancer, and the Delaney Amendment.

Vander concludes the book with a plea for more extensive research into environment-health issues.   No shortcuts are possible; real understanding of disease origins depends upon a thorough knowledge of basic science. He thinks in time solutions will be found to many current questions, but meanwhile scientists must share their ignorance as well as their discoveries with the public.

571.   Wertheim, Alfred H. **The Natural Poisons in Natural Foods.** Secaucus, NJ: Lyle Stuart, Inc., 1974. 198p. bibliog. index. $7.95. LC 73-90775. ISBN 0-8184-0169-9.

This book is unlike most "health" food or "natural" food books. The author examines fallacies of many of the fad diets that are currently popular and points out that there are many natural poisons in "natural" foods. He is not a scientist, but has had an interest in farming and gardening and has edited a "natural" foods newsletter. Wertheim speaks of his personal experience with "natural" foods. He says he became enthusiastic about the subject, then realized he had become a fanatic and a bore to his friends. He hopes his book will serve four purposes: 1) to make consumers aware that although foods may be "natural" they may contain naturally occurring poisons; 2) to demonstrate that a food should not automatically be considered good just because it is "natural" or because people have been eating it for a long time; 3) to show that because the science of nutrition is still in its infancy, the consumer should be cautious in choosing any one plan or diet; 4) to place foods in proper perspective in relation to other factors that affect health.

The presentation is in two parts. The first part deals with poisons occurring in foods; the second considers implications and ponders other aspects of the subject.

Some topics discussed and conclusions reached include the following: 1) Natural poisons in foods are usually small in quantity, but are dangerous for some individuals; 2) Shellfish may be poisonous at certain times of the year due to their ingestion of toxic planktons; 3) Oxalic acid poisoning in livestock occurs when the animals eat certain weeds. Plants used for human food, such as spinach and rhubarb, also contain the substance, but in small amounts; 4) Goiter may be produced by substances found in cruciferous plants; 5) Vitamin intoxication results from excessive doses of vitamin preparations; 6) Legumes contain deleterious substances; 7) The human body can cope with small amounts of poisonous substances, but unlucky combinations of substances may result in serious hazards; 8) There are many food allergens; 9) Natural radiation is ever present, and medical procedures account for a large share of the total one may receive; 10) Many natural materials contain stimulants, depressants, or hallucinogens, e.g., coffee beans, tea leaves, cocoa beans, coca leaves, jimson weed, mescal buttons, and the marijuana plant; 11) Certain elements are essential to diet, but excessive quantities are harmful, e.g., lead, zinc, cadmium, and selenium; 12) Some foods are overrated in their alleged benefits; 13) There is no perfect food; 14) Leaders and pioneers in the health field may live no longer than others; 15) There is no "fountain of youth"; 16) Brown or "raw" sugar and white sugar contain essentially the same amount of sucrose; 17) Raw foods are not necessarily healthful; and 18) Food faddists are not the healthiest, happiest individuals; eat a varied diet.

The book contains much good, reliable, and realistic advice.

572.   Whelan, Elizabeth M., and Frederick J. Stare. **Panic in the Pantry: Food Facts, Fads, and Fallacies.** New York: Atheneum, 1975. 231p. illus. bibliog. index. $8.95. LC 75-7952. ISBN 0-689-10671-8.

Whelan's preface says it all began with the banning of cyclamate sweeteners in 1969. That's when she began to wonder if eating was hazardous to her health. The authors of the book believe we have all been sold a bill of goods by the self-appointed "consumer advocates," the health food industries, and irresponsible reporters. Whelan and Stare debunk food faddism, vitamin use, fear of packaged or "treated" foods, and the "back-to-nature binge." They are well qualified to write such a book; both have advanced degrees in suitable fields, have been in academic positions at noted institutions, and Stare is also a physician.

The book puts food additives in proper perspective. In the introduction, written by Ralph A. Nelson, Head of the Section of Clinical Nutrition at the Mayo Clinic, it is pointed out that toxicants in foods that are life-threatening are naturally occurring, and he wonders why the fuss about food additives.

The book traces the history and development of food additives and the origins of food cults. Fallacies in the philosophies of these groups are pointed out. Problems with food additives are admitted, but the authors believe they are under control. The Delaney Clause of the federal Food, Drug, and Cosmetic Act (dealing with cancer-causing substances) is discussed and its impact explained. The dangers of large vitamin and mineral supplements to the diet are dealt with.

Chapter headings are: 1) From "What's for Dinner?" to "Name Your Poison"; 2) Eating Naturally through the Ages; 3) The Garden of Eden: 1970's Style; 4) Beware! It's Natural; 5) What Have Additives Done for You Lately?; 6) The Delaney Dilemma! 7) Come and Get It (Before They Ban It)!; 8) Regulating Our "Inner Environment"— Rationally!

In conclusion, these recommendations are made: 1) The frequent panics about various substances "causing cancer" do nothing but slow down the scientific quest for facts. We need reporting and general health education that gives a balanced account of the facts. Additionally, we must have administrators who will not feel compelled to act on rumor. 2) We need food legislation that allows us to judge the things we eat not by whether they are "natural" or "artificial" or by the effects they may have when used in unrealistic quantities. Foods should be judged on their individual benefits, safety, and acceptability. 3) We must struggle against the deleterious effects of food faddism, the health food charlatans, and the rumors about the hazards of specific foods. We must put our faith in scientific research to determine what is hazardous and what is acceptable.

The book provides an excellent treatment of the subject.

573.   Whole Foods Natural Foods Guide: What Happens to Natural Food Products from Farm to Consumer. Berkeley, CA: And/Or Press, 1979. 310p. bibliog. index. $8.95 pa. LC 79-19013. ISBN 0-915904-46-2.

This is a compilation of material from *Whole Foods* magazine, a publication of the "natural" foods business (see entry 125). The guide provides an inside look at food products and production methods in the natural foods industry. Articles reproduced are those presumed to be of particular interest to the consumer.

Included are detailed descriptions of the manufacture of products, and also discussions of retailing, wholesaling, and advertising. The aim is to give the reader accurate information so an informed choice of food can be made. The natural food industry's intent is said to be to provide food with a minimum of processing and a maximum of disclosed information about what goes into the product. Chemical additives are presumably not used, although the editors do admit that the industry is not able to avoid the complex machineries of food technology. A little information is provided about growing "organic" food, and an attempt is made to define the term. It is obviously very difficult to grow food without chemicals of some sort, natural or synthetic.

Herbs are said to be the fastest growing category of products in the natural foods industry, and there is a substantial section on them. It is pointed out that there is no clearly defined national policy for herb regulation, although safety and efficacy must be proved for drugs sold through usual channels. Herb companies are indirect about the qualities of their products.

The material is presented under the following section heads: 1) From the ground up; 2) Rules and regulations; 3) Snacks and sweets; 4) Grains and beans; 5) Soyfoods; 6) Herbs; 7) Cosmetics; 8) Edible oils; 9) Made-up foods; and 10) Natural foods as a business. Most sections contain a "Consumer's Guide."

A low-key approach is used throughout the work. While the authors obviously believe in the superiority of "whole," "natural," and "organic" products, extravagant claims are not made. They do not want the credibility of the industry threatened.

574.   Williams, Roger J. **Nutrition Against Disease: Environmental Prevention.** New York: Pitman Publishing Corp., 1971; repr. Bantam Books, 1973. 370p. bibliog. index. $1.95 pa.

The author of this book, a biochemist, takes the view that the "microenvironment of our body cells is crucially important to our health." That is, our bodies must have complete, proper nutrition to combat disease. He is critical of the medical profession for neglecting the relationship between nutrition and disease. Williams also says some of his conclusions are unconventional.

Following are chapter headings: 1) The Flaw in Medical Education; 2) The Nutrition-Heredity Factor; 3) A New Hope for Better Health; 4) Stillborn, Deformed, and Mentally Retarded Babies; 5) Protecting the Hearts We Have; 6) The Fight against Obesity; 7) Prevention of Dental Disease; 8) The Nutritional Approach to Arthritis and Related Disorders; 9) How Can We Delay Old Age?; 10) Environmental Control of

Mental Disease; 11) The Battle against Alcoholism; 12) How Is the Cancer Problem Related?; 13) Food Fads; 14) What the Food Industries Can Do; 15) New Developments in Basic Medicine. Appendices present tables of food values.

Few would quarrel with the author's basic premise, and he makes many good points. However, the book implies that proper nutrition can prevent or cure the diseases mentioned above, all complicated conditions for which there are no simple cures. The claims made seem extravagant.

575.   Worstman, Gail L. **The Natural Fast Food Cookbook.** Seattle, WA: Pacific Search Press, 1980. 142p. index. $5.95pa. LC 80-19474. ISBN 0-914718-52-5.

The view of the author of this cookbook is that people want alternatives to fast food chain hamburgers and French fried potatoes. They also need to prepare nutritious meals that can be fixed ahead of time and in a hurry because of busy schedules. More than 150 recipes for beverages, appetizers, snacks, cereals, breads, sandwiches, salads, main dishes, crepes, quiches, and desserts are given. These dishes are based on "natural" foods, or are made up completely of "natural" ingredients for developing a totally "natural" diet. A few international recipes are included, such as Mexican, Japanese, or Italian dishes.

576.   Wynne-Tyson, Jon. **Food for a Future: The Complete Case for Vegetarianism.** New York: Universe Books, 1979. 160p. bibliog. index. $8.50. LC 78-65622. ISBN 0-87663-334-3.

The author of this book makes a case for vegetarianism on economic, nutritional, ecological, and humanitarian grounds. His approach is radical, if not hysterical. He calls our attitudes toward food animals merciless and maintains that meat eating has brutalized our nature and turned us into the most cruel species the world has ever known. In addition, he thinks man's chemistry is not designed to cope with "the toxic properties of decomposing flesh" and believes we should rely on nuts, fruits, and grains to the exclusion of meat.

There is a chapter on the history of vegetarianism. A chart has been included listing the amounts of water, protein, fat, and carbohydrates present in foods. Each chapter begins with a quotation pertaining to vegetarianism.

Perhaps the most sensible point the book makes is that plant protein could play an increasingly important part in solving the world's food problem.

16

VITAMINS
AND MINERALS

Although virtually all nutritionists agree that a properly balanced diet will furnish all necessary vitamins, many books promote vitamin supplements, often in doses far in excess of recommended daily allowances. Furthermore, megadoses may be toxic and dangerous, according to experts. Several books listed below make a case for treatment of certain conditions with large vitamin doses, particularly the work by Adams and Murray and the controversial book by Nobel Prize winner Linus Pauling.

The supposed value of vitamin E for a number of diseases is discussed in several recent books; some are included in this chapter. Scientists are still undecided about what, if any, role the vitamin plays in human nutrition. The title by Di Cyan, suitable for the layperson, assesses what is known about vitamin E, and Machlin's book is a highly scientific and technical work for the expert.

"Natural" food proponents have for some time stressed that natural vitamins are superior to synthetically made ones, but, according to researchers, the human body can tell no difference.

The book by Kutsky and the one by Levy and Bach-y-Rita will help readers make rational judgments about the use of vitamins.

* * * * *

577.   Adams, Ruth, and Frank Murray. **Body, Mind and B Vitamins**. New expanded ed. New York: Larchmont Books (25 W. 45th St., New York, NY 10036), 1976. 317p. bibliog. index. $1.75. LC 79-109758.

A popular work, this book discusses 11 vitamins of the B complex. Claims are made that they are effective against physical ills, mental illness, alcoholism, depression, and stresses of modern life. Charts show the best food sources of the vitamins and the recommended daily dietary allowances for each vitamin.

578.   Adams, Ruth, and Frank Murray. **Megavitamin Therapy**. New York: Larchmont Books, 1973. 277p. bibliog. index. $1.75. LC 75-110853.

The viewpoint taken in this book is that massive doses of certain vitamins, along with proper diet, can return an ailing patient to good health. Evidence is presented that alcoholism, schizophrenia, hyperactivity in children, and even drug addiction are often the result of improper diet. Case histories are used to substantiate claims.

Megavitamin therapy has its proponents, but the matter is controversial.

579.   Bock, Raymond F. **Vitamin E: Key to Youthful Longevity**. New York: Arco Publishing Co. (219 Park Ave. South, New York, NY 10003), 1977. 62p. $3.60pa. LC 76-26591. ISBN 0-668-04078-5.

This small book, written by a practicing gynecologist, presents a case for the use of vitamin E (alpha tocopherol) as a kind of cure-all and an important factor in retarding the aging process and maintaining health, when taken in "adequate" doses. Bock speaks almost entirely from his own experience as a physician and with little reference to scientific studies. The book is popular in approach.

Vitamin E has been used enthusiastically but uncritically to treat a variety of diseases, particularly those for which there is no specific cure. Real scientific evidence of its effectiveness is lacking, but many have given testimony to its benefits. This book is another such testimony.

580. Bosco, Dominick. **The People's Guide to Vitamins and Minerals, From A to Zinc.** Chicago, IL: Contemporary Books, 1980. 325p. bibliog. index. $12.95; $6.95pa. LC 79-8743. ISBN 0-8092-7140-0; 0-8092-7139-7pa.

This work provides information, based on scientific evidence, about vitamins and minerals known to be essential for proper nutrition. Although intended for the lay public, it is a rather thorough treatment.

In the introduction, "Can Vitamins Make You Healthier?," the author stresses that he is not encouraging vitamin faddism, but that vitamins and minerals are effective in improving health.

The first section discusses 16 vitamins, while section 2 covers 16 minerals. The last section, "Partners, Outlaws, and Questions," contains miscellaneous material. First, the role of bioflavonoids is outlined; then vitamins B_{15}, B_{17}, Q, and U are discussed. They are called "outlaw vitamins" because none has been generally recognized as a vitamin, and one, B_{17} (laetrile), has been outlawed by the federal government as an ineffective and toxic cancer cure. The view taken is that at least some of these substances have been granted more credit than is deserved, but perhaps more study of them is desirable.

Also included in the last section are answers to "The Eight Most Asked Questions About Vitamins and Minerals." The answer given to the query "are natural vitamins better than synthetic?" is that there is no evidence to support this common claim.

On the whole, the book presents a balanced account of the subject.

581. Di Cyan, Erwin. **Vitamin E and Aging.** New York: Pyramid Books, 1972. 176p. bibliog. index. $1.25pa. LC 72-80402. ISBN 0-515-02761-8.

Vitamin E was discovered in 1922, but it has been largely ignored by scientists until recently. It is now believed that the vitamin has a role in slowing the process of aging. The objectives of this book, written by a drug researcher, are to make available certain information on the vitamin (which has appeared in scientific literature since about 1960) and to assess the material. The author points out that Vitamin E is controversial; one group has high praise for it, and another thinks it is worthless. Di Cyan stands in between, but believes the substance should be properly assessed.

Contents of the book is as follows: 1) What is Vitamin E?; 2) What does "aging" mean?; 3) Other faces of aging; 4) Malabsorption; 5) Polyunsaturated fatty acids and the liver; 6) Respiration and pollution; 7) Circulation in the legs; 8) Vitamin E and muscle; 9) Vitamin E and blood; 10) Vitamin E in nutrition; 11) Trace metals; 12) Vitamin E in foods; 13) Several other uses of Vitamin E; and 14) Some aspects of research on biological or biochemical effects of Vitamin E. Also included is a supplement that summarizes papers delivered at the International Conference on Vitamin E and Its Role in Cellular Metabolism, New York Academy of Sciences, December 6 and 7, 1971.

Findings of the researchers include: 1) Vitamin E plays a role in some diseases; 2) There are substances that can replace some of the functions of the vitamin, but most are not safe to take; 3) Scientists differ on how Vitamin E works; and 4) Much more research on the substance is necessary and worthwhile.

582.   Ellis, John M., and James Presley. **Vitamin B₆: The Doctor's Report.** New York: Harper and Row, 1973. 251p. illus. bibliog. index. $6.95. LC 72-9753. ISBN 0-06-011171-2.

The senior author of this book is a physician who is an authority on vitamin B₆, and the other author is a journalist and free-lance writer. They present an account of the history of the vitamin and report on research and experimentation that shows the substance to be valuable in the treatment of arthritis, rheumatism, certain kinds of heart disease and nervous disorders, diabetes, edema, and some gynecological problems. Much of the evidence reported is in the form of case histories, although there are source notes with references to scientific and clinical publications. Many patients reported dramatic improvement after vitamin B₆ therapy, according to the book.

The authors do not claim that vitamin B₆ relieves diabetes or prevents heart disease. They do believe, however, that it is helpful to a patient with these diseases and that it may be a factor in prevention of the illnesses. A plea is made for proper nutrition and the proper teaching of it in schools and to the public.

583.   Fried, John J. **The Vitamin Conspiracy.** New York: Saturday Review Press, E. P. Dutton and Co., 1975. 212p. $8.95. LC 74-23321. ISBN 0-8415-0366-4.

The author of this work, who is a science writer, says he set out to write the book with no preconceptions. He found paranoia and suspicion rampant on both sides of the vitamin controversy. He wrote the book in spite of, and not because of, those associated with the promotion of, or the demystification of, vitamins.

Following are chapter headings: 1) Introduction; 2) Vitamin E: Snake Oil for the Heart; 3) From Saskatchewan—An Answer for Schizophrenia; 4) The Greening of Nicotinic Acid; 5) Counterattack; 6) Everyman's Vitamin; 7) Vitamin C vs. the Common Cold; 8) Not Letting Facts Interfere with a Good Story; and 9) Is the Daily Vitamin Necessary?

The book looks at people who are investigating vitamins and those who are using them to treat patients. The conclusions drawn are distressing. The author thinks the lay public needs a new understanding of nutrition. He believes most physicians cannot advise patients properly on how to eat well. Many nutritionists believe that no amount of education will do any good anyway. However, Fried notes that health and food faddists have managed to get their views across to millions of people who turn a deaf ear to conventional nutrition experts. They have been successful because the nutrition community has forfeited the public to them, the author concludes.

584.   Holmes, Marjorie. **God and Vitamins: How Exercise, Diet, and Faith Can Change Your Life.** Garden City, NY: Doubleday, 1980. 365p. bibliog. (A Doubleday-Galilee Original). $9.95. LC 80-911. ISBN 0-385-15249-3.

Holmes is the author of several books and has contributed columns to the *Washington Star* newspaper and *Woman's Day* magazine. She is known as a religious writer. Her viewpoint in this book is that proper diet, exercise, and faith can promote good physical and spiritual health. She explains the role of each vitamin and mineral in the body and emphasizes the value of "natural" foods.

585.   Kutsky, Roman J. **Handbook of Vitamins and Hormones.** New York: Van Nostrand Reinhold Co., 1973. 278p. bibliog. index. $7.95pa. LC 70-190499. ISBN 0-442-24550-5.

The purpose of this handbook is to make readily available in one place basic information on vitamins and hormones. Emphasis is placed on the relationship between chemical reactions of the substances in the test tube and their metabolic reactions in the human body. All common vitamins and hormones (13 vitamins and 23 hormones) are discussed except the plant and insect hormones; a chapter is devoted to each substance. The information is treated from several different approaches: the pharmacological and medical, nutritional, chemical, physiological, and biological. Consequently, the book will be of use to various individuals, including researchers and students, physicians, pharmacologists, nurses, and dieticians. The educated layman will also find use for it, particularly to aid in making rational judgments regarding vitamin claims. This handbook is the first of its kind.

586.   Levy, Joseph V., and Paul Bach-y-Rita. **Vitamins: Their Use and Abuse.** New York: Liveright, 1976. bibliog. index. $7.95. LC 75-44347. ISBN 0-87140-616-0.

The authors of this book are biomedical professionals on the faculty of a university. They wrote the book because they were alarmed at the confusion, conflicting information and claims, and fraudulent husksterism that existed in the field of vitamins. Their objective is to establish a better understanding of vitamins. Many individuals consume vitamins in amounts far exceeding recommended minimum allowances for good health. Responsible nutritionists agree that a well-balanced diet provides all necessary vitamins for the normal person, although supplements may be needed in special situations. Self-medication can lead to excessive vitamin intake and toxicity.

The first section of the book deals with vitamins in daily life. An attempt is made to define a vitamin, and their role in nutrition is explained. Recommended dietary allowances are defined. Section 2 examines some common beliefs, including the use of vitamin C and the common cold; vitamin E and human fertility and sexuality; natural versus synthetic vitamins; and orthomolecular medicine and megavitamin therapy. The third section is on vitamins in special circumstances; pregnancy, aging, weight reduction, alcoholism, and cancer are among topics considered. Section 4 covers frequently overlooked factors such as vitamins in relation to other substances, vitamin dependency, placebo effects, vitamin toxicity, antivitamins, and factors influencing potency. The fifth section takes up other aspects of nutrition, namely, water, energy, acids, and minerals. An appendix includes a good list of literature sources, a glossary, a table of recommended dietary allowances, and a short discussion of recent vitamin legislation.

The book provides a realistic and authoritative view of the subject and is suitable for the general reader.

587.   Machlin, Lawrence J., ed. **Vitamin E: A Comprehensive Treatise.** New York: Marcel Dekker, Inc., 1980. 660p. illus. bibliog. index. (Basic and Clinical Nutrition, vol.1). $79.50. LC 80-12467. ISBN 0-8247-6842-6.

The preface of this highly scientific and technical work states that there is more myth and controversy concerning vitamin E (tocopherol) than any other nutrient, mainly because there are many gaps in knowledge about the substance. There is still disagreement on how the vitamin functions at the cellular and molecular level, on its role in nutrition, and on the therapeutic usefulness of it. This book was produced to provide a source of current information on the subject. It is particularly intended for the scientific audience: nutritionists, biochemists, students, clinicians, and others who are interested. Contributors are noted researchers.

Chapter headings are: 1) The First Two Decades of Vitamin E History; 2) Chemistry of Tocopherols and Tocotrienols; 3) Assay Methods; 4) Tocopherols in Foods; 5) Biochemistry; 6) Role of Vitamin E in Plants, Microbes, Invertebrates, and Fish; 7) Pathology of Vitamin E Deficiency; 8) Disease Resistance: Immune Response; 9) Vitamin E as an *In Vivo* Lipid Stabilizer and Its Effect on Flavor and Storage Properties of Milk and Meat; 10) Counteraction of Environmental Effects; 11) Human Health and Disease; and 12) Epilogue.

In summary, despite many claims that vitamin E will cure an endless number of maladies and all the popular and scientific literature on the subject, there is still no clear definition of its role in human health. Many questions remain to be clarified by further research.

588.   Mindell, Earl L. **Earl Mindell's Vitamin Bible: How the Right Vitamins and Nutrient Supplements Can Help Turn Your Life Around.** New York: Rawson, Wade Publishers, 1979. 292p. bibliog. index. $12.95; $5.95pa. LC 76-64203. ISBN 0-89256-106-8; 0-89256-114-9pa.

Mindell is a pharmacist who was converted to the use of vitamins because they reportedly helped him cope with a 15-hour workday in the pharmacy. He does not advocate the use of megavitamins, however, just a moderate dose only slightly in excess of FDA recommendations.

Mindell includes a great deal more in his book than a discussion of vitamin use. He is critical of the overuse of tranquilizers, certain fad diets, and excessive use of salt, sugar, alcohol, and tobacco.

The author also makes some recommendations that have little basis in accepted scientific fact. He recommends use of bioflavonoids, vitamin E, RNA-DNA tablets, and a number of "vitamins" such as B_{10}, B_{11}, B_{13}, B_{17}, H, L, P, T, and U. He believes many more are yet to be discovered. In addition, Mindell claims certain vitamins relieve alcohol craving, protect the liver from cirrhosis, and relieve symptoms of angina and asthma. A table of drugs said to impair vitamin utilization has been included.

589.   Passwater, Richard A. **Selenium as Food and Medicine.** New Canaan, CT: Keats Publishing, 1980. 240p. illus. bibliog. index. $10.95; $2.95pa. LC 80-82325. ISBN 0-87983-237-1; 0-98983-229-0pa.

The author of this work, who holds a Ph.D. degree, has written a number of popular books relating to health, diet, and nutritional therapies. This one is about nutritional needs of people for selenium, a trace element. Without it, according to the author, the body's immune system is weakened, and heart disease, cancer, arthritis, and a number of other conditions become more likely.

Passwater's view is that environmental factors, such as glaciers that scraped the northeastern United States and pollution-induced acid rains, have removed selenium from the soil of the country making it unavailable to plants and to animals and people who eat the plants. Selenium supplements should be added to the diet to promote optimal health. Documentation is provided for these opinions.

Chapter headings are: 1) Introducing the Selenium Spectrum; 2) Selenium against Cancer; 3) Selenium Builds a Healthy Heart; 4) Slowing Down the Aging Process with Selenium; 5) Arthritis; 6) Selenium Strengthens Your Immune System; 7) The Growing Danger of Radiation; 8) Cystic Fibrosis; 9) Muscular Dystrophy; 10) Cataract; 11) Sexual Function; 12) Selenium Detoxifies Pollutants; 13) The Experts Speak Out; 14) Recommended Daily Allowances; 15) We Need More Selenium; 16) Selenium Supplements; 17) Toxicity; 18) Man Does Not Live by Selenium Alone; and 19) Perspective.

The book was evidently written for popular use, but a good deal of scientific material is included.

590.   Pauling, Linus. **Vitamin C and the Common Cold.** San Francisco, CA: W. H. Freeman and Co., 1970. 122p. bibliog. index. $1.95pa. LC 76-140232. ISBN 0-7167-0160-X.

When Pauling, a noted holder of two Nobel prizes, wrote this book the scientific community was quite critical of it. It appeared to many that he did not have sufficient evidence for his views, and that the book would have escaped notice if the author had not been so well known. Pauling's noted contributions have been in chemistry rather than life sciences. This book is for the general public.

Pauling takes the position that common colds can be controlled through nutrition, specifically through large doses of Vitamin C (ascorbic acid). Other aspects of Vitamin C are also considered.

Chapter headings are as follows: 1) The Common Cold; 2) Scurvy; 3) The Discovery of Vitamins; 4) The Properties of Ascorbic Acid; 5) Ascorbic Acid and the Common Cold; 6) Vitamin C and Evolution; 7) Orthomolecular Medicine; 8) Human Biochemical Individuality; 9) Vitamin C and Drugs Compared; and 10) How to Control the Common Cold. Appended materials include: 1) How to buy vitamin C; 2) Multi-vitamin food supplementation; 3) Other studies of ascorbic acid and the common cold; and 4) Possible governmental restriction of the sale of ascorbic acid.

Pauling has written another related book, *Vitamin C, the Common Cold, and the Flu.*

591.   Shute, Wilfrid E. **Your Child and Vitamin E.** New Canaan, CT: Keats, 1979. 153p. bibliog. index. $2.25pa. (A Pivot Original Health Book). LC 79-88120. ISBN 0-87983-202-9.

Shute has written several books on the benefits of Vitamin E therapy. This one extols the value of the substance in children's diets to insure maximum growth, health, and development, and also for treatment of certain diseases such as rheumatic fever. Case histories are provided as evidence of the healing powers of the vitamin.

Many people believe that wild plants have been neglected as a source of food, and the recent back-to-nature movement has sparked an interest in foraging for the plants. Although medicinal and a few other uses for certain plants are mentioned in some works included in this section, the emphasis is on the use of the plants for food. A number of the works are suitable to be used as field guides, and most are illustrated, some very handsomely. In addition, recipes for using the plants are frequently included.

Some works, such as those by Gibbons, have a good deal of charm, probably because of the personal accounts included. A few books deal with aquatic plants, and several are concerned with plants usually classed as weeds.

The largest number of books are about mushrooms. Mushroom hunting is increasingly popular, and there are many guides available to assist the forager. Mushrooms present problems, though, because a number of the species are poisonous, some deadly. Proper identification is very important, and, as several books point out, there is no easy rule-of-thumb to distinguish poisonous from edible types.

Many books listed in this chapter cover specific geographical regions, most located in the United States.

* * * * *

592.   Benoliel, Doug. **Northwest Foraging: A Guide to Edible Plants of the Pacific Northwest.** Lynnwood, WA: Signpost Publications, 1974. 171p. illus. index. $4.95pa. ISBN 0-913140-13-9.

Most plants included in this work are common to the northeastern United States and Canada as well as to the Pacific Northwest, so the book can serve as a good personal pocket guide for a wide area. The line drawings are realistic, and, as an added attraction, eight pages of recipes have been provided.

593.   Cazort, Mimi, ed. **Mr. Jackson's Mushrooms.** Ottawa: National Gallery of Canada/National Museums of Canada; distr. University of Chicago Press, 1979. 161p. illus. (col.). bibliog. index. $35.00. ISBN 0-88884-364-X.

Almost half of this folio-size book is made up of 42 beautiful watercolor illustrations of fungi painted by Henry C. Jackson, a noted commercial artist and amateur mycologist who lived from 1877 until 1961. The original watercolors are in the National Gallery of Canada.

The book also contains excerpts from Mr. Jackson's notebooks, covering from 1931 through 1954. Material is included on mushroom collecting activities, along with the social and environmental changes of the time in the Quebec area. Jackson's love of nature is evident throughout.

The work is attractive in all respects. The text is printed on heavy textured paper, and the plates are exceptionally well reproduced, most in actual size. The book is well worth the asking price.

594.   Clarke, Charlotte Bringle. **Edible and Useful Plants of California.** Berkeley, CA: University of California Press, 1979. 280p. illus. (part col.). bibliog. index. (California Natural History Guides: 41). $5.95pa. LC 76-14317. ISBN 0-520-03261-6.

More than 220 species of plants are included in this book, arranged alphabetically by common name under broad geographical categories where they are commonly found in California, e.g., foothills and mountains, deserts, urban and cultivated areas. Ornamentals is the single non-geographic category.

Each entry (usually covering one or two pages) gives other common names, the scientific name, a description, the distribution and habitat, past and present uses, and culinary recipes. Some recipes are a bit unusual, for instance, pyracantha marmalade. However, many sound quite good. Medicinal uses are mentioned, but specific formulations and dosages are not given. Six pages of glossy color photographs of selected plants are included.

A list of California botanical gardens, reading lists, a table of phylogenetic relationships, a glossary, and an index make this book a useful reference tool.

The author states that the book is written for the person with no knowledge of botany and it is meant to be useful to the camper, vegetarian, and survival instructor. Although these plants are found in California, many are also found throughout the United States, so this is a useful book for everyone interested in the subject.

595.   Coker, William Chambers, and John Nathaniel Couch. **The Gasteromycetes of the Eastern United States and Canada.** Together with a supplementary article, **The Gasteromycetae of Ohio: Puffballs, Birds'-Nest Fungi and Stinkhorns** by Minnie May Johnson. New York: Dover Publications, 1974. 1v. (various paging). illus. bibliog. index. $5.00pa. LC 73-91490. ISBN 0-486-23033-3. (The former title originally published in 1928 by the University of North Carolina Press; the latter in the **Ohio Biological Survey Bulletin** 22, v.IV, No.6, p.271-352).

The class of fungi covered in this standard work includes puffballs, stinkhorns, and birds'-nest fungi. Some listed are not known to most amateur collectors. However, the material is of interest to mycologists on all levels. Finding keys, line drawings, photographs, habitat, good descriptions, literature references, and comparisons are provided.

Some species of this class are edible, and none are known to be poisonous.

596.   Coon, Nelson. **Using Wayside Plants.** 4th rev. ed. New York: Hearthside Press, 1969. 288p. illus. bibliog. index. $5.95. LC 70-76158. (This work was reprinted by Dover Publications, New York, in 1980 with a new title **Using Wild and Wayside Plants** and an updated bibliography.)

The author of this useful work believes wayside plants should be used more often and appreciated more fully. His book is a guide to useful plants of the U.S., particularly the northeastern area. The presentation is in two sections. The first section contains chapters that give general information on wild plants, observations on food plants (with some good old-fashioned recipes), use of plants in children's play, plant crafts, dyeing with roadside plants, plant remedies, and wild plants in and out of doors.

The second section, called "Notes on the Plants," contains the following contents: useful trees, useful shrubs, herbaceous plants, plants of wet places, lichens and fungi, poisonous plants, wayside plants in your backyard, and the naturalistic camper. For the most part, these chapters present material in short monographs plant by plant. There is usually a picture, a map of the U.S. showing the geographic area where the plant is found, common and scientific names, descriptions, uses, and comments.

This classic work has been popular with naturalists, campers, and hikers, and is a good selection for libraries.

597.   Elliott, Douglas B. **Roots: An Underground Botany and Forager's Guide.** Old Greenwich, CT: Chatham Press, 1976. 128p. illus. bibliog. index. $5.95pa. LC 75-46234. ISBN 85699-132-5.

The author of this guide also drew the black-and-white sketches for it. They are an outstanding feature of the book. The introduction to the presentation includes a brief general discussion of plant roots. Wild plants that have useful roots are listed next, such as those that may be used for food, beverages, dyes, medicines, dentrifices, and shampoos. The material is divided into four sections: roots of shade-loving forest plants, roots of sun-loving field plants, roots of aquatic and marsh plants, and other roots. Appended is a short discussion on harvesting roots and a method of detailed examination of root systems. A glossary is also included.

Information provided about each plant usually includes: common and scientific names, habitat, description, uses of the root, historical background and anecdotes, cautions about use, preparation, and an illustration. Roots included are, for the most part, those of familiar herbal plants, such as ginseng, golden seal, Solomon's seal, American sarsaparilla, jack-in-the-pulpit, and many more.

598.   Findlay, W. P. K. **Wayside and Woodland Fungi.** With color illustrations by Beatrix Potter and others. London, New York: Frederick Warne and Co., Ltd., 1967. 202p. illus. (part col.). bibliog. index. LC 68-10154.

This book begins with the comment that fungi play an important role in the life of man, being both beneficial and harmful. Fungi are scavengers, destructive agents, food, dangerous poisons, sources of valuable drugs, and the cause of a few ailments.

The first several chapters discuss the following topics: fungi and man, the nature and naming of fungi, the role of the amateur in mycology, collection and identification of fungi, ecology and habitats of fungi, and classification. The remaining chapters (about three-fourths of the book) discuss the various types of fungi group by group. Good descriptions, habitat, edibility, toxicity, and keys to identification are provided. There is a short glossary. Illustrations, particularly the color paintings, are very fine.

599.   Freitus, Joe. **160 Edible Plants Commonly Found in the Eastern U.S.A.** Lexington, MA: Stone Wall Press, 1975. 1v. (unpaged). illus. $2.95pa. LC 74-31874. ISBN 0-913276-17-0.

A New England teacher interested in nature study wrote this small booklet that serves well as a field guide to edible plants throughout most of the U.S. The following information is provided for each plant: vernacular and scientific name, description, a line drawing, habitat, range, notes on edibility, time of harvest, and cooking instructions. There are cautions provided if the plant is toxic and must be cooked rather than eaten raw.

600.   Furlong, Marjorie, and Virginia Pill. **Edible? Incredible! Pondlife.** Happy Camp, CA: Naturegraph Publishers, Inc., 1980. 95p. illus. (col.). bibliog. index. $8.95; $4.95pa. LC 79-27779. ISBN 0-87961-084-0; 0-87961-083-2pa.

Common edibles found in and around ponds of the United States are described and illustrated in this small book. Brief information about how to hunt the plants (and a few animals) are provided. The work is divided into these sections: grasses and herbs, trees and shrubs, animals, and recipes. About 25 plants are listed by common name with family, synonymous and Latin names also given. A description, habitat, and information about preparation for eating are provided in each monograph.

Following are some of the plants listed: cattail, mint, nettles, watercress, wild rice, cranberry, gooseberry, rushes, wild rose, and willow.

The book is nicely done with good recipes.

601.   Furlong, Marjorie, and Virginia Pill. **Wild Edible Fruits and Berries.** Photography by Marjorie Furlong. Healdsburg, CA: Naturegraph Publishers, 1974. 62p. illus. (col.). index. $7.95; $3.95pa. LC 74-32015. ISBN 0-87961-033-6; 0-87961-032-8pa.

Most of this book is made up of color photographs and descriptions of about 40 berry and wild fruit plants that may be found growing in easily accessible areas, usually not far from a road. The plants are native to the Pacific states, but many can also be found in other areas of the United States.

The book contains recipes (in a separate section) for beverages, cakes and muffins, candy and desserts, jams and jellies, pies, relishes and meat sauces, and syrups.

The reader is advised to take the book along on trips to the woods in order to compare the photo and text with the plant discovered.

602.   Gibbons, Euell. **Stalking the Good Life: My Love Affair with Nature.** Illustrated by Freda Gibbons. New York: David McKay, 1971. 247p. illus. index. $7.95. LC 77-146480. ISBN 0-679-50276-9.

This work deals mainly with the eating of wild plants. It is not a scientific work but a popular one for enjoyable reading as the author relates his own experiences in finding and using edible wild plants. The book does not serve well as an identification guide, but it isn't intended to be one. Edible wild plants can be found in the wilderness and in one's own back yard.

Gibbons uses both common and scientific names when discussing the plants. A better botanical description can be found elsewhere if the reader is not familiar with the plant. Although the work is mainly about wild plants, the author also goes into living in harmony with nature, the beauty of nature, and the life cycle and food chain. Not much is said about wild plants being any more healthful than other foods, but there is a chapter on "wild winter vitamins" and one on "wild health foods." An autobiographical chapter is included, telling how the author became interested in eating wild plants.

603.   Gibbons, Euell. **Stalking the Healthful Herbs.** With drawings of plants by Raymond W. Rose. Field Guide Edition. New York: David McKay Co., 1970. 303p. illus. index. $3.95pa. LC 66-17354. ISBN 0-679-50235-1.

This guide has been quite popular and has been reprinted a number of times. Although this edition is called a field guide edition, it is probably not very satisfactory for that purpose, although there are some line drawings of plants to assist in identification. The charm of the book lies in the writing. It contains lore and personal accounts of the author's experiences with plants and nature. If a particular experiment with a wild food is not successful, Gibbons cheerfully says so.

The title perhaps suggests that this is a book of herbal remedies. This is not quite true; Gibbons most often gets carried away into discussions of the use of the plants for food and tells how they may be prepared. Supposed medicinal value of the plants is mentioned, however, as well as other uses, such as for cosmetics.

Gibbons says he is not a food faddist in any sense of the term. He loves to gather and prepare the plants though, and they are an ornament to his cuisine. He says he has a love affair with nature.

604.   Gibbons, Euell. **Stalking the Wild Asparagus**. With illustrations by Margaret F. Schroeder. New York: David McKay Co., 1962. 303p. illus. index. LC 62-13703.

This enjoyable book was written by one who has gathered wild food as a hobby. Gibbons says people can live solely on the bounty of nature in many parts of the U.S., and he hopes his book will arouse the interest of others in this pursuit.

A wide range of wild plant materials are covered: fruit, nuts, leaves, roots, tubers, bulbs, and seeds. Plants are emphasized, but there are also chapters on fish, crayfish, frog legs, turtles, terrapins, and wild game.

Some food plants discussed are: crab apples, Jerusalem artichokes, wild asparagus, sweet birch, blackberries, dewberries, huckleberries, great burdock, cattails, wild cherries, chickory, wild cranberries, elderberries, wild grapes, ground cherries, maple sugar, may apple, milkweed, mulberries, mushrooms, wild mustard, wild onion, pawpaw, sassafras, wild strawberries, sunflowers, walnuts, hickory nuts, wild rice, and wild honey. Recipes for tasty dishes are included throughout the book.

There is a short chapter on herbal medicine from wild plants. Some history is included and a few recipes, e.g., cough syrups, some distilled medicines, witch hazel, and distilled teas.

The author presents personal accounts of foraging trips taken alone or sometimes with family and friends. The book is very nicely done and has been deservedly popular.

605.   Glick, Phyllis G. **The Mushroom Trail Guide**. New York: Holt, Rinehart and Winston, 1979. 247p. illus. bibliog. index. $9.95; $5.95pa. LC 18424. ISBN 0-03-018306-5; 0-03-018301-4pa.

About 400 edible and poisonous mushrooms that grow in the United States are described in this pocket-sized guide. Emphasis of the work is on edibility, and instructions for cooking the food mushrooms are included.

After brief introductory remarks on how to collect, identify, cook, and preserve mushrooms, the book is divided into two sections, the gilled and the nongilled mushrooms. Each part is preceded by a picture key to the common genera or groups; the text is then arranged by family. For each genus or group there is a short discussion of field characters and the edibility of the species. Species are described and illustrated by sketches by the author.

The book is attractive and well designed. It has been criticized, however, as have many other mushroom hunters' field guides, in that it really does not tell the amateur hunter enough to make sure distinctions between edible and certain poisonous mushrooms. A microscope must be used in some instances to determine edibility.

606.   Groves, J. Walton. **Edible and Poisonous Mushrooms of Canada**. Ottawa, Canada: Research Branch, Canada Department of Agriculture, 1962. 298p. illus. (part col.). bibliog. index. (Publication 1112).

Mushrooms appeal to individuals in a number of ways, according to the author of this book. The biologist, for instance, is interested in the variety of species, their place in nature, and their relationship with other forms of life; the artist is interested in them because of their form and color; the researcher looks to them as a source of drugs; and ordinary people may be most interested in them as a source of food. Ordinary people often face an important problem: How to tell edible from poisonous mushrooms. Groves makes it clear that there is no simple way to distinguish the two types. He also points out that it has been mainly through trial and error that knowledge has been built up of which plants are edible and which poisonous. He suggests that unrecognized species of mushrooms should not be eaten, and that because of the very great danger from the deadly species of *Amanita*, the characters of this genus particularly should be learned and its species avoided.

The introductory material of the book includes short sections on parts of a mushroom, collecting them, food value, mushroom poisoning, identification, nomenclature, classification, and keys to the genera. The monographs about mushrooms are arranged with various species of a genus grouped together. Some general information is given about each genus, then specific information about each species follows. The following information is included: a description, habitat, fruiting season, edibility, and distinguishing features. Many photographs, some colored, and a glossary are provided.

607.   Guba, Emil Frederick. **Wild Mushrooms—Food and Poison.** Waltham, MA: The author (36 Marianne Road, Waltham, MA 02154), 1970. 118p. illus. bibliog. index.

The author of this book is a professor emeritus of plant pathology and mycology. He has produced a guide with rules on collecting wild edible mushrooms, and, in addition, has provided information on food value, poisonous and unpalatable species, mushroom toxins, and therapy for mushroom poisoning. Guba has emphasized the troublesome poisonous species and treatment for the poisoning because he thinks the amateur mushroom hunter should learn to recognize these species first and avoid tragedy. Other material presented includes mushroom recipes and ways to preserve them.

Species are described in detail, grouped by type (poisonous, suspected, unknown, or safe). Black and white illustrations are provided.

The book should be valuable to collectors and the medical profession.

608.   Haard, Karen, and Richard Haard. **Foraging for Edible Wild Mushrooms.** Rev. ed. Photography by Lee Mann and Richard Haard, illustrations by Cindy Davis. Seattle, WA: Cloudburst Press, 1978. 156p. illus. (part col.). index. $11.95; $5.95pa. ISBN 0-88930-015-1; 0-88930-017-8pa.

Although most mushroom manuals cover from 100 to 200 species of fungi, and there are perhaps 1,500 to 2,000 occurring in any single area, this book deals with 36 species of edible fungi. The limited number is dealt with because they are easy to identify; they can be collected from spring through fall; and they have a variety of flavors. The book is for the rank beginner. Suggestions on how to collect, identify, and distinguish the mushrooms are given, along with information about preserving and cooking the plants.

The authors of this work have also produced a companion volume, *Poisonous and Hallucinogenic Mushrooms*, which helps identify questionable species.

About half of this book is made up of species descriptions. Arrangement is by species name with the popular name, description (including size, surface, flesh and gill features, stem, spore print, and habitat), distinguishing features, remarks, and name derivation given. Good photographs illustrate the mushrooms. A glossary has been provided.

609.   Hard, Miron Elisha. **Mushrooms, Edible and Otherwise: Habitat and Time of Growth.** With a new appendix on nomenclatural changes by Martina S. Gilliam. New York: Dover Publications, Inc., 1976. (Republication of 1908 edition). illus. bibliog. index. $7.95pa. LC 75-41595. ISBN 0-486-23309-X.

This work is a general guide to mushrooms that grow in the midwestern and eastern United States. More than 500 species are described and illustrated (with photographs) to assist amateur mushroom hunters. Care is taken to help people distinguish edible from non-edible species.

Chapter 1 is a general introduction. Chapters 2 through 17 present individual monographs of about one-half page on various mushrooms by types as follows: 2) the white-spored agarics; 3) the rosy-spored agarics; 4) the rusty-spored agarics; 5) the purple-brown-spored agarics; 6) the black-spored agarics; 7) polyporaceae, tube-bearing fungi; 8) fungi with teach; 9) thelephoraceae; 10) clavariaceae—coral fungi; 11) tremellini; 12) ascomycetes—spore-sac fungi; 13) nidulariacae—bird's nest fungi; 14) group gastromycetes; 15) lycoperdaceae—puff balls; 16) sphaeriaceae; 17) myxomycetes. Each monograph gives scientific name, common name, description, habitat, and information about edibility.

Also included are chapters on recipes for cooking mushrooms and how to grow them, a glossary, a brief history of mycologists, and a nomenclatural appendix.

610.   Harris, Ben Charles. **Eat the Weeds.** Barre, MA: Barre Publishers, 1969. 223p. bibliog. index. $3.95pa. LC 69-12302. ISBN 0-517-51730-2.

Harris believes that many familiar wild and field plants have been neglected as a source of food, and, in his introductory chapter, he discusses many plants that are edible and tasty as well as nutritious. Sections are included on identifying herbs, collection and preservation, a chapter on preparation of plants for cooking or preserving, and a chapter on herbs as soil builders.

The rest of the book (about two-thirds of the bulk) is made up of short monographs about each plant. About each is usually given: common name, scientific name, synonyms, habitat, parts used, when to collect, and preparation and use. Recipes are included throughout.

The book is nicely done. Authentic information is presented without exaggerated claims.

611.   Hatfield, Audrey Wynne. **How to Enjoy Your Weeds.** London: Frederick Muller Ltd., 1969. 116p. illus. bibliog. index. SBN 584-10130-9.

The author of this small book tells how various plants, usually considered weeds, can be put to use. Both historical and practical information is provided.

A rather long (25 pages) introduction presents general information, history, notes on plant cultivation, and information on wine making. The plants are then discussed individually. Relatively few plants are included, but each is treated in some detail. Descriptions, uses, and recipes (particularly for wines) are given. There is a chapter on weed control and a list of "Weeds to Relieve Your Aches, Pains, Boils and Blanes."

612.   Hitchcock, Susan Tyler. **Gather Ye Wild Things: A Forager's Year.** Illustrated by G. B. McIntosh. New York: Harper and Row, 1980. 182p. illus. bibliog. index. $10.95. LC 79-2622. ISBN 0-06-011904-7.

A handsome, readable, and fascinating book, this guide to foraging stands out among other books devoted to the same subject. It presents 52 short essays, one for each week of the year, telling what wild things to look for each week. Some of the things described are: greens for salads, roots to harvest, tree bark for a spring tonic, wild herbs for flavor, a plant for making soap, and fruits from abandoned orchards. Included are odd bits of folklore, traditions, formulas, recipes, and instructions for preserving wild foods. Drawings that illustrate the book are especially nice.

613.   Hotchkiss, Neil. **Common Marsh, Underwater and Floating-Leaved Plants of the United States and Canada.** New York: Dover Publications, Inc., 1972. 124p. illus. index. $3.00pa. LC 74-187019. ISBN 0-486-22810-X.

This book is a republication of two publications of the Bureau of Sport Fisheries and Wildlife, United States Department of the Interior, *Common Marsh Plants of the United States and Canada* (Resource Publication 93, December 1970) and *Underwater and Floating-Leaved Plants of the United States and Canada* (Resource Publication 44, May 1967). It offers information to assist in field identification of North American marsh and water plants. Both publications list the plants, provide brief descriptions, and include common, scientific, and alternative names.

The first publication identifies emergent and semiemergent plants most likely to be found in inland and coastal marshes. The plants are discussed in seven groups. Within each group, the kinds that resemble one another most closely are placed next to each other. Plants in this part of the book are important for food and shelter for wildlife.

The second publication describes wild flowering plants, ferns, liverworts, and Characeae in which the foliage is habitually under water or floating. The plants are discussed in 12 groups, each group beginning with northern inland plants and continuing through southern inland to strictly coastal ones. Although sometimes considered weeds because they get in the way of boating, swimming, or fishing, many of these plants are important food sources for ducks, geese, muskrats, and other animals. They also protect bottoms from currents that stir up mud and sand.

614.   Kavaler, Lucy. **Mushrooms, Molds, and Miracles: The Strange Realm of Fungi.** New York: John Day Co., 1965. 318p. illus. bibliog. index. LC 65-13747.

The author of this book has attempted to give an idea of the large number, diversity, and ubiquitous nature of fungi and explain their importance to mankind. Fungi are both beneficial and harmful, and both aspects are dealt with in this work. Several fields of science are involved, including mycology, agriculture, medicine, psychiatry, genetics, and food processing.

The book is divided into these sections: 1) Fungi and mankind; 2) Fungi as food; 3) Fungi and your health; 4) Fungi and our crops; 5) Fungi and the things you use; and 6) Fungi and the conquest of space. Following are some specific topics dealt with: poisonous mushrooms, mushroom growing and preparing for the table, truffle hunting, molds and yeasts, fungus diseases, penicillin, ergot and LSD, hallucinogenic mushrooms, fungicides, and the search for life on other planets.

615.   Kavina, K. **Atlas of Fungi.** London: Lincolns-Prager Limited, 1947. 95p. illus. (part col.).

This book is concerned with only a small number of the higher fungi, those that come readily to notice. The intent of the work seems to be to encourage the study of mushrooms.

More than half of the book is made up of excellent photographs of mushrooms, 40 in black and white and 24 in color. In addition, line drawings appear with the brief text. The text covers the following topics: 1) about fungi, mycology and mycologists; 2) something about the shape of fungi; 3) how fungi reproduce themselves; 4) how fungi grow; 5) the nutrition of fungi; 6) fungi as a chemical factory; 7) the sensitivity of fungi; 8) the symbiosis of fungi with other organisms; 9) the classification of fungi; 10) edible and inedible fungi; 11) two kinds of fungus collectors; 12) in praise of mycology.

The author concludes that mycology is both a science and a sport.

616.   Kibby, Geoffrey. **Mushrooms and Toadstools: A Field Guide.** Illustrated by Sean Milne. Oxford, England: Oxford University Press, 1979. 256p. illus. (part col.). bibliog. index. $23.00. ISBN 0-19-217688-9; 0-19-286004-6pa.

There is an ever-increasing interest in accurate identification of mushrooms, particularly since the late 1960s. This practical guide provides fine color illustrations of more than 400 fungi of Great Britain and Europe.

The introduction to the book discusses the larger fungi from the botanical, taxonomic, and economic points of view, giving specific information on structure, useful and harmful species, fungi as food, poisonous fungi, and collecting and studying the plants. A simplified key to identification and a glossary are provided.

The main part of the book, a guide to species, divides the fungi into these groups: gill fungi, boletes and allies, brackets and allies, jelly fungi, puffballs and allies, cup fungi, and flask fungi. Information given about each species includes: a description, habitat, season and frequency of occurrence, details of the fruit body and spores, simple chemical tests, and a note on edibility.

The guide is suitable for the amateur collector. The illustrations are very attractive as well as helpful for identification purposes.

617.   Lange, Morten, and F. Bayard Hora. **Collins Guide to Mushrooms and Toadstools.** With color plates from **Flora Agaricina Danica** by Jakob E. Lange, with additions by Ebbe Sunesen and P. Dahlstrøm. London: Collins, 1963. 257p. illus. (part col.). bibliog. index.

This field guide is adapted from the Danish work *Illustret Svampeflora* by Jakob E. Lange and Morten Lange. The 96 color plates that illustrate the gill fungi in the book are reproduced from *Flora Agarcina Danica* by Jakob E. Lange.

The introductory section of the book contains information on the general structure, biology, and seasonal appearance of fungi. Edible and poisonous species are discussed in general. Also, a key to identification and a glossary are provided.

The second section of the book is a listing of the fungi. Arrangement is by plant family. Information provided includes details of size, structure, frequency, edibility, habitat, date of appearance, and special characteristics about growth, appearance, or taste. The color illustrations are nicely done paintings. Microscopical details of the spores of each species are given in the index, and chemical tests are described in some cases. The book also included general information on mushroom collecting.

618.   Largent, David L. **How to Identify Mushrooms to Genus, I: Macroscopic Features.** Illustrations by Sharon Hadley, key by Daniel E. Stuntz. 2d ed. Eureka, CA: Mad River Press (Route 2, Box 151 B, Eureka, CA 95501), 1977. 86p. illus. bibliog. index. $3.50. ISBN 0-916-422-00-3.

It is important that mushroom hunters learn to tell poisonous from edible species. The author of this book believes that an amateur learns to identify mushrooms by becoming good at recognizing features; then he must also be able to correlate several combinations of features to identify them with any degree of certainty. Mushrooms with similar features are grouped together in this presentation, which is the first of a series of books on mushroom identification. It covers only macroscopic features of the fruiting body. (For other volumes of the set see entries 619, 620, 641, 645).

Material is presented in four parts: 1) Macroscopic features of the basidiocarp; 2) Stature types of fruiting bodies; 3) Generic identification by stature type; and 4) Key to genera of mushrooms using only macroscopic features. Black and white figures and plates included in the book show the specific features the author wishes to emphasize.

619.   Largent, David, and David Johnson. **How to Identify Mushrooms to Genus, III: Microscopic Features.** Roy Watling, consultant: Kathryn Simpson, illustrations. Eureka, CA: Mad River Press (Route 2, Box 151 B, Eureka, CA 95501), 1977. 148p. illus. bibliog. index. $7.25. ISBN 0-916-422-09-7.

In classifying certain mushrooms, particularly the agarics and boleti, microscopic features are usually emphasized. The authors of this work felt there was a need for an inexpensive book that discussed and illustrated these features, and they produced this book as a source of information. It is a companion volume to other works (see also entries 618, 620, 641, 645).

The presentation begins with a review of terminology. Other sections are as follows: 1) Laboratory techniques; 2) Chemical reagents; 3) Hyphae; 4) The pellis or cortex; 5) Trama; 6) Cystidia; 7) Basidium and Basidiole; and 8) Basidiospores. There is a short bibliography and a section that combines an index, glossary, and examples of features. Illustration are line drawings and photomicrographs.

620.   Largent, David L., and Harry D. Thiers. **How to Identify Mushrooms to Genus, II: Field Identification of Genera.** Eureka, CA: Mad River Press (Route 2, Box 151 B, Eureka, CA 95501), 1977. 32p. bibliog. index. $2.50. ISBN 0-916-422-08-9.

One of the purposes of this book, the second of a series (see entries 618, 619, 641, 645), is to explain how the authors recognize various mushroom genera in the field. A second purpose is to introduce several segregate genera, particularly those that can be recognized using only macroscopic features. Segregate genera are those that have definite similarities that make them distinctly different from other species classified in that genus.

The mushrooms are listed alphabetically by genus name. Information provided includes key characters, a discussion of features, and a list of segregate genera.

The material is rather technical, suitable for a serious collector. The authors assume that readers become more expert as they progress from one volume to the next in this series.

621.   Lucas, Jannette May. **Indian Harvest: Wild Food Plants of America.** Illustrated by Helen Carter. Philadelphia, PA: J. B. Lippincott, 1945. 118p. illus. (part col.). bibliog.

This is a nice narrative account of the native plants the American Indians used for food. The way the plants were prepared for eating is discussed. Illustrations of the book are particularly attractive, and the text is suitable for young readers. A wide area of the country is covered, including the arid West. Many plants mentioned are also considered medicinal plants, and some are considered poisonous, as the author points out.

The book ends with the comment that "a new group of people are becoming interested in nature's foods." At the time the book was written, this interest was brought out primarily because of World War II when all sources of foods were becoming strained and depleted.

622.   McIlvaine, Charles, and Robert K. Macadam. **One Thousand American Fungi: Toadstools, Mushrooms, Fungi: How to Select and Cook the Edible: How to Distinguish and Avoid the Poisonous.** With a new essay on Nomenclatural Changes by Robert L. Shaffer. New York: Dover Publications, Inc., 1973. 729p. illus. (part col.). index. $6.95pa. LC 72-87763. ISBN 0-486-22782-0. (A republication of the 2d rev. ed. of 1902 of the work originally published in 1900 by Bowen-Merrill Co. with a new essay and table of nomenclatural changes).

The author of this work says he personally tested the mushrooms listed to determine whether they are poisonous. He published this book to report what he found. One finding (usually accepted as true) is that there is no general rule to distinguish between edible and poisonous mushrooms. He made his tests by eating small portions, or at least tasting them.

Introductory material in the book includes instructions to students, abbreviations of names of authors of species, names or principle reporters of American species, and nomenclatural changes (1973). The main section (about 600 pages) lists species by families. About each is given a description, habitat, fruiting season, information about edibility, cooking suggestions, and references to literature and reports on species. At the end of the book there are chapters on toadstool poisoning and its treatment, recipes for cooking and preparing for the table, a glossary, information on raising mushrooms at home, and indexes to genera and species. Illustrations are line drawings, photographs, and color plates.

This is a nicely written book with many personal touches.

623.   McKenny, Margaret. **The Savory Wild Mushroom.** Rev. and enl. by Daniel E. Stuntz, with contributions by Varro E. Tyler and Angelo M. Pellegrini. Seattle, WA: University of Washington Press, 1971. 274p. illus. (part col.). bibliog. index. $8.95. LC 78-160288.

This is a revised and enlarged edition of a popular 1962 publication. More than 150 species of mushrooms are covered, each illustrated in black and white, and some also in color. The book is intended for the mushroom hunter, including the beginner.

Species are arranged by major groups: boletes, chanterelles, gilled mushrooms, puffballs, polypores, spine fungi, coral fungi, jelly fungi, cup fungi, helvellas, and morels. The largest group, gilled mushrooms, are arranged first by spore color and then by other conspicuous features. There is a short monograph (about one-half page) on each species with such information as color and description, when and where found, and remarks given.

Also included in this work is a very good chapter on "Mushroom Poisons" by Varro E. Tyler, and one on "The Hunt, the Quarry, and the Skillet" by Angelo M. Pellegrini where cookery is discussed. Also, a few recipes are included.

This is an attractive, useful book, suitable for use as a field guide.

624.   McPherson, Alan, and Sue McPherson. **Edible and Useful Wildplants of the Urban West: Medicinal, Edible, Dye, and Landscape Uses for the Wildplants of Denver and Other Western Cities.** Boulder, CO: Pruett Publishing, 1979. 330p. illus. bibliog. index. $7.95pa. LC 79-20899. ISBN 0-87108-533-X.

For individuals who are interested in useful plants of the western cities of the United States, this book provides information to assist in the identification of them. Also included are examples of how to use the plants with recipes given for edible species. Quite a few dye plants are included in the work with an indication of the colors obtained using various mordants. The text often includes origins and derivations of plant names. There are good photographs illustrating the plants, indexes with multiple common names and Latin names, and an extensive bibliography.

625.   McPherson, Alan, and Sue McPherson. **Wild Food Plants of Indiana and Adjacent States.** Bloomington, IN: Indiana University Press, 1977. 215p. illus. bibliog. index. $12.50; $4.95pa. LC 76-48528. ISBN 0-253-19039-8; 0-253-28925-4pa.

Since Indiana has a variety of topographies, climates, and soils, a wide variety of plants grow there. The authors have divided the state into eight natural areas: the Dunes, the Lake Area, the Prairie, the Tipton Till Plain, the Lower Wabash Valley, the Southwestern Lowlands, the South-Central Mixed Woods, and the Southeastern Till Plain. Each area supports its own distinctive plant communities. The authors point out, however, that many species have vanished from the state as the earth was harnessed for agriculture. The book contains sensible cautions about protecting unique areas such as the Indiana Dunes National Lakeshore.

The first chapter is a plant perspective of the state. Included are two maps, one showing natural areas and the other a county map. Also, there is a seasonal guide to wild plant foods. The remainder of the book presents sections on individual plants. A detailed description and drawing are given for each plant or plant family, and the usual habitat and distribution within the state is indicated. Hints for locating the plants, how to prepare them, and recipes are given. A good deal of regional lore is included, with numerous comments about how the Indians used various plants.

This is a delightful book, authentic, and a real pleasure to read. Most of the 80 plants discussed are familiar, at least to native Hoosiers. However, some recipes, such as violet pudding, day lily fritters, and rose butter sandwiches are completely unfamiliar.

626.   Mabey, Richard. **Plantcraft: A Guide to the Everyday Use of Wild Plants.** Plates and line drawings by Marjorie Blamey. New York: Universe Books, 1978. 176p. illus. (part col.). bibliog. index. $10.00. LC 77-82824. ISBN 0-87663-303-3. (Issued in Great Britain as **Plants with a Purpose**).

Wild plants were once the chief raw materials in the household economy. This book is an attempt to revive some early skills in using these plants and to describe ways the commoner plants of Europe and North America have been, and still can be, put to use.

The introduction provides history and discusses raw materials and basic techniques. Five basic classes of use are identified as follows: medicinal herbs, dyes, scents, woods, and weaves.

The main part of the book discusses a great many and a wide variety of things that can be made from wild plants. Plants themselves are described as well as the uses made of them. Following are some of the section headings: 1) Ashplants and walking sticks; 2) Balsams; 3) Bamboo pipes; 4) Flax and fibers; 5) Gums and glues; 6) Hop pillows; 7) Lichens as litmus; 8) Reeds and rushes; 9) Toadstools; and 10) Wicker.

Material in the book is interesting history as many curious items are mentioned. Much information is not very practical, however. For instance, a better water jug than one made from fine willow twigs no doubt could be found; few people have need for woven eel traps; and, in the United States, at least, sticky fly paper has not been widely used for 40 or 50 years.

627.   Major, Alan. **Collecting and Studying Mushrooms, Toadstools and Fungi.** Illustrated by Barbara Prescott. New York: Arco Publishing Co., 1975. 268p. illus. (part col.). bibliog. index. $12.00. LC 74-19896. ISBN 0-668-03725-3.

There are said to be over 200,000 species of fungus in the world. More than 290 are described in this book with 200 line drawings and eight color plates for illustration. British, European, and North American species are included. The author points out that fungi have an aura of mystery and fear about them, and, for that reason, he has attempted to show how fascinating they can be.

Chapter 1 is on fungi and their development; Chapter 2 tells how to collect them. The main part of the book lists examples of the plants. About each is given: common name, geographic location, habitat, scientific name, and description. Also provided are a quick glossary of text terms, a spore color aid to classification, and a habitat aid to identification.

This book would serve well as a field guide.

628. Marteka, Vincent. **Mushrooms, Wild and Edible: A Seasonal Guide to the Most Easily Recognized Mushrooms.** New York: Norton, 1980. 290p. illus. (part col.). bibliog. index. $19.95. LC 13910. ISBN 0-393-01356-1.

This is a well-written and nicely illustrated guide to some of the most common edible, and a few poisonous, mushrooms of the United States. (It is important that poisonous species are recognized.)

The book is arranged by collecting season. Included are good recipes for mushroom dishes provided by the author's wife. There are also chapters on preserving mushrooms, finding fungi in stores, and growing mushrooms. In addition, there are lists of amateur mycological societies and sources of supply for growing the fungi.

The book has a good deal of popular appeal.

629. Miller, Orson K., Jr. **Mushrooms of North America.** New York: E. P. Dutton and Co., Inc., 1972. 360p. illus. (part col.). bibliog. index. (A Chanticleer Press edition). $17.95. LC 72-82162. ISBN 0-525-16165-1.

This fine work was prepared by a professor of mycology to satisfy the needs of all types of users, casual observers, amateur mycologists, and students of biology. He has included more than 680 mushroom species, with full descriptions of 422. More than 280 species are illustrated with excellent color photographs, usually in the natural habitat. Also included are simplified drawings that serve as keys to major groups to assist in identification.

After an introductory chapter, individual descriptions are presented, grouped by family. Each section begins with basic information about the family. About each species is usually given: a description including size, shape, texture and color of cap, stalk, gills, ring, veil, and spores; information about growth habitat, chemical reaction of spores, edibility, hallucinogenic properties, frequency, distribution, season of occurrence; alternate names, related species, and notes about taste and cooking (if an edible species). Warnings are given regarding toxic species. Also included are a few recipes, a glossary, and a list of authors who have written about fungi and who are mentioned in the monograph section.

The work, although rather large for a field guide, should be very useful in helping to identify mushroom species. It is important that species be identified correctly as poisonous and edible types often look similar.

630. Orr, Robert T., and Dorothy B. Orr. **Mushrooms and Other Common Fungi of Southern California.** Berkeley, CA: University of California Press, 1968. 91p. illus. (part col.). bibliog. index. (California Natural History Guides: 22). $1.75pa. LC 68-13021.

The geographical area covered by this handbook/guide includes San Luis Obispo, Kern, San Bernardino, Santa Barbara, Ventura, Los Angeles, Riverside, Orange, San Diego, and Imperial counties. The book is designed to assist the amateur in identifying some common woody and fleshy fungi that occur in this area.

The first section discusses characteristics of fungi. A short section on sac fungi follows. The last and longest section covers club fungi. Material presented is condensed, sometimes with only one paragraph devoted to a species. Descriptions are well written, however, and a number of color photographs are included, making identification of common species reasonably easy. Information about habitat, fruiting season, and edibility is included. A short glossary and a checklist to genera and species have been provided. The latter serves as an index.

631.   Orr, Robert T., and Dorothy B. Orr. **Mushrooms of Western North America.** Berkeley, CA: University of California Press, 1979. 293p. illus. (part col.). bibliog. index. (California Natural History Guides: 42). $12.95. LC 77-93468. ISBN 0-520-03656-5.

An extensive geographical area is covered by this work, the Pacific Coast from southern California east through the Rocky Mountains to the western edge of the Great Plains, and north to British Columbia, western Alberta, the Yukon Territory, and Alaska. Full descriptions for 300 species of mushrooms are given, and another 123 are described by comparisons adequate for identification. Color photographs are included for 96 species, and line drawings are also provided.

The first section of the book contains general information on characteristics of fungi, occurrence and habitat, how to collect, nomenclature and classification, and comments on edible, toxic and hallucinogenic mushrooms. The main part of the work is a listing of various fungi by family. The genus is described, then the species. About each is usually given: the name of the person who described the species, distinguishing features, fruiting season, habitat, and edibility. The book also includes a glossary, names of describers of fungi, and a list of western mycological collections and societies.

The book serves well as a field guide, although the authors admit that mushroom hunters frequently find specimens that fail to fit any description in a reference book. This is because some genera contain hundreds of species, and new species, and even genera, are being found all the time. Special monographs will often identify them for the serious student.

632.   Parker, Loni, and David T. Jenkins. **Mushrooms, a Separate Kingdom.** Illustrations and calligraphy by Loni Parker, text by David T. Jenkins. Birmingham, AL: Oxmoor House, 1979. 101p. illus. (col.). bibliog. $16.95. LC 79-88459. ISBN 0-8487-0501-7.

This very fine book is most noteworthy for its artistic features, although the text, which was written by a professor and expert in the taxonomy and nomenclature of mushrooms, is quite authoritative.

The book is illustrated with watercolor paintings of great delicacy that are also biologically accurate. In addition, the text is produced in a script lettering called *fraktur*, which is based on a German Renaissance style.

The text is divided into these sections: 1) The natural history of the mushroom; 2) The edible and the poisonous; 3) Of science and mythology. Emphasis is given to mushrooms in mythology, folklore, and superstition, but general information is also included, such as suggestions for hunting and cooking the plants. Poisonous types are pointed out.

The book has been criticized because it is not clear what function and what audience are served by it. It doesn't help much in identifying and classifying species.

633.   Peterson, Lee. **A Field Guide to Edible Wild Plants of Eastern and Central North America.** Boston, MA: Houghton Mifflin Co., 1978. 330p. illus. (part col.). bibliog. index. (Peterson Field Guide Series). $8.95. LC 77-27323. ISBN 0-395-20445-3.

The author of this valuable guide is the son of Roger Tory Peterson, the bird expert and creator of the field guide approach to studying wild life. It is intended that the user of these guides will take the books into the field to observe or make some use of the wild life. Peterson's view is that one can use wild foods to varying degrees, ranging from living on them entirely to occasionally supplementing regular meals with them. In addition, collecting edible plants gives the forager greater insight into the processes that are taking place around him.

The guide is in three principal sections: 1) The visual and descriptive text; 2) Finding edible plants; and 3) Food uses. The first and largest part contains information necessary for identification, location, and use of plants covered. Each species is illustrated (with a line drawing) on the right-hand page, and a description faces it on the left. Arrangement is by category such as flowering plants, woody plants, and miscellaneous. Flowering plants are organized according to flower color and subdivided into plates according to other characteristics such as shape and position of leaves. Woody plants are arranged according to leaf types.

The second section describes habitats found in eastern North America in rough successional sequence, listing by season the food plants for each habitat. The last section, on food uses, provides general information on food preparation and lists by season the species that fall within each major food-type category.

Nearly 400 species have been included in this outstanding work. There are a number of special features of note. Common poisonous plants that resemble edible ones are pointed out; a glossary has been provided; and the descriptions and illustrations (some colored plates as well as line drawings) are excellent.

634.   Pond, Barbara. **A Sampler of Wayside Herbs: Discovering Old Uses for Familiar Wild Plants.** Illustrated by Edward and Marcia Norman. Riverside, CT: The Chatham Press, 1974. 126p. illus. (part col.). bibliog. index. $17.50. LC 73-89773. ISBN 0-85699-096-5.

The author of this work points out that many plants now called weeds were deliberately brought into this country by our ancestors because of their herbal uses. The book gathers together nearly 100 common herbs that are, for the most part, natives of England or the Continent and that were imported to America and later allowed to grow wild. All can be found in the northeastern United States, and many are prevalent in the mid- and far-western states. There is an index of both common and scientific names.

The book is very attractive, particularly the illustrations of plants in flower. There are 32 full-page watercolor paintings and 60 fine-line pencil drawings. The text gives the history of the plant, its role in literature and legend, and its herbal use in the past. There are recipes for dandelion wine, rose hip jelly, candied sweetflag root, and the like. In addition, information is given on the making of scents, dyes, cosmetics, flavorings, and herbal remedies.

The author has been involved in the commercial production of herbal plants and products.

635.   Smith, Alexander H. **A Field Guide to Western Mushrooms.** Ann Arbor, MI: University of Michigan Press, 1975. 280p. illus. (col.). bibliog. index. $16.50. LC 74-25949. ISBN 0-472-85599-9.

The introduction to this work is a general essay on mushrooms, including systematic classification, techniques of collecting, edibility, poisoning, and habitat. In regard to the latter, the author points out that western United States contains a great diversity of species of fleshy fungi as compared to the rest of the world. Smith, who is a professor of botany and a foremost expert on mushrooms, presents a "key" to selected major groups of fungi. Such a key enables one who is unfamiliar with a particular group of organisms to eliminate, in orderly fashion, all species except one. Other keys to particular genera are included throughout the work.

The main part of the guide presents, by major groups, monographs on various species. For each is given: a color photograph, scientific name of the plant, field identification marks, observations, edibility, when and where to find the plant, and microscopic characters. A glossary has been provided.

This is an excellent presentation, suitable for the beginner as well as for the experienced mushroom hunter. It is particularly valuable for the information on how to sort out edible from inedible or poisonous mushrooms.

636.   Smith, Alexander H. **Mushrooms in Their Natural Habitats.** New York: Hafner Press, 1973. (Repr. of 1949 ed.). 626p. illus. bibliog. index. $14.95. LC 73-76648. ISBN 02-852420-9.

This reprinted work is one volume of a two-volume set. It was written especially to be used with color photographs that were not included in the reprinting. It was felt that the text material, a serious introduction to the study of mushrooms, was needed. There are many popular works with illustrations, photographs particularly.

The author of the book is a noted authority on fleshy fungi. The problem of distinguishing species is primarily dealt with, and very complete descriptive data has been provided in technical fashion. It is important to distinguish edible from inedible or poisonous species.

The introductory chapters are as follows: 1) Mushroom in Relation to Other Living Organisms; 2) The Fruiting Habits of Fleshy Fungi (includes lists of edible and poisonous species); 3) How to Collect Mushrooms and Prepare Speciments; 4) Parts and Characteristics of the Mushroom Fruiting Body Which Can Be Studied without a Microscope; 5) Laboratory Techniques and the Study of Microscopic Characters of Importance; 6) How Mushrooms Are Named; 7) Mycophagy (includes preparing and cooking, recipes, mushroom poisoning, and growing mushrooms); and 8) Short Key to Groups of Fungi. The bulk of the book is a classification of the fungi. Arrangement is by class. About each species is given: a general discussion; edibility; habit, habitat, and distribution; technical description. Also included with the monographs are literature references. A glossary of terms has been provided.

637.   Smith, Alexander H., and Nancy Weber. **The Mushroom Hunter's Field Guide: All Color and Enlarged.** Ann Arbor, MI: University of Michigan Press, 1980. 336p. illus. (col.). bibliog. index. $14.95. ISBN 0-472-85610-3.

First published in 1958, this field guide has been very popular. Smith, who is a leading expert on mushrooms, for years refused to write such a guide because he felt that field characters alone were not sufficient for accurate recognition of the native mushroom species. This is true still, but Smith changed his mind about the matter because he realized many people would persist in fungi collecting for food anyway and a guide might help prevent poisoning. The book includes mushrooms that are easily identified by their pictures, and emphasis is on illustration and field characteristics. When and where to find the species is given as are comments about edibility, quality, and caution.

This is an excellent guide.

638.   Smith, Alexander H., Helen V. Smith, and Nancy S. Weber. **How to Know the Gilled Mushrooms.** Dubuque, IA: Wm. C. Brown Co., 1979. 334p. illus. bibliog. index. (The Pictures Key Nature Series). $8.95. LC 78-69782. ISBN 0-697-04772-5; 0-697-04773-3pa.

This book is a companion volume to one called *How to Know the Non-Gilled Fleshy Fungi.* The senior author is a well-known expert on the subject. Basic techniques of collecting, studying, and preserving fungi are discussed in the other volume and are not repeated in this one in detail. Only a fraction (about 800 species) of gilled mushrooms known from North America are covered in the volume. The authors say selections have been made, for the most part, to include those that can be recognized at sight. They also point out that mushroom flora of North America are not completely known; there are more species in the field than can be found in any work yet written.

There are several introductory chapters as follows: 1) The Parts of a Mushroom; 2) Collecting and Identifying Mushrooms; 3) Mycophagy and Mycotoxins; 4) General Considerations.

The main part of the book presents descriptions of families and species with pictures. Habitat and edibility are indicated. A key or code has been provided for each family, genus and species. An appendix on "Identifying Mushroom Genera by Macroscopic Characters" has been provided as has a glossary (with the index).

639.   Spencer, Edwin Rollin. **All About Weeds.** Illustrated by Emma Bergdolt. New York: Dover Publications, 1974. 333p. illus. bibliog. index. $3.00pa. LC 73-91485. ISBN 0-486-23051-1. (A republication of the expanded edition of the work as published by Charles Scribner's, New York, in 1957 under the title **Just Weeds**).

The author says he wrote this book because there are few weed books that are of any use to the layperson, and many individuals will want to learn something of these plants. He has succeeded in making a mundane subject quite interesting as well as informative.

About 100 common weeds found throughout the U.S. are covered, including some that are used for food or medicine, some that are the bane of hayfever sufferers, poisonous ones, and particularly those that crowd out cultivated plants.

The weeds are discussed in two section: weeds that are grasslike and weeds that are not grasslike. Preceding these two main sections is an "index" of habitat and seasons arranged as follows: weeds of the lawn and yard, weeds of the garden and truck patch, weeds of the meadow and pasture lands, weeds of the corn and cotton fields, weeds of winter wheat and clover fields, weeds of the farm lots, worst weeds of wayside and waste places, weeds of moist and wet places, weeds of spring time, weeds of summer, weeds of autumn, and weeds of winter. There is a final section on weed control.

About each weed the following information is provided: common name; scientific name; synonymous names; a line drawing; a description about a page in length including such information as value (if any); habit and season of growth; how to eradicate the weed; and a technical description.

640.   Stubbs, Ansel Hartley. **Wild Mushrooms of the Central Midwest.** Illustrated with color photographs and with drawings by Chester E. Moore. Lawrence, Manhattan, Wichita, KS: University Press of Kansas, 1971. 135p. illus. (part col.). bibliog. index. $6.95. LC 76-107330. ISBN 0-7006-0067-1.

This small book can serve as a field guide to edible mushrooms of the central midwest. The language is non-technical and descriptions are confined to external characteristics. The author wishes to help rid individuals of unreasonable fear of mushrooms. Many varieties that are used for food bear no resemblance to any poisonous fungi, he says. He hopes Americans will become better acquainted with mushrooms.

The species are grouped by family. A drawing, description, habitat information, and methods of preparation are given for each. In addition, general information is included, and there is a section of recipes and a chart of characteristics to be used for identification purposes.

641.   Stuntz, Daniel E. **How to Identify Mushrooms to Genus, IV: Keys to Families and Genera.** Editorial changes by David L. Largent and Roy Watling. Eureka, CA: Mad River Press (Route 2, Box 151 B, Eureka, CA 95501), 1977. 94p. index. $4.50. ISBN 0-916-422-10-0.

This is a volume in a set of books designed to assist in mushroom identification (for the other volumes see entries 618, 619, 620, 645). It contains two "keys" to assist the student in classification of genera. The first key is called "Relation of Friesian Genera to Singer's Classification"; the second, "Families and Genera Accepted in Modern Classification in Agarics." Along with the key published in the first volume of this series, these keys should prove very useful.

642.   Thiers, Harry D. **California Mushrooms: A Field Guide to the Boletes.** New York: Hafner Press, 1975. 261p. illus. bibliog. index. $15.95. LC 74-11002. ISBN 0-02-853410-7.

The author of this book is a professor of biology and a mycologist. He says Californians are especially interested in mushrooms, some because of the pharmaceutical properties of the plants and others because of culinary characteristics. Thiers thinks fleshy fungi of California had been neglected before his book was produced. The book is designed to assist the amateur and the professional mycologist in identifying boletes in the field without use of a microscope. Most of this group of mushrooms are edible, and 80 species are described.

The presentation is in three parts: 1) About boletes; 2) Taxonomic keys and species descriptions (the bulk of the book); and 3) Field key to California boletes. About each species is given: a detailed description of each part of the mushroom, chemical reactions, habit, habitat, distribution, material studied, observations, and edibility. Documentation is provided, along with lists of places where illustrations appear. A unique feature of the book is its illustrations. A microfiche of 54 color photographs of some of the most important species is inserted in a pocket inside the cover. The reader may use it in the field with a hand lens, or it can be used in a microfiche reader.

643.   Von Frieden, Lucius. **Mushrooms of the World.** With 186 color plates by Laura Maggiora. Translated by Ronald Strom, American edition edited by Carol Sturm Smith. Indianapolis, IN: Bobbs-Merrill, 1969. 439p. illus. (part col.). bibliog. index. $12.95. LC 68-11153. (First published in Italy under the title **I Funghi di Tutti i Paesi**).

This attractive, practical guide identifies 186 mushrooms of the world. Most grow in the United States. Each species is illustrated by an excellent full-color plate.

Introductory material includes how mushrooms live; how to distinguish an edible mushroom; gathering, keeping, and cooking mushrooms; and recipes. Suitable warnings and precautions are given regarding poisonous species. Also, information is provided on naming mushrooms, and a list of mycologists referred to in the book is given.

The main part of the guide lists mushrooms alphabetically by scientific name. Information about each usually includes: edibility (excellent, good, edible, edible with caution, suspect, not advisable, inedible, poisonous, or deadly), a detailed description, habitat, other species possibly confused with the one under consideration, and special notes.

The guide is intended for the amateur mushroom hunter, the naturalist, and the gourmet.

644. Walters, Anthony B., ed. **Mushrooms and Man: An Interdisciplinary Approach to Mycology.** Albany, OR: Linn-Benton Community College, 1978. 310p. illus. (part col.). bibliog. index. $23.50. (Proceedings of the Mushrooms and Man Symposium, held November 4-7, 1977).

This symposium made it possible for a number of groups interested in mushrooms to share knowledge. These groups included mycologists, medical researchers, culinary artists, fungal folklorists, commercial mushroom producers and processors, forest mycological researchers, botanical illustrators, taxonomists, and psychoactive mushroom experts.

Seventeen interesting papers are presented in this book, some by distinguished authorities, e.g., James A. Beard speaking on the culinary uses of mushrooms. Beard also provides recipes for mushroom dishes.

Papers and their authors are as follows: 1) Development of classification of the macrobasidiomycetes (Daniel E. Stuntz); 2) Some difficulties encountered in identifying agarics (Daniel E. Stuntz); 3) Folk uses of mushrooms—medicoreligious aspects (Varro E. Tyler); 4) Mushroom toxicity and medical treatment (Lynn R. Brady and Philip Catalfomo); 5) The use of psychoactive mushrooms in the Pacific Northwest: an ethnopharmacologic report (Andrew T. Weil); 6) The legalities of mushroom experimentation (Richard E. Triska); 7) Getting to know mushrooms and wildflowers—canvas or camera for botanical illustration (Ronald H. Havard); 8) Forest pathology: fungi, forests and man (Everett M. Hansen); 9) The taxonomy, ecology, economics, edibility and toxicity of the boletes (Harry D. Thiers); 10) Ectomycorrhizal fungi and forest practice (Randolph J. Molina); 11) Ectomycorrhizal fungi: interactions of mushrooms and truffles with beasts and trees (James M. Trappe and Chris Maser); 12) The nutritional value of mushrooms (Edward J. Trione and Thomas J. Michaels); 13) Commercial mushroom production (Mickey R. Foley); 14) Prospects for commercial cultivation of alternative mushrooms in the United States (William C. Denison); 15) Foraging for mushrooms (John E. Kelley); 16) The culinary uses of mushrooms (James A. Beard); and 17) Mushroom recipes (James A. Beard).

645. Watling, Roy. **How to Identify Mushrooms to Genus V: Cultural and Developmental Features.** Eureka, CA: Mad River Press (Route 2, Box 151 B, Eureka, CA 95501), 1981? 159p. illus. bibliog. index. $6.95pa. ISBN 0-916422-17-8.

A companion volume to four other titles (see entries 618, 619, 620, 641) this work takes up cultural characters as an aid in the classification and identification of mushrooms and toadstools known as agarics. It documents cultural techniques and discusses such matters as descriptions of asexual stages, poorly known before.

The first part of the book gives recipes for reagents, media, and other materials used in the techniques described, and includes methods of preparation of food materials and basic laboratory technology. The second part describes how to prepare cultures of the fungi, and the third indicates the characteristics exhibited when the mushrooms are in culture. The last section is limited to a discussion of mushrooms and toadstools that carry out their life cycle under artificial conditions.

The book is intended as a student's field guide and as an aid to teachers wishing to study the fungi in the laboratory.

646.   Weldon, L. W., R. D. Blackburn, and D. S. Harrison. **Common Aquatic Weeds.** New York: Dover Publication, 1973. 43p. illus. bibliog. $2.00pa. LC 73-76598. ISBN 0-486-20009-4. (A republication of the 1969 U.S. Department of Agriculture, Agriculture Handbook No. 352).

This book discusses about 50 common aquatic plants that have become weeds in one situation or another in the United States. Some are beautiful, such as the hyacinths, waterlilies, and American lotuses; others are aquarium plants; and still others are edibles. They are found most often in ditches, small ponds, and along lake shores. The plants are rapidly becoming a major problem, although some are desirable in one situation and not in another.

The intent of this work is to aid in identification of the species. The 116 illustrations included are mostly photographs, but some are drawings showing distinguishable characteristics.

Plant monographs are presented in five groups: free-floating plants, aquatic grasses, emersed plants, submersed plants, and algae. About each plant is given: common names, scientific name, description, habitat, distribution, and importance.

647.   Wilkinson, R. E., and H. E. Jaques. **How to Know the Weeds.** 2d ed. Dubuque, IA: Wm. C. Brown Co., 1972. 232p. illus. index. (Pictured Key Nature Series). LC 75-167729. ISBN 0-697-04881-0; 0-697-04880-2pa.

The purpose of this book is to make it easy to identify common weeds of the United States. Although the book does not emphasize the fact, many common weeds are considered by other authors to be herbs and/or edible plants. Slightly less than 400 species of plants are dealt with in this book.

The first section deals with plant names; plant parts; weed reproduction, origins, and dissemination; weed control; and how to use the keys offered in the book to identify weeds. The main section presents short descriptions of plants with key statements, habitat, and a line drawing. Arrangement is by plant family, and scientific and common names are provided. Distribution maps are included in some instances. The last section arranges the weeds in botanical order. The index is unique: it is also a pictured glossary.

A new third edition of the book will soon be available.

648.   Wilson, Charles Morrow. **Roots: Miracles Below.** Garden City, NY: Doubleday and Co., 1968. 234p. illus. bibliog. index. LC 68-17806.

The author of this unusual book is a journalist. He discusses many aspects of plant roots. The aim seems to be to show the vital place roots have had in life from early prehistoric times to the present. Various plants that have valuable roots, particularly those that supply food and those that have unusual root systems, are covered specifically. For the most part, however, roots are discussed in a general way.

Chapter headings are: 1) Miracles beneath Our Feet; 2) Roots Are also for Eating; 3) A Closer Look; 4) Roots of Yesteryear; 5) Scholar with Pick and Shovel; 6) A Table of

Roots; 7) Wanted: Healthier Roots; 8) Better Breeding: Better Roots; 9) Roots and Light; 10) Roots and Chemistry; 11) Roots: Battleground or Sanctuary; and 12) Roots of Tomorrow.

This is a nice book, but more sentimental than scientific.

18

SPICES

Spices and herbs are similar. This chapter lists books that deal with substances that are commonly called spices or flavorings. The history and accounts connected with them have considerable popular appeal. Several works include material about the spice trade, an important aspect of the subject. Recipes are provided in some works.

The work by Furia is especially outstanding as a comprehensive scientific reference work. Parry's books are classics of their kind.

* * * * *

649.   Brobeck, Florence. **Old-Time Pickling and Spicing Recipes.** New York: M. Barrows, 1953. 126p. illus. index. LC 52-5034.

This work contains recipes for the "smaller households," those with little time or space for large quantities of spices and pickles. "In the small kitchen of a busy young mother, business woman, or bachelor cook, the secrets of success (shining filled jars), is to make only a small amount at a time when fruits and vegetables are at their best." One could, however, undoubtedly increase the quantities if desired.

The book begins with general suggestions on pickling and spicing and a list of items needed in the kitchen. There are separate sections of recipes on butters, catsups, chutneys, brandied fruits, pickled and spiced fruits, pickled and spiced vegetables, relishes, sauces, and vinegars. Each section begins with a description and general discussion of the product covered.

650.   Cooper, Elizabeth K. **And Everything Nice: The Story of Sugar, Spice, and Flavoring.** Illustrated by Julie Maas. New York: Harcourt, Brace and World, Inc., 1966. 80p. illus. index. $5.50. LC 66-12588. ISBN 0-15-203498-6.

The author of this charming work is a noted writer of science books for children. She tells the history and stories connected with popular flavorings such as chocolate, vanilla, sugar, pepper, and mustard. Also included are a few simple recipes a youngster could follow.

Following are chapter titles: 1) Ice Cream, Gingerbread, Cinnamon Buns, and Candy; 2) Chocolate, Cocoa, and Cacao Trees; 3) The Mystery of Vanilla; 4) Pepper—Black, White, and Red; 5) The Cinnamon Monsters; 6) Little Nails from the Spice Islands (cloves); 7) The Little Nut Tree (nutmeg); 8) Mustard for Hot Dogs; 9) Gingerbread and Ginger; 10) The Most Expensive Spice in the World (saffron); and 11) Sugars from Plants, Trees, and Bees. Illustrations included are nice delicate line drawings. The book should appeal especially to young people from grades three to seven.

651.   Furia, Thomas E., and Nicoló Bellanca, eds. **Fenaroli's Handbook of Flavor Ingredients.** 2d ed. Adapted from the Italian language work. Cleveland, OH: CRC Press, 1975. illus. bibliog. index. 2v. $129.90. LC 72-152143. ISBN 0-87819-533-5.

The subject treated in these large volumes is viewed by many as a mystery, at times suggestive of alchemy. However, sophisticated analytical techniques are fully utilized by chemists in the field to resolve flavor components and to elucidate structures, and also as product control measures. The flavor (and fragrance) industry is highly interdisciplinary and includes analytical, organic, physical, and natural products chemistry; botany; food technology; and several other fields, even the artistic efforts of the flavorist.

There are about 1,200 flavor ingredients used in the United States. Approximately 200 are well-characterized products of natural origin, and about 1,000 others are precisely defined synthetics. The scope of this publication is to present an authoritative, current description of natural and synthetic flavor ingredients with their characteristics and application in food.

The first part of volume 1 is a 264-page section of "General Considerations," presenting some highly technical material. In a historical section, the evolution of flavor ingredients is summarized as follows: 1) the direct addition of dried herbs and spices to food; 2) the extraction and concentration of active ingredients of dried herbs and spices and the blending of these to imitate natural flavors; 3) the formulation of compounded flavorings; 4) the combining of extracts and synthetic products to imitate additional natural flavor ingredients and to formulate non-existing types; and 5) the rebuilding of natural flavor ingredients and precursors through identification and synthesis of components.

The second section of volume 1 lists natural flavors alphabetically with the following information given: other names, botanical source, botanical family, foreign names, description, part of plant used, physical-chemical characteristics (essential oil, derivatives), organoleptic characteristics, uses, and regulatory status (safety). Products listed are familiar to people interested in herbs and spices.

Volume 2 of the set lists synthetic flavors and includes chemical data such as formula, structure, physical-chemical characteristics, synthesis, and regulatory status. The last section is on uses of flavor ingredients in foods.

Long bibliographies are provided throughout this excellent, highly technical scientific work.

652.   Hayes, Elizabeth S. **Spices and Herbs Around the World.** Illustrations by J. M. Yeatts. Garden City, NY: Doubleday, 1961. 266p. illus. bibliog. index. LC 61-12527. (Reprinted under the title: **Spices and Herbs, Lore and Cookery.** New York: Dover Publication, 1980. $3.50pa. LC 80-66063. ISBN 0-486-24026-6).

This is a readable work for the home user of spices, herbs, and other seasonings. Emphasis is on food seasoning rather than on medicinal uses.

There are separate sections for spices, herbs, beverages (coffee, tea, and cocoa), salt, and sugar. Fifteen spices and 77 herbs are covered. Each entry includes both the common and scientific name, an interesting history on trade, perhaps a reference to Gerard's *The Herbal or General History of Plants* (see entry 150; one chapter includes the dedication of the *Herbal*), a description of the plant, parts of plant used, its uses, and a simple line drawing. Of special interest are recipes that are scattered throughout the work. At the end of each section there is a list of the herbs and spices, giving again their uses. At the close of the herb section is a guide to growing herbs, some garden designs, and material on harvesting and preserving.

653.   International Symposium on Spices and Medicinal Plants. **First International Symposium on Spices and Medicinal Plants, Freising-Weihenstephan, Fed. Rep. Germany, 31 July - 4 August 1977.** The Hague: International Society for Horticultural Science, 1978. 341p. illus. (Acta Horticulturae; Technical Communication of ISHS, No. 73).

This work contains the proceedings of the first symposium of the working group 'Spices and Medicinal Plants' of the International Society for Horticultural Science. The stated goal of the working group is to "improve the cultivation of such plants, to increase the contents of active substances, and to contribute to the continuous supply of high quality drugs."

There were approximately 90 participants from 20 different countries at the symposium. More than 40 papers were presented, most in English. Since participants were horticulturists, the main emphasis of the papers is on breeding and production of plants. Effects of fertilization, irrigation, selection, and weed and pest control on the yield of certain compounds from specific plants are typical subjects covered. This work is of most interest to the professional horticulturist.

654.   Parry, J. W. **The Spice Handbook: Spices, Aromatic Seeds and Herbs.** Brooklyn, NY: Chemical Publishing Co., 1945. 254p. illus. index.

This work was written to provide an informative handbook on the description and identification of spices, aromatic seeds, and herbs for those involved with the trade. Part 1 consists of two chapters of extracts from the pure food laws and regulations of the U.S. and Canada. Much of this material is now out of date. Parts 2 to 4 of the book are descriptive sections on spices, aromatic seeds, and herbs, respectively. Each description includes: common names, botanical name, family, nativity and cultivation, botanical description, properties, uses, adulteration, grinding, packing, starch content, essential oils, government standards, and black and white photographs. Plants described under spices are allspice, cinnamon, cassia, clover, ginger, mace, nutmeg, black and white pepper, red pepper, cayenne, chillies, paprika, and turmeric. The aromic seeds include anise, cardamom, caraway, celery, cumin, coriander, dill, fennel, fenugreek, mustard, poppy, sesame, and star anise. Herbs discussed are laurel leaves, marjoram, mint, origanum, parsley, rosemary, sage, savory, sweet basil, and thyme. Garlic and onion powders are listed separately. Part 5 is on spice formulae such as curry powder, mincemeat spice, pumpkin pie spice, and frankfurter seasoning. Included in the appendix are materials of interest in the spice trade such as contracts of the American Spice Trade Association, a table of distances between ports, differences in standard time, a glossary, and foreign weights.

Although some material included in the work is out of date, much of it is basic and still of value.

655.   Parry, John W. **Spices. v.1, The Story of Spices; The Spices Described.** New York: Chemical Publishing Co., 1969. 235p. illus. bibliog. index. $15.00.

This small volume is in two sections. The first section is an account of the history of spices and spice trading from ancient times to the present. Topics covered are spices in the ancient world, the Bible, the ancient Middle East, Arabia, Ancient Greece and Rome, the early Christian era, the Middle Ages, and Portugal. Also discussed are the contributions of Marco Polo, John Cabot, Magellan, Sir Francis Drake, the British, the Dutch, and America in the pepper trade. Uses of spices in the modern world are covered.

The second part of the book describes 37 spices individually. Photographs are provided. About each spice is given: plant source, description, countries producing, method of preparation or production, cultivation, description of taste, and uses.

The book has been well received and is suitable for general use. Botanical terms have been avoided as much as possible. Emphasis is on commercial spices available. There is not much information to help the amateur grow or gather spices and herbs. Volume 2 of the two-volume set is on morphology, histology and chemistry.

656. Rosengarten, Frederic, Jr. **The Book of Spices.** Rev. and abridged for this edition. New York: Pyramid Books, 1973. 475p. illus. (part col.). bibliog. index. $1.95pa. ISBN 0-515-03220-4.

This non-technical work was written by an executive of a spice-producing firm. Information is given on about 40 products, including their history, folklore, and place in the modern world. Medicinal uses of the products are mentioned, and the fact that some have had former uses is indicated.

The book begins with a section of about 100 pages of historical material. The main part of the book is an alphabetically arranged listing (by common name) of spices. Each monograph is several pages and includes scientific name of the plant, names in 11 different languages, an illustration of the plant and/or parts of it, and a rather complete discussion of the spice. In addition, several recipes are included with each listing.

The book gives comprehensive coverage of various spices and is quite nicely done in all respects. All important and common spices are included, most which are familiar to the average cook. The recipes are particularly appealing.

657. Verrill, A. Hyatt. **Perfumes and Spices: Including an Account of Soap and Spices.** Boston, MA: L. C. Page and Co., 1940. 304p. illus. (part col.). index.

Although an older work, this book still has a great deal of appeal. It is "the story of the history, source, preparation, and use of the spices, perfumes, soaps, and cosmetics which are in everyday use." The author says of all the material discussed spices are the most interesting and romantic because no other article of commerce has had such a romantic history or such an important part in international trade, exploration, and the spread of civilization. The perfume industry, though, is probably more technical and diversified.

Contents of the book is as follows: 1) The romance of spices; 2) A good deed well done (a true story of the New England spice trade); 3) Spices and what they are; 4) Hot stuff (on pepper and other hot spices); 5) Spices of the New World; 6) The spice that is not a spice (vanilla); 7) Perfumes past and present; 8) Perfume side lights; 9) Fields of fragrance (perfume plants); 10) What is a perfume?; 11) Mysterious ambergris; 12) How perfumes are made; 13) Synthetic and artificial perfumes; 14) The perfume of the gods (incense); 15) Beautifiers and cosmetics; 16) Cosmetics and what they are; 17) The dawn of soap; 18) Soapy fact; and 19) Soap in the making. An appendix defines the terms used in connection with perfumes, spices, cosmetics, and soaps.

19
COSMETICS

There has been recent interest in cosmetics made at home from herbs and other "natural" materials. It is possible to manufacture simple, usable cosmetics in the kitchen, although it is unlikely that they will have the elegance of commercial products. The cosmetics industry is highly developed.

This chapter contains a mixture of scientific or technical books and popular do-it-yourself works on cosmetic production. Perfumes are covered as well as other cosmetic products. Some books contain a good deal of history.

* * * * *

658. Aguilar, Nona. **Totally Natural Beauty: The Natural Beauty Treatment Book.** New York: Rawson Associates Publishers, Inc., 1977. 289p. index. $10.95. LC 76-53296. ISBN 0-89256-009-6.

This book presents material about health and how to improve one's appearance. It includes, in addition, over 100 recipes for beauty products said to be "natural" (built around "natural" foods and other "natural" substances). The presentation is in several sections: 1) Skin; 2) Hair; 3) Diet; 4) Eyes; 5) Hands and feet; 6) Mouth and teeth; and 7) Body-all.

Most products described are not appealing. Nearly all contain foods, for example, oatmeal, tomatoes, lemon, buttermilk, mayonnaise, vinegar, and eggs. Claims made for the concoctions are doubtful; the evidence provided is not convincing or sensible in many instances. References are frequently made to works of little merit, popular rather than scientific. There are better books on home-made cosmetics than this one.

659. Arctander, Steffen. **Perfume and Flavor Materials of Natural Origin.** Elizabeth, NJ: the author, 1960. 736p. illus. (part col.). index.

The author of this dictionary-handbook is a perfumer and flavorist who produced the work with the assistance of the University Extension Division, Rutgers, the State University of New Jersey and the perfume and flavor industry.

The book is in dictionary format in two separate sections. The first section, "Definitions and Methods of Processing," is the shortest (47 pages). The second section, "Monographs on Raw Materials," makes up most of the book. Odors and flavors of the raw materials of nature are described. Use of the materials, appearance, source, evaluation, constituents, the replacement of one material for another, proportional strength, availability, processing, world production figures, and other miscellaneous information is provided in the definitions. Many substances are included, and the treatment is rather comprehensive. Literature sources are usually not given; the author says he checked information personally and provided only practical material—perhaps a weakness of the book since it includes a good deal of data, for instance, production figures.

There are several tables on world production and location of centers of production. Also, there is a list that groups natural materials according to odor type and suggested use. A general index and a "French-German-Spanish Condensed Index" similar to a polyglot foreign language dictionary is appended. The book is illustrated with good photographs of production machinery and of plants, some in color and in flower.

As the author correctly points out, the perfume and flavor trade has been veiled and concealed for many decades, if not for centuries. Perfumers have preferred to keep their art to themselves. Arctander hopes his book will contribute to a wider knowledge of perfumes and flavors from nature. It is, in any case, a fascinating compilation.

660.   Billot, Marcel, and F. V. Wells. **Perfumery Technology; Art: Science: Industry.** New York: Halsted Press, a Division of John Wiley and Sons, 1975. 353p. illus. bibliog. index. $49.95. LC 75-5768. ISBN 0-470-07298-9.

This is a rather comprehensive compendium of information on the nature and practice of perfumery. It was the intent of the authors, who are leading authorities in France and Great Britain, to treat the subject in such a way as to appeal to the interested layperson as well as to the experienced perfumer. They have succeeded. There is a balance between the practical and the theoretical in this book. Perfumer's raw materials are classified and described, and formulas provided serve as guidelines to individual effort.

Contents of the book is as follows: 1) The study and practice of perfumery; 2) Historical and biographical (perfume in the ancient world is discussed as is the Japanese incense cult); 3) The perfumer's raw materials: products of natural origin (discusses concrete oils, absolute oils, essential oils derived from distillation, essential oils obtained by expression, isolates from essential oils, natural odorants as tinctures, balsams and resins, rose and other natural odorants); 4) Products of natural origin (continued) (an alphabetically arranged list of essential oils, terpeneless oils); 5) Products of natural origin (continued) (discusses tinctures, resins, balsams); 6) The perfumer's raw materials: products of synthetic origin (includes descriptions and an alphabetically arranged list); 7) Classification of odours and odorants; 8) Creating a perfume; 9) Formulary section: flower perfumes (describes and provides formulas for rose bases and perfumes, jasmin perfumes, orangeflower and neroli, violet bases and perfumes. Also lists flower perfumes arranged alphabetically); 10) Formulary section: sophisticated or fantasy perfumes (includes formulas with discussion); 11) Colognes: eaux de toilette; perfumes for men; 12) Olfaction and gustation; 13) Perfumes for many purposes (includes perfumes for soap, disinfectants, the air, cosmetics, aerosols, medicine, and flavors as perfumes); 14) Packaging and marketing; and 15) Perfumery as a career.

The book can serve as a reference work for the professional perfumer and is also valuable as a text for the trainee.

661.   Buchman, Dian Dincin. **The Complete Herbal Guide to Natural Health and Beauty.** Garden City, NY: Doubleday and Co., Inc., 1973. 221p. illus. index. $2.95pa. LC 73-79653. ISBN 0-385-08815-9.

This book contains a large number of recipes for cosmetic products' that the author says she has collected from her grandmother, the works of famous herbalists, and diaries of great beauties such as Marie Antoinette, the Duchess of Alba, and Lady Hamilton.

Chapter headings are: 1) How to Use Herbs (contains a chart on ways of using dried herbs); 2) Skin; 3) Bathing; 4) Hair; 5) Eyes; 6) Mouth and Teeth; 7) Hands; 8) Feet; 9) Sleep; 10) Perfumes; 11) Collecting and Drying Herbs; 12) Sources; and 13) Botanical, Pharmaceutical, Food Usage Chart.

This is a better collection of cosmetic recipes than is often found in such books. Exaggerated claims are not made regarding usefulness, and most cosmetics are likely of value for the purpose stated. Modern commercial cosmetics are similar in many instances. Ingredients needed may be difficult to obtain, so a list of manufacturers, shops, and other sources have been provided in chapter 12. The book is well written and can be recommended for those interested.

662.   Cooley, Arnold J. **The Toilet and Cosmetic Arts in Ancient and Modern Times: With a Review of All the Different Theories of Beauty and Copious Allied Information, Social, Hygienic, and Medical.** London: Robert Hardwicke, 1866; repr. New York: Burt Franklin, 1970. 804p. index. (Research and Source Series. No. 511). $43.00. LC 78-80248. ISBN 0-8337-0653-5.

The intent of the author of this volume was to present a useful and practical work rather than a learned, showy, or sensational one, and to address society at large rather than any special group. The subject is covered comprehensively, beginning with historical information and concluding with formulas for producing cosmetic products. The formulas were (and still are) suitable for those uninitiated in chemical manipulations.

Chapter headings are as follows: 1) Introductory Remarks; 2) Early Ages; 3) The Jews; 4) Egypt, Assyria, Babylonia, Persia, etc.; 5) Greece, Carthage, Sicily, Rome; 6) Middle Ages; 7) Modern Nations—England; 8) France, Germany, Italy, the East, Turkey, Persia, Russia, China; 9) Semicivilized Nations—Savage Tribes—Conclusion; 10) Beauty: Its Constituents and Sources—Hypotheses and Opinions—Personal Beauty—Ideal Beauty—German Art and Sculptures, etc.; 11) Promotion and Preservation of the Personal Appearance and Beauty—Common Errors—Influence of Health, etc.; 12) Clothing—Dress—Jewelry; 13) Cleanliness—Ablution—Bathing—Baths, etc.; 14) The Skin: Its Beauty, Uses, Construction, Management, etc.; 15) The Hair: Its Estimation, Structure, Growth, Management, etc.; 16) The Head, Face, Trunk, Limbs, etc., and Their Subdivisions, Separately Considered; 17) Cosmetics: Their Classification, Preparation, etc.—Formulae, Directions, Cautions; 18) Perfumes, Perfumery, Formulae, Directions, etc.; and 19) Certain Substances Employed in Cosmetics, Perfumes, etc.—Supplemental Notices, and Formulae Previously Referred to—Miscellaneous Formulae, etc.—Conclusion.

663.   Gjerde, Mary. **Organic Make-Up.** Los Angeles, CA: Nash Publishing, 1971. 124p. $1.95pa. LC 79-172421. ISBN 0-8402-8003-3.

The purpose of this book is to point out "organic" beauty preparations that can be found in the kitchen, "natural" materials for beauty. Statements are made that commercial cosmetic products are made of synthetic ingredients that are harmful, that "organic" materials contain substances that cannot be duplicated by chemistry, and that "natural" substances are made up of botanical and biological materials that are neither toxic nor irritating. All of these statements are false or are at least misleading. The term "organic" has been used incorrectly; it means something else to a chemist or any other scientist. Many organic materials can be synthesized. "Natural" substances are not necessarily less toxic than synthetics, and commercial products do not necessarily use synthetic ingredients.

The book contains material on skin care, recipes for creams, cleansers, fresheners, eye lotions and washes, hair dye, perfumes, depilatories, and insect lotions. Herbs and vitamins are discussed briefly.

The book contains a good deal of nonsense with some good advice.

664.   Huxley, Alyson. **Natural Beauty with Herbs.** Foreword by Muriel, Lady Dowding. Illustrated by Linda Diggins. London: Dartman, Longman and Todd, 1977. 95p. illus. (part col.). (Herbwise 5). $3.00pa. LC 78-310924. ISBN 0-232-51388-0.

After an interesting discussion of the history of herbal cosmetics, the major part of this book is dedicated to herbal cosmetic preparations.

Specific formulas and directions for making cosmetics at home are given for the following uses: hair, eyes, teeth-mouth-lips, face, body, sunbathing, hands and nails, feet, floral waters and colognes, and sleep. Included are all kinds of soaps, oils, and lotions.

Other brief sections on drying and storing herbs, and on terminology and processing methods are also included. British Commonwealth herb suppliers (with addresses) are listed. The work is a brief, practical introduction to herbal cosmetics.

The author uses no animal products as ingredients in her recipes because she believes such products are often obtained in cruel ways. Also, she believes plant products are superior (a view not necessarily founded on scientific evidence). She is opposed to any testing that requires the use of laboratory animals. This is unnecessary anyway, she says, because people have experimented on themselves throughout history.

665.   James, Ronald W. **Fragrance Technology: Synthetic and Natural Perfumes.** Park Ridge, NJ: Noyes Data Corporation, 1975. 305p. index. (Chemical Technology Review No. 42). $36.00. LC 74-21492. ISBN 0-8155-0558-2.

The review of this book has been included to put perfumery in proper perspective. The work supplies detailed, descriptive information on the manufacture of synthetic and natural perfumes based on U.S. patent literature since 1964. It presents an advanced and technically oriented review of commercial fragrances and helps provide background for individuals contemplating research in the field.

The introduction to the book points out that only some 50 years ago perfumes were restricted to the rich and sophisticated. Today, through great progress by the chemical research community, fine perfumes are available to all. This advance has been made possible because components of many natural fragrances have been identified and duplicated synthetically at relatively reasonable cost. Also, today the supply of fragrances is almost limitless with less than five per cent coming directly from natural sources, and the perfumer can develop fragrances far in excess of those found in nature.

The book describes over 240 processes relating to all phases of the manufacture of perfume. The chemistry presented will not be understandable to the general reader, but the view of the field is enlightening and interesting. Material is arranged to reflect the major types of perfumes. The contents is as follows: 1) Woody fragrances (sandalwood, cedarwood, vetiver, ambergrisionones, and woody-general); 2) Mush fragrances (naphthalene and indene derivatives, dihydrocoumarins, Cedarwood oil derivatives, ambrette oil, and other processes; 3) Floral fragrances (jasmine, rose, rose oxide, violet, lily of the valley, lilac, lavender, geranium, and general floral); 4) Other fragrances (fruit-like, watermelon, apple, peach, citrus, camphor, minty, tobacco, peppermint, caramel, and miscellaneous specific fragrances); 5) General processes; and 6) Product application (detergents and cleaning products, odor prolongation, and other product applications). There are company, inventor, and U.S. patent number indexes.

666.   Jesse, Jill. **Perfume Album.** 2d ed. New York: Beauty Data (45 W. 9th St., New York, NY 10011), 1965. 188p. illus. bibliog. index.

This book discusses materials from all over the world from which perfumes are made. Anecdotes and historical information are provided as well as more practical information. The work is definitely intended for the general reader; probably the author has gone a bit too far in attempting to make the work popular in appeal. Some material is chatty and frivolous and adds nothing to the knowledge of perfume.

Contents is as follows: 1) Flowers (rose, jasmin, orangeflower, ylang ylang, violet, narcissus, jonquil, hyacinth, tuberose, acacia, cassie, mimosa, gardenia, carnation, muguet, lilac, and frangipani); 2) Grasses (lemongrass, citronella, gingergrass, and palmarosa); 3) Spices and herbs (ajowan to vanilla, costus and clary sage, lavender and rosemary); 4) Citrus products (orange, bergamot, lemon, lime, and petitgrain); 5) Woods (Sandalwood, cedarwood, and rosewood); 6) Leaves and roots (patchouli, geranium, vetivert, and orris); 7) Gums and balsams (labdanum, myrrh, galbanum, olibanum, benzoin, opopanax, storax, balsam Peru, and balsam Tolu; 8) Lichen (oakmoss); 9) Animal products (castoreum, civet, musk, ambergris). Appended are a glossary and a chart of perfume raw materials.

667.   Krochmal, Connie. **A Guide to Natural Cosmetics.** New York: Quadrangel/ The New York Times Book Co., 1973. 227p. illus. bibliog. index. $8.95. LC 73-77028. ISBN 0-8129-0362-5.

This book is made up almost entirely of formulas for cosmetic preparations that consist primarily of "natural" ingredients. There are two preliminary chapters on the history of cosmetic use and development, and methods and materials used by the author in compounding her products. Fifteen chapters follow, each on a different category of product, including: lotions, bath preparations, creams, colognes and perfumes, complexion washes, face preparations, hair preparations, conditioners, massage creams, nail preparations, sachets, shaving preparations, soaps, suntan lotions and creams, and toothpastes, powders, and mouth washes. In addition, there are several short appended sections: descriptions of natural materials used in formulas, essential oils, animal products, some sources of materials, definitions, preparing alcohol of varying strengths, and some astringent plants.

The work is intended as a recipe book for the preparation of cosmetic products by the layperson. Formulas use familiar household measurements and utilize kitchen equipment. Ingredients are reasonably familiar products.

The book is of interest as a historical work, perhaps, but many products are probably too primitive for people accustomed to modern cosmetics. In addition, the work has been criticized because ingredients are listed that are known to cause allergic reactions, sensitivities, or irritation and are seldom used now in commercial products. The author seems to have few qualifications for compiling such a book other than a hobby interest in the subject.

668.   Nature's Gate, A Division of Levlad, Inc. **Herbal Cosmetics and Herbal Glossary.** Chatsworth, CA: Nature's Gate (9740 Cozycraft Ave., Chatsworth, CA 91311), 1980? 20p. illus.

This small publication lists cosmetic products manufactured by Nature's Gate, products which are said to be authentic herbal creations, containing pure and natural, fresh-cured extractions of herbs and plants blended for a particular hair or skin application, and all naturally fragrant, organic, pH balanced, and biodegradable. About half the publication is a glossary of ingredients, listing and defining materials used in the company's products. A note on the use of preservatives says that only "natural" preservatives are used in the products, but that it is necessary to use such materials to prevent bacterial contamination.

669.   Rose, Jeanne. **The Herbal Body Book.** New York: Grosset and Dunlap, 1976. 400p. illus. bibliog. index. $8.95; $4.95pa. LC 75-27402. ISBN 0-488-12260-X; 0-448-12242-1pa.

A rather thorough guide to making herbal cosmetics, this work contains hundreds of recipes for the skin, hair, nails, face, and body.

The book is in four main parts: 1) Directions (plants and their external uses, descriptions of plants, collecting and storing cosmetic plants and equipment, etc.); 2) The recipes (divided into separate sections according to the part of the body involved); 3) "The extra-special make-your-body-feel-good day"; and 4) "Cosmetics used in magic."

In the first part about 400 herbal plants are described and illustrated with information on cosmetic applications. Sources for buying basic ingredients are included in the book.

670.   Rose, Jeanne. **Kitchen Cosmetics: Using Herbs, Fruits, and Eatables in Natural Cosmetics.** Botanical drawings and cover art by Annetta Gunter. San Francisco, CA: Panjandrum/Aris Books, 1978. 128p. illus. bibliog. index. $4.98pa. LC 77-17077. ISBN 0-915572-25-7.

Only "natural" ingredients should be used in order to have beautiful, wholesome looking skin, the author of this book maintains. And, of course, many ingredients to create this attractive skin are found in the kitchen among foods.

Simple recipes are provided for a range of products. Also given are instructions for making herb teas and soups that are said to help in beautifying the skin through internal avenues. The text, which is illustrated with line drawings of various herbs and plants, is presented in sections pertaining to various parts of the body.

671.   Sanderson, Liz. **How to Make Your Own Herbal Cosmetics: The Natural Way to Beauty.** New Canaan, CT: Keats Publishing, 1979. 109p. illus. bibliog. index. $4.95pa. LC 78-65301. ISBN 0-87983-190-1.

Brief articles on how to prepare herbs (e.g., tinctures, infusions) how to dry and keep herbs, and the ways herbs are used for cosmetic purposes introduce the reader to this book.

Following these initial articles, specific herbs and recipes are given along with exact applications of each. "Old time" uses and some historical notes are also included under each category. (Many of the uses have been included mainly as curiosities.) Categories range from face creams to slimming, with 21 categories in all. All information given is practical, and most ingredients used are readily available.

Herbs mentioned in the recipes are also listed alphabetically by common name. With each entry is included the scientific name, some historical notes, cultivation hints, and general uses other than for cosmetic purposes.

A list of herb suppliers (with addresses) has been provided. Generally speaking, this is a nice introduction to herbal cosmetics, although, as is the case with many similar publications, there are quite a few concoctions mentioned one would not care to try.

672.   Traven, Beatrice. **The Complete Book of Natural Cosmetics.** Cosmetic formulations by Robert L. Goldemberg. New York: Simon and Schuster, 1974. 154p. illus. $7.65. LC 74-3247. SBN 671-21769-0.

The intent of this book is to instruct on how to make "natural" cosmetics, defined here as those that do not contain certain emulsifiers and preservatives other than alcohol.

Chapter headings are: 1) Equipment; 2) Ways and Means; 3) Fine and Picky Points to Ponder; 4) Fruit and Vegetable Cosmetics; 5) Teas and Herbs; 6) The Richness of Oils; 7) Nuts and Seeds and Grains; 8) Milk, Cream, Butter, and Yogurt; 9) Beauty and the Bees; 10) Good-Earth Products; 11) Gums and Thickeners, or How to Make Milk into "Cream"; 12) Other "Mothers"; and 13) Natural Perfumes. A glossary of 26 pages is included.

There are about 60 basic recipes for a variety of products such as perfumes, cold creams, bath oils and powders, astringents, hair conditioners, soaps, baby oils, lotions, facial masks, shampoos, and other products. Basic materials used for the cosmetics include honey, flower petals, herbs, cocoa butter, fruits, lanolin, various oils, and spices.

Traven is an author and dramatist; Goldenberg is a cosmetic chemist. For those interested in the subject, this is a good book.

673.   Traven, Beatrice, with the assistance of Ferenc Tibor. **Here's Egg on Your Face.** Old Tappan, NJ: Hewitt House, 1970. 192p. index. $5.95. LC 73-112452.

This is a how-to-do-it book on making cosmetics. The senior author is a cosmetic user, and Dr. Tibor is a cosmetic chemist who has tested the recipes given. Included are recipes for making perfume (from flowers and herbs), colognes, aftershaves, and refreshers; masks and oatmeal scrubs; eye creams, foundations, and moisture creams; shampoos, deodorants, and suntan lotions. Ingredients called for are said to be readily available, which seems to be true. There are chapters on tools of the trade, tricks of the trade, and a note about preservatives. The last chapter is on base stocks, such as soap stock, beeswax base, paraffin wax base, suspension jelly, and mother bases. An appendix lists cosmetic ingredients that may be mentioned in the book.

The work does not make extravagant claims for the virtues of home or "natural" cosmetic products. Lower price is mentioned frequently, however. Recipes do not contain added preservatives, but some contain materials that serve as preservatives (such as alcohol). It is pointed out that like foods, the products listed will tend to spoil eventually, and fresh batches should be made frequently.

20

Material in many of these books reads like something written a century or so past. Indeed, much material was revived from early works, and the treatments sound quite primitive when compared to modern medical practices and techniques.

The recent popular interest in unconventional (often called "alternative") medical systems has grown up at least partly because the media have been so critical of our health care institutions and practitioners. Many unconventional systems emphasize self-treatment, and, in addition, the prevention of disease is stressed.

Many systems discussed in the books of this chapter rely on herbal medicine or other systems called "natural." A prevailing philosophy that permeates much of the thinking seems to be that some spiritual as well as physical good comes from the use of herbal plants and other "natural" therapies.

Systems of medicine treated in the following works include: water therapy, herbal medicine, acupuncture, holistic (wholistic), natura, Thomsonian, homeopathic, iridology, chiropractic, naturomatic, biochemic, and some merely called "natural."

Holistic medicine has perhaps received the most attention as an "alternate" or "natural" system. It focuses on the "whole" individual by considering body, mind, and spirit. Many books have religious overtones; faith healing is considered; and a recurring theme is that ordinary people are responsible for health, not doctors, nurses, or hospitals. Use of plant remedies and home remedies is often encouraged.

The concept of holistic medicine is not well understood by the public. Some think of it as traditional medicine with a back-to-basics slant, treating the whole patient instead of just the disease. Others think of it as a medical fad, on par with foot reflexology or iridology. The books listed here show that both groups are somewhat correct. It isn't quite clear just what the "holistic" label means.

It is interesting that there has been a resurgence of interest in homeopathic medicine. Kaufman's book is a good assessment of the movement that began in the 1820s and was doomed to disappear by the 1960s, according to Kaufman's calculations.

Acupuncture, an ancient Chinese practice, has attracted interest among both lay and professional groups. There is agreement that it holds some promise in medicine, particularly in anesthesia, but its underlying basis of action is not understood at this time.

Other systems treated in this chapter, with the exception of the herbal and chiropractic, have not received as much attention as holistic medicine and acupuncture.

* * * * *

674.   Buchman, Dian Dincin. **The Complete Book of Water Therapy**. Illustrated by Blanche Fried. New York: Dutton, 1979. 240p. illus. index. $12.95; $8.95pa. LC 78-18243. ISBN 0-525-93092-2; 0-525-93093-0pa.

Subtitled "500 Ways to Use Our Oldest Natural Medicine," this book outlines ways water may be used therapeutically. Internal and external uses are covered as is the combination of water with herbs. Step-by-step instructions are included with various therapies as are illustrations to clarify treatments. Among the conditions said to be improved by water therapy are acne, arthritis, headaches, insomnia, nervousness, and fatigue.

675.   Cerney, J. V. **Handbook of Unusual and Unorthodox Healing Methods**. West Nyack, NY: Parker Publishing Co., 1976. 217p. illus. index. $8.95. LC 75-23270. ISBN 0-13-382739-7.

Each chapter of this book is devoted to a method of treatment considered unconventional in medicine today. Following are chapter titles: 1) "Z" Zone Alarm Points (trigger point therapy); 2) New Health through Herbs; 3) Magic Minerals Called "Cell Salts"; 4) Raw Juices and Concentrated Liquid Health; 5) Fasting; 6) Somatherapy and the Magic of Soft-Tissue Manipulation to Relieve Pain; 7) Cupping and Skin-Rolling for Pain Relief; 8) Concussion, Percussion and Vibration; 9) Healing with White Clay Packs; and 10) Aquatonics, the Water Way to Health.

The only evidence usually given for the effectiveness of these treatments is a case history or personal testimony.

676.   Chai, Mary Ann P. **Herb Walk Medicinal Guide**. Provo, UT: The Gluten Co., Inc. (Box 482-G, Provo, UT 84601), 1978. 127p. illus. bibliog. index.

The purpose of this book is "to present a foundation upon which ordered healing may be logically explained, accurately determined, and consistently validated. It will of necessity, involve the reader to very likely view himself and his universe by standards he has heretofore been unaware of, or organized in." In order to accomplish the above, the author has provided in the first chapter a "brief stimulative presentation of the philosophy of the nature and purpose of man." Included is a philosophy chart that makes a comparison among "the three major healing philosophies" of today. These are allopathic medicine (conventional medicine), eclecticism philosophy, and holistic philosophy. The author prefers the latter and has provided a reading list of supportive literature.

Chapter 2, on modifying factors, deals with biological rhythms, chemical pollution, social interactions, personal management, and congenital defects. Chapter 3, on physiology and therapeutic action, defines terminology and discusses nine systems of the body with diagrams to show their location. The next two chapters provide guidelines on gathering or buying herbs and for administering and formulating herbal medicines. Chapter 6 is an herb list with correlated therapeutic actions. Chapter 7 is on first aid (using herbs), and the last chapter is a glossary.

The book could conceivably serve as a self-care manual for those interested in an alternative, holistic, herbal medical treatment system.

677.   Christopher, John R. **School of Natural Healing**. Provo, UT: BiWorld Publications, Inc. (P. O. Box 62, Provo, UT 84601), 1976. 653p. bibliog. index. $39.95. ISBN 0-89557-010-6.

Intended for the teacher, student, or herbal practitioner, the contents of this volume was originally part of a series of lectures given by the author to groups interested in natural healing.

Christopher's introduction is liberally sprinkled with references to God, the scriptures, and doctrine of the Mormon Church. He suggests going back to the old forms of healing—"in the natural manner as the Lord intended."

The first chapter of 50 pages lists common diseases with symptoms, cause, herbal aids, and useful herbs named. A few diseases sound a bit old-fashioned, for instance, ague, catarrh, dyspepsia, hysteria, quinsy, and scrofula. Most remaining chapters present herbal remedies grouped by general use. Included are: the alternative herbs, the anthelmintic herbs, the astringent herbs, the cathartic herbs, the diaphoretic herbs, the diuretic herbs, the emmenagogue herbs, the expectorant and demulcent herbs, lobelia, the nervine and antispasmodic herbs, the stimulant herbs, and the tonic herbs. In addition, there are chapters on collecting herbs, the cleansing program, the regenerative diet, and herb alternatives. The latter category groups herbs that may be substituted for one another.

Much material is included in the book. Monographs on herbs, each several pages long, provide common and scientific names, identifying characteristics, part of plant used, collection, therapeutic action, medicinal uses, preparation instructions and formulas, dosage, administration, special notes, and related plants.

678.   Chu, Luke S. S., Samuel D. J. Yeh, and Denise D. Wood. **Acupuncture Manual: A Western Approach.** Illustrated by David R. Purnell. New York: Marcel Dekker, 1979. 256p. illus. bibliog. index. $15.00. LC 79-13978. ISBN 0-8247-6798-5.

The authors of this work hold positions of some prominence in medicine in the U.S. Their book is intended for physicians, dentists, medical students, and others involved with acupuncture, research in the field, and pain studies. It is called a manual, but in addition to providing a set of instructions, it is a monograph useful to those interested in the field. The authors believe that acupuncture has advanced to the point where training in this ancient Chinese practice is necessary for Western practitioners. The book presents an account of the old concepts, current techniques, and research findings with physiological and neurochemical background. Descriptions of anatomical points are provided with many illustrations.

There are chapters on the history and philosophy, basic concepts, technique, treatment, acupuncture points and their location, new methods and developments, acupuncture as a method of surgical anesthesia, and current acupuncture research. Included is an index of acupuncture points and three appendices as follows: 1) Tables summarizing points in specific anatomic regions; 2) Regulations governing the practice of acupuncture in New York State: a model for state regulation and licensing; and 3) Sample forms for patient records.

The book basically attempts to make the ancient practice of acupuncture thoroughly modern.

679.   Clark, Linda. **How to Improve Your Health: The Wholistic Approach.** New Canaan, CT: Keats Publishing, Inc., 1979. 149p. bibliog. index. $8.95; $4.95pa. LC 78-61329. ISBN 0-87983-181-2; 0-87983-180-4.

A number of unconventional approaches to good health are described in this book. For the most part, they are do-it-yourself methods. Chapters on the following subjects are included: 1) How to Improve Your Health (all therapies should be allowed to work together for the "wholistic" approach); 2) Self Care—Is It Wise? (yes, it's a necessity); 3) Nutrition (eat "natural" foods); 4) What Else Helps Nutrition? (exercise, positive thinking, and lack of discouragement); 5) Color Healing (included are color formulas for various disease conditions); 6) Herbs and Health (some discretion is suggested in the use of herbs); 7) Homeopathy Can Help You (the author believes homeopathic physicians are being welcomed back to their rightful place in the healing community); 8) Press for Health (discusses manipulative therapies, chiropractic, osteopathy, and pressure therapy; 9) Using Sound for Healing (sound vibrations and "toning"); and 10) Other Ways to Healing (dream therapy, the rule of three, spiritual vs. psychic healing, Kahuna prayer and healing, and the star exercise).

A list of sources for products and therapies mentioned in the book is provided.

680.   Clifford, Terry. **Cures.** Designed by Sam Antupit; illustrated by Charles B. Slackman. New York: Macmillan Publishing Co., 1980. 146p. illus. bibliog. index. $8.95. LC 80-21232. ISBN 0-02-526200-9.

A note at the beginning of this book states that the "cures" contained therein are not meant to replace necessary professional medical treatment. The author is not prescribing cures, but simply reporting their use in folk medicine and nontraditional healing systems. Cures from around the word are collected in the volume. Surprisingly, perhaps, disparate sources often recommend the same remedy.

The book first points out basic types of holistic cures and discusses them briefly. These are nature, energy, and mind cures. The main part of the work lists disease conditions alphabetically and then presents various cures that have been used for them in various cultures of the past and present. Such therapies as reflexology, Shiatsu massage, acupuncture, yoga, Indian Ayurvedic medicine, Pennsylvania Dutch remedies, naturopathic remedies, and many other curative methods are included. It is quite a bizarre collection of remedies. An appendix presents general directions for taking the cures, and includes sections on herbs and plants, honey, color treatment, fasts, gems used therapeutically, a holistic health diet.

681.   Clymer, R. Swinburne. **Nature's Healing Agents: The Medicines of Nature (or The Natura System).** Additional copy by The Humanitarian Society. Quakertown, PA: The Humanitarian Society (Box 77, Quakertown, PA 18951), 1973. 230p. index. $6.95. LC 62-21710.

Although this work carries a recent copyright date, almost all of it seems to be taken from a 1905 publication. The author was born in 1879. The book contains an advertisement for the Clymer Health Clinic complex, comprised of the clinic, a guest house, and health foods store, and devoted to "healing, regaining, or maintaining of health through Natural Therapy." The facility has been in operation since 1969.

The book begins with an explanation of the natura physician's basis of procedure. The chapter headings for this section are as follows: 1) The Natura Physician's Basis of Procedure; 2) The Thomsonian or Physio-Medical Treatment of Disease; 3) Basic Principles of the Natura System; 4) Emetics in the Elimination of Disease; 5) Steam, or Vapor, and Pack Baths; 6) The Internal Bath; and 7) The Natura System. The next three chapters (eight through 10) contain short monographs on individual herbs with common names, scientific names, uses, instructions for preparation, and dosages given. The next chapter, "The Natura Treatment of Disease," lists diseases and gives formulas for cures. Disease names uncommon now, such as ague, catarrh, croup, dementia, dropsy, dyspepsia, hysteria, and la grippe, are included.

In a separate section of 25 pages at the back of the volume, "Dr. Schuessler's Twelve Tissue Biochemic Remedies, the Natural Cell-Salts" are described. These substances are said to be nature's way of body-building by biochemistry, supplying natural mineral elements lacking in the system.

There is possibly some material of current usefulness in the book, although it seems hopelessly out of date. Like most of its kind, this book is of most value as a curiosity and remnant of times past.

682.   Colby, Benjamin. **A Guide to Health: Being an Exposition of the Principles of the Thomsonian System of Practice, and Their Mode of Application in the Cure of Every Form of Disease; Embracing a Concise View of the Various Theories of Ancient and Modern Practice.** Nashua, NH: Charles T. Gill, 1844. 144p. index. (A reprint of the 1864 revised and enlarged edition is available from BiWorld Publishers, P. O. Box 62, Provo, UT 84601. $5.95. ISBN 0-89557-013-0).

The subtitle of this early work provides a brief description of its contents. The author's views were at odds with those of the conventional medical profession of the nineteenth-century, and his book expounded the Thomsonian system of medicine that employed herbal medicines. The book was dedicated "to the human race of both sexes. . .to render them familiar with the means of being their own physicians, and thereby avoiding the miseries entailed on them by learned and ignorant quacks."

The book is in three main sections. The first section deals with the history and development of medical theories prevalent in the author's day. Another section presents descriptions of herbs and herbal formulas, and another lists diseases with treatment recommended.

Colby's viewpoints and remedies are of interest today because they are similar to those proclaimed by persons who call themselves modern herbalists.

683.   Coulter, Harris L. **Homeopathic Medicine.** St. Louis, MO: Formur, Inc., Publishers (4200 Laclede Ave., St. Louis, MO 63108), 1972. 73p. $1.65pa. LC 74-190020. ISBN 0-89378-072-3.

An essay setting forth homeopathic rules and philosophies, this work also contrasts homeopathy and allopathy (a term homeopaths use to indicate conventional medical practice). Chapter titles are: 1) Assumptions about Health and Disease; 2) Epistemological Assumptions; 3) Homeopathic Therapeutic Method; 4) The Place of Pathological Diagnosis in Homeopathy; 5) The Search for a Scientific Therapeutics; and 6) Homeopathy and Modern Medicine.

The author concludes that the time is ripe for those familiar with homeopathic therapeutic principles to press for their general acceptance.

684.   Goldwag, Elliott M., ed. **Inner Balance: The Power of Holistic Healing: Insights of Hans Selye, Elisabeth Kübler-Ross, Marcus Bach, and others.** Englewood Cliffs, NJ: Prentice-Hall, 1979. 360p. illus. bibliog. index. (A Spectrum Book). $13.95; $4.95pa. LC 79-14525. ISBN 0-13-465609-1; 0-13-465591-5pa.

The editor of this work says it developed out of his conviction that the health care system of today is on the brink of a rebirth. He thinks present methods of treatment are counterproductive to the long-term health of the individual and that new ideas about illness prevention will dramatically lower health costs. Chapters presented here, several by well-known individuals, highlight the view that a better approach to healing can be achieved through methods of controlling stress and through integration of body, mind and spirit (or holistic health).

Chapter titles are: 1) The Dilemma in Health Care, by Elliott Goldwag; 2) Stress: The Basis of Illness, by Hans Selye; 3) Self-Regulation: The Response to Stress, by Hans Selye; 4) Voluntary Self-Regulation of Stress, by Charles F. Stroebel; 5) Meditation: Achieving Internal Balance, by Syed Abdullah; 6) Stress, Self-Regulation, and Cancer, by O. Carl Simonton and Stephanie Matthews-Simonton; 7) Peer Healing and Self-Healing in Children, by Gerald G. Jampolsky and Patricia Taylor; 8) Self-Regulation through Nutrition, by William J. Goldwag; 9) Spiritual Power in Holistic Healing, by Marcus Bach; 10) Spiritual Help in Health Care, by Julian Byrd; 11) Spiritual Psychotherapy and Self-Regulation, by James A. Knight; 12) The Global Aspects of Health:

Role of Medical Education, by Robert A. Liebelt and Valory Murray; 13) Where Do You Go for Help? by Donald M. Hayes; 14) The Future Starts Now, by Elliott Goldwag; and 15) Epilogue, by Elisabeth Kübler-Ross. Two appendices are included: A) A city of health: model of a holistic health center; and B) Brompton's Mixture for relief of pain in terminal disease.

In spite of the unconventional views underlying much material presented in this book, it is a rather scholarly work on a considerably higher level than most holistic writings.

The epilogue (by Kübler-Ross) deals primarily with considerations of the dying patient. The appendix on Brompton's Mixture is evidently included because use of the mixture (a time-honored, conventional remedy for relief of terminal cancer pain) is encouraged by Kübler-Ross. Brompton's Mixture (or Cocktail as it is sometimes called) contains morphine, cocaine, flavoring, and alcohol.

685.   Griffin, LaDean. **Eyes: Windows of the Body and the Soul.** Provo, UT: Bi-World, 1976. 208p. illus. (part col.). bibliog. index. $9.95. ISBN 0-89557-007-6.

It is said that iridology (or iro-diagnosis) has its roots in ancient Middle East medicine. About 50 years ago, Bernard Jensen pioneered in the field and wrote some works about it. The author of this book has made a study of the "science" and has compiled a lay guide to it. She believes the eyes are the "windows of the body and the soul" and that by reading the iris health problems within the body can be recognized. Griffin has related iridology with the use of herbs and a mild food diet.

The book contains detailed eye charts, before and after treatment pictures of the eye, and many pages of testimonials supporting the author's views. There are strong religious overtones throughout the book.

686.   Griffin, LaDean. **Is Any Sick Among You?** Provo, UT: Bi-World Publishers (P. O. Box 62, Provo, UT 94601), 1974. 228p. illus. bibliog. index. $7.95. ISBN 0-89557-001-7.

The author of this best seller has few qualifications, formal or other, as an authority on medicine. She says she has discovered that "disease can be eliminated and wonderful health maintained when the body is clear of debris and properly fed." She has also found that "there can be almost total cleansing and reconstruction through fasting and semi-fasting foods." She has experimented on herself; she once lived for two years on fruit and nuts alone. Griffin is a devout Mormon, and the inspired writings and beliefs of her religion are scattered liberally throughout the book along with her personal beliefs about "natural" remedies. Faith healing, also, is worked in.

Contents of the book is as follows: 1) Herbs to drugs and back to herbs (a history of medicine from ancient Egypt to the present); 2) Fasting—the Garden of Eden to the millennium (about a restricted diet more than about fasting); 3) Color, sound and the aura choice vs. conditioned reflex (about the effects of surroundings on the individual); 4) Antidotes—the herbs, and home remedies (diseases are listed with remedies); 5) More antidotes—the vitamins (lists foods and herbs high in vitamin and mineral content; also lists symptoms of vitamin and mineral deficiencies); 6) Iridology—the eyes are the windows of the body (explains how the eyes provide clues for what is wrong in the body); 7) The hormone balance: nature's own insulin, natural-type cortisone, natural estrogen, natural ACTH, and natural thyroid (tells how to find "natural" hormones in plants); and 8) Conclusion.

The book is controversial and has reportedly been banned from a Mormon-owned book store chain in Utah. The reasons are not entirely clear. Perhaps the Mormons do not wish to endorse the "cures" (including one for cancer) given in the book.

The remedies are based on little more than the author's notions and personal testimonies. The book contains many inaccuracies, and standard scientific terminology is not used. The author defines some of her terms in the foreword to the book as follows: "When I speak of 'drugs' I mean anything made from inorganic sources, except when I speak of the young people taking hard drugs as I realize marijuana is an herb. Many herbs are considered to be drugs. Many herbs are an essential part of the inorganic, man-made drug products on the market. They are a mixture of plant and inorganic chemicals. When they are both, I will call them chemical or drug. When they are entirely chemical, they will be referred to as drug. When they are herbs or plants only, I will call them herbs. All through history, herbs have been called drugs as well as herbs and were, of course, not made of inorganic substances until Paracelsus and others of his time began to introduce inorganic substances (chemicals) into the bodies of men. Do not be confused by the strange concoctions added to the herbs in the apothecary; they will not be referred to as either drug or herb." As further examples, Griffin refers to herbal remedies and vitamins as "antidotes," and cayenne and ginger are "catalysts."

687.   Griffin, LaDean. **No Side Effects: The Return to Herbal Medicine.** Provo, UT: Bi-World Publishers, 1975. 212p. bibliog. index. $7.95. LC 76-380133. ISBN 0-89557-002-5.

The author of this work shares a common misconception among authors of herb books that herbal remedies have no side effects. She says she was convinced while searching through old medical books in a library (evidently at Brigham Young University) that the old books contained valuable information about herbs. Her work contains many quotations from these old books, some dating back to the fifteenth-century. Also biblical quotations are included throughout the book, which is perhaps more about faith than about medicine or herbs.

The book is curiously organized. The first three chapters present the author's views and discuss the old books. The main listing of herbs is in chapter 4, which contains a list of "herbal functions" such as "for relief of pain," "counteracts putrifaction," or "against poisons." Under each function is a list of herbs. Then there is a list of herbs with medicinal uses indicated; one finds, for instance, that burdock purifies blood and cures syphilis, cancer, leprosy, and tuberculosis.

Chapter 5, entitled "Art of Relaxation; Make Peace with Yourself: Be of Good Cheer," presents the author's religious philosophy. A few biographical sketches of the authors of the old herbals are included as are Mishnah Herbal References and Biblical References.

If the book has value it lies in the review of the old herbals and perhaps in the author's expression of faith. Suggested remedies cannot be taken seriously today.

688.   Haldeman, Scott, ed. **Modern Developments in the Principles and Practice of Chiropractic.** Based on a conference sponsored by the International Chiropractors Association, Anaheim, California, February, 1979. New York: Appleton-Century-Crofts, 1980. 390p. illus. bibliog. index. $28.50. LC 80-12312. ISBN 0-8385-6350-3.

Covering diverse approaches of spinal manipulation, this work provides an up-to-date reference work of value to chiropractors. Included are many illustrations to serve as visual guides to performing the spinal adjusting techniques. Each of the 16 chapters is by a different author, presumably one skilled in the area discussed.

The book is in three sections. The first section, on social aspects, covers the evolution of this form of alternative medicine with medical and social protest in America stressed. In addition, the present and future role of the chiropractor is considered. The second section of the book is on principles of chiropractic, and the third on practice.

689.   Hastings, Arthur C., James Fadiman, and James S. Gordon, eds. **Health for the Whole Person: The Complete Guide to Holistic Medicine.** Boulder, CO: Westview Press, 1980. 529p. bibliog. index. $30.00; $12.95pa. LC 79-25285. ISBN 0-89158-883-3; 0-89158-884-1pa.

A comprehensive work on holistic medicine, this publication is based on a report prepared by the Institute of Noetic Sciences for the National Institute of Mental Health. The foreword, by Senator Edward M. Kennedy, remarks that the book "tells us a good deal about why our present health care system is not adequate to meet the needs of the American people, and better yet, it tells us some of the directions we might pursue to improve our health." The book presents attitudes, information, and tools for what is called a holistic approach to medicine, health, and mental health. Contributing authors have defined three aspects of the holistic approach: 1) It expands the focus to include the many personal, familial, social, and environmental factors that promote health, prevent illness, and encourage healing; 2) It views the patient as a person, not as a symptom-bearing organism; and 3) It tries to make wise use of the many diagnostic, treatment, and health modalities that are available in addition to the standard materia medica—including alternate medical and healing systems as well as psychological techniques and physical modalities. Many of the latter are not generally accepted and can be considered unconventional practices.

Each chapter of the book, written by a different author, surveys a specific topic and is followed by an extensive annotated bibliography. Some topics covered include: biofeedback; autogenic therapy; hypnosis; meditation; psychic healing; the placebo effect; touch; chiropractic; Eastern spiritual disciplines; the therapeutic use of plants, music and sound in health; the use of light and color; alternative in childbirth; holistic approaches to oral health and dentistry; stress; programs for the elderly; dying and death; homeopathic medicine; Chinese medicine; and alternate forms of diagnosis.

The book covers the subject quite completely, and it will answer numerous questions about what is involved in holistic medicine. However, readers may not be convinced of the value of many of the unconventional practices.

690.   **Homeopathic Primer.** St. Louis, MO: Luyties Pharmacal Co., 1976. 31p. illus. bibliog.

The Luyties Pharmacal Company, a manufacturer of homeopathic remedies, has published this pamphlet. The publication includes these sections: 1) An introduction to homeopathy; 2) Homeopathic remedies still cure people; 3) Single remedies (lists and describes some plant and a few other remedies. The plants are pictured); 4) Dr. Schuessler's biochemic theory (describes 12 Schuessler remedies which are "mineral salts"); 5) Combination remedies; and 6) Homeopathy in common ailments.

The booklet points out that homeopathy gives the layperson the opportunity to treat himself.

691.   Homola, Samuel. **Doctor Homola's Natural Health Remedies.** West Nyack, NY: Parker Publishing Co., 1973. 250p. illus. index. $6.95. LC 73-7552. ISBN 0-13-216945-2.

The author of this book is a Doctor of Chiropractic. He has outlined basic home-treatment methods for dealing with a wide variety of common ailments that, in most cases, can reasonable be self-treated. Dr. Homola calls his remedies "Naturomatic Healing."

These are chapter headings: 1) How to Extend Your Life with Naturomatic Healing of Heart and Blood Vessel Diseases; 2) Naturomatic Healing Methods for

Coughs, Colds, Sore Throat, and Other Respiratory Ailments; 3) How to Cope with
Disease More Successfully by Relieving Everyday Stress and Tension with Naturomatic
Healing; 4) How to Relieve Daily Aches and Pains with Good Body Mechanics and
Proper Foot Care; 5) First Aid Nature's Way for Bruises, Sprains, and Muscle Injuries;
6) How to Relieve Neck, Arm, and Shoulder Pain with Drugless Methods of Naturoma-
tic Healing; 7) How to Get Prompt Relief from Backache, Arthritis and Leg Pain with
Naturomatic Healing; 8) Tested Naturomatic Healing Methods for Headache, Constipa-
tion and Hemorrhoids; 9) How to Relieve the Pain and Misery of Stomach Ulcers,
Colitis and Other Digestive Troubles with Naturomatic Healing, 10) How to Care for
Your Teeth, Gums, Bones and Joints with Naturomatic Healing Methods; 11) How to
Treat Simple Skin Disorders with Naturomatic Healing; 12) How to Relieve Fatigue
and Rejuvenate Your Body with Massage and Naturomatic Tonics; 13) How to Reverse
the Causes of Premature Aging and Remain Younger Longer with Naturomatic Healing; 14) How to Boost Your Sex Life and Ease the Strain of the Menopause and the
Male Climacteric; and 15) Miscellaneous Naturomatic Remedies for a Variety of Injuries
and Ailments.

    With some possible exceptions, suggested remedies in the book make sense
and might be recommended by a physician. The "Naturomatic" label applied to the
remedies adds little and is perhaps used mainly to attract attention.

692.   Inglis, Brian. **Natural Medicine.** London: Collins, 1979. 255p. bibliog.
index. £6.50. ISBN 0-00-216145-1.

    Journalistic rather than scholarly, this work relates the history and develop-
ment of "natural" or "alternative" medicine. Such systems as acupuncture, chiropractic, faith and spirit healing, herbalism, homeopathy, naturopathy, osteopathy, and the
like are discussed as reasonable alternatives to conventional (sometimes called "allopathic") medicine. The author claims neutrality in the matter of conventional versus
"natural" medicine, but the selection of material included makes that claim doubtful.

693.   Kaufman, Martin. **Homeopathy in America: The Rise and Fall of a Medical
Heresy.** Baltimore, MD: Johns Hopkins Press, 1971. 205p. bibliog. index. $10.00.
LC 79-149741. ISBN 0-8018-1238-0.

    Written by a historian, this book traces the relationship between homeo-
pathic and conventional medicine from 1820 to 1960. The book is an outgrowth of
the author's research for an academic dissertation.

    Kaufman remarks that the period from 1780 to 1850 has been called the age
of heroic medicine. Conventional physicians prescribed blood-letting and huge doses
of drugs for most ailments. In response to such harsh therapeutics, unconventional
medical sects arose, the most important being the homeopaths. The treatment they
prescribed was highly diluted doses of drugs that, if given in large doses to healthy persons, would produce the same symptoms as the patient's disease. Since such treatments
were safer than the conventional, many physicians converted to homeopathy. However, since homeopathic medicine was based on a questionable if not false theory, the
regular medical profession reacted with ridicule.

    Medical license laws were repealed in the mid-1800s, and quacks and char-
latans invaded the field. Conventional physicians united to form the American Medical
Association in the hope of improving standards, and homeopaths were barred from
many hospitals.

    After 1860, the book relates, conventional medicine abandoned heroic prac-
tices in favor of more effective and safer therapeutics. Homeopaths accepted conventional medical practices, and the American Medical Association grew more tolerant.

This acceptance weakened homeopathy, and many homeopathic schools whose graduates did not meet new standards shut down.

Kaufman concludes that by the 1960s this important sect, which had forced conventional medicine to moderate during the nineteenth-century, was doomed to disappear. He further points out the parallel between the history of homeopathy and that of osteopathy, the largest unconventional medical section of the twentieth-century. In 1967 the American Medical Association's house of delegates was authorized to negotiate the conversion of schools of osteopathy to conventional colleges. While the American Osteopathic Association did not wish to vote itself out of existence by merging with the AMA, one can expect, Kaufman feels, that the osteopaths will decline in number as more graduates of their college seek to advance in professional status by joining the AMA. Those who remain loyal to osteopathy will likely be fighting a losing battle.

This well-written and interesting account sheds a good deal of light on the emergence and decline of unconventional sects in medicine.

694. Kent, James Tyler. **Lectures on Homoeopathic Materia Medica, Together with Kent's 'New Remedies' Incorporated and Arranged in One Alphabetical Order.** Introduction by Jugal Kishore. First Indian ed. (enlarged). New Delhi, India: Jain Publishing Co. (2787, Rajguru Road, New Delhi - 110055), 1980 reprint. 1031p. index.

A reprint of a 1904 work, this book is basically a course of lectures on homeopathic materia medica delivered at a school of homeopathic medicine. Remedies are discussed individually, with attention given to the symptoms that suggest the remedies. The book also includes a life sketch of the author (a Professor of Materia Medica at the Hahnemann Medical College, Chicago) and a 1971 introduction by Kishore.

695. Kloss, Jethro. **Back to Eden.** Santa Barbara, CA: Woodbridge Press (P. O. Box 6189, Santa Barbara, CA 93111), 1975. 684p. illus. index. $9.95; $5.95pa. LC 75-585. ISBN 0-912800-33-X; 0-912800-12-7pa. (Original edition copyright 1939 by Jethro Kloss).

This work is claimed to be a "classic" in the natural health and healing movement, "the world's best known guide," "the standard," and "an essential guidebook" in the area of herbals and home remedies. It is not just a list of herbs used for curing diseases; it is a total guide to healthful living, focusing on the use of "natural" foods and proper diet in the prevention of diseases.

There are chapters on soil and its proper cultivation for growing healthful foods, the history of medicine, fresh air and exercise, fasting, aluminum utensils, cooking under steam, water and its cures, baths, massage, trees, enemas, and nursing. These are all covered in addition to chapters on herbs and other foods, which include preparation, recipes, and uses.

Emphasis is on "inexpensive" recipes that "can be made in any home." The author wants to take people back to the basics and believes that "the fundamental principle of true healing consists of a return to the natural habits of living." The book is interesting as a curiosity, but like many of its kind there is little scientific evidence available to substantiate the statements made about foods and herbs mentioned.

696. LaPatra, Jack. **Healing: The Coming Revolution in Holistic Medicine.** New York: McGraw-Hill, 1978. 235p. bibliog. index. $9.95. LC 78-19013. ISBN 0-07-036359-5.

Self-treatment has become popular recently, particularly since the media have been telling us that health care institutions and practitioners are not entirely trustworthy.

Many books have been written that attempt to set the record straight on matters of health, and various views have been taken. This work analyses the issue and offers the holistic movement in medicine as an answer to the problem. Holism, or "whole body healing" considers psychological and social aspects of the patient's problems as well as the physical. Also, the patient uses his/her own healing powers, that is, treats himself/herself and attempts to prevent illness by diet, exercise, use of herbs, and alternative or unconventional therapeutic systems.

LaPatra divides his work into four categories of healing: body, mind, spirit, and hybrids. Among other "systems" the following are discussed: the eckankar movement (purports to heal by "soul travel or by mail"), color therapy (the patient is irradiated with a colored light after diagnosis and drinks water exposed to the same light), graphology (connects handwriting and disease), and sleep therapy. A number of case histories are presented throughout.

As is the case with most books on this subject, the rapid advances and constructive changes that are taking place in conventional medicine and health care are ignored.

697.   Malstrom, Stan D. **Own Your Own Body**. New Canaan, CT: Keats Pub., 1977. 398p. illus. bibliog. index. (A Pivot Health Book). $2.95pa. LC 76-58968. ISBN 0-87983-215-0pa.

The view taken by the author of this book is that one should assume responsibility for his/her own good health, and he sets out to tell how to do this. He suggests proper nutrition (use "natural" foods) and "natural" treatments for ailments, such as fasting, exercise, diet, herbs, and massage.

698.   Mauskopf, Seymour H., ed. **The Reception of Unconventional Science**. Boulder, CO: Westview Press for the American Association for the Advancement of Science, 1979. 137p. bibliog. (AAAS Selected Symposium No. 25). $13.25. LC 78-19735. ISBN 0-89158-297-5.

This work provides a context for the serious study of heterodox science and scientific theories. It contains four studies, each of which considers the response of a scientific community to an unconventional theory or claim. Titles of the studies are: 1) The reception of an acausal quantum mechanics in Germany and Britain; 2) The reception and acceptance of continental drift theory as a rational episode in the history of science; 3) Reception of acupuncture by the scientific community: from scorn to a degree of interest; and 4) The controversy over statistics in parapsychology 1934-1938. In addition, there is a final general discussion on the reception of unconventional scientific claims.

The section on acupuncture is of special interest. It concludes that acupuncture was shunned for many decades by the scientific community. The Chinese have shown its strengths and weaknesses. American practitioners should try to improve the method, not by adding to the mythology but by exploring the nature of the factors involved.

The conclusion to the final discussion points out that within a group, deviance, such as adherence to unconventional scientific ideas, is seldom positively greeted by those benefiting from conformity. Science, however, is dependent upon such innovations for growth, and there is a need for tolerance.

699.   Meyer, Clarence. **Vegetarian Medicines**. Glenwood, IL: Meyerbooks, 1981. 92p. illus. bibliog. index. $5.95pa. ISBN 0-916638-06-5.

Meyer believes that every household should be familiar with the medicinal properties of food plants. Their proper selection can help prevent many physical ailments. All of the plants mentioned in this book have specific healing properties, according to Meyer. His compilation was gleaned from old German and English herbals.

The work is in two parts. The first part provides information on the medicinal value of 18 foods. Part 2 is an encyclopedic arrangement of common ailments and home treatments suitable for the conditions. Recipes for products that can be used to treat common complaints are provided.

700.   National Analysts, Inc. **A Study of Health Practices and Opinions**. Final Report. Conducted for: Food and Drug Administration, Department of Health, Education, and Welfare. Springfield, VA: National Technical Information Service, 1972. 340p. (PB 210-978; Report No. FDA-PA-72-01). $6.00.

This publication reports on a national survey designed to determine the nature and prevalence of fallacious or questionable health beliefs and practices, and susceptibility to them. The presentation is in two parts. The first part includes the background of the study, its methodology, extensive summaries of findings, and action implications derived. Part 2 presents findings of the major survey portion of the study in full detail.

The following beliefs and/or practices were investigated: use of vitamins and other nutritional supplements without a physician's guidance; use of "health food"; weight reduction practices; use of laxatives or other aids to bowel movements; self-diagnosis of ailments; self-medication for serious ailments; practices in the diagnosis and treatment of arthritis; practices in the diagnosis and treatment of cancer; health practitioners used; hearing aids and medication; "aids" to quitting smoking; and general health-related attitudes and opinions.

A few of the findings: three-fourths of the public believe that extra vitamins provide more pep and energy, the most common of the misconceptions investigated; one-fifth agreed that even such diseases as arthritis and cancer are caused, at least in part, by vitamin or mineral deficiencies; about half the users of self-medication were satisfied that the products did what they had hoped, and the higher the expectations, the higher the satisfaction reported; one-tenth had eaten food advertised or labeled as 'organic' or 'natural', and a majority of them really expected to be helped by the food. An important conclusion, though, is that many questionable health practices are better accounted for by a kind of "rampant empiricism" than by specific false beliefs, i.e., anything is worth a try.

701.   **The New Healers: Healing the Whole Person**. Edited by Larry Geis and Alta Picchi Kelly; with Aidan Kelly. Compiled by the New Dimensions Foundation. Berkeley, CA: And/Or Press (P. O. Box 2246, Berkeley, CA 94702), 1980. 147p. illus. (A New Dimensions Series Book). $5.95pa. LC 80-12100. ISBN 0-915904-49-7.

The preface of this book says that modern health care focuses on the body as the key to good health and considers mind and spirit as afterthoughts. The so-called modern-day healers, who present the material in this book, "see body, mind, and spirit as integral parts of a contiguous whole, each as important as the other." Another theme the book presents is that each person is responsible for his/her own health.

The presentation is in five sections: 1) Basics of holistic health; 2) Physical awareness and healing; 3) Mental awareness and healing; 4) The life cycle; and 5) Spiritual awareness and healing. Each section contains several chapters by various authors on such subjects as biofeedback, vitamins, intuitive massage, thinking healthily, holistic childbirth, growing older, helping the dying person, spiritual therapy, and spiritual healing.

Perhaps the best-known contributors are Nobel Prize winner Linus Pauling (writing on vitamins and orthomolecular medicine), and Ruth Carter Stapleton, sister of ex-president Jimmy Carter (writing on spiritual healing).

702.   Otto, Herbert A., and James W. Knight, eds. **Dimensions in Wholistic Healing: New Frontiers in the Treatment of the Whole Person.** Chicago, IL: Nelson-Hall, 1979. 543p. illus. bibliog. index. $22.95; $12.95pa. LC 78-27071. ISBN 0-88229-513-6; 0-88229-697-3pa.

Concerned with basic principles and concepts of wholism, this book presents an overview of the subject in its 31 diverse chapters. The wholism therapeutic system is directed toward treating the whole person and includes mental, emotional, physical, social, and spiritual dimension. Emphasis is given to therapies that the patient can make use of himself. Subjects treated include biofeedback, nutrition, ultrasonics, acupuncture, and faith healing. Contributors to the volume are from various branches of medicine, psychology, and parapsychology.

703.   Perry, Edward L., comp. **Luyties Homeopathic Practice: A Homeopathic Medical Book for Family Use.** St. Louis, MO: Formur, Inc. Publishers (4200 Laclede Ave., St. Louis, MO 63108), 1974. 153p. index. $1.65pa. ISBN 0-89378-052-9.

This work was originally published in 1924 by F. August Luyties of the Luyties Pharmacy Company of St. Louis, one of the few companies in the United States manufacturing homeopathic medicines. This edition has been reprinted several times since 1974 because of recent interest in the subject.

The theory of homeopathy is explained by Perry. Briefly, homeopaths believe the body is helped to cure itself by administration of very dilute doses of medicines that excite the body to produce its own antidotes. These drugs, if given in larger doses, produce symptoms similar to those initially suffered by the patient.

The main section of the book lists diseases alphabetically with symptoms given. Then a number of products (mostly plant remedies) are listed with preparation method and dosage provided. Also included is a paragraph or so on "general measures." Appended is a short list of homeopathic remedies (a condensed materia medica) arranged alphabetically by the name of the product and giving uses.

The book emphasizes that homeopathic medicines are safe and not unpleasant to take. This is true because the doses are so dilute. The question is whether they are of any value.

704.   Sahni, B. **Transmission of Homoeo Drug-Energy from a Distance (A New Discovery).** Patna, India: Sahni Homoeo Pharmacy and Publication (Boring Canal Road, Patna-1), 1970. 108p. bibliog. $3.00pa.

This is an unusual book to say the least. The foreword says it a pioneering effort in an area practically unknown in India, although conventional homeopathy is evidently known. The novel approach to treatment described is called an "augury" in homeopathic science. Dr. Sahni believes "drug-energy" can be transmitted through the patients uprooted hair, making use of "radiesthesia." Radiesthesia is defined as an instrument or device that "detects the radiations given off by human organism and finds out the diseased organ and helps the ailing beings."

Several chapters cover the background of the treatment. There is a chapter with 61 case reports of instantaneous cures using the method. The method consists of touching the detached hair of the patient with a globule of a suitable remedy. Distance is no bar to treatment. In the first case of Transmission a distance of only five feet was covered. Gradually, homeopathic drug-energy can be transmitted to any corner of the world, the moon, or other planets, according to the author.

The bibliography contains 38 references, most of them incomplete and most to homeopathic literature.

705.   Schneider, L. L., in association with Robert B. Stone. **Old-Fashioned Health Remedies That Work Best.** West Nyack, NY: Parker Publishing Co., 1977. 227p. illus. index. $8.95. LC 76-56734. ISBN 0-13-633701-5.

The author of this work evidently holds degrees in chiropractics, naturopathy, and physical therapy and is interested in acupuncture. He calls his remedies "low cost natural time-tested health boosters you can use at home for successful self-care." The remedies have, like so many, been handed down from generation to generation.

Chapter headings are: 1) Old-Fashioned Health Remedies Are Winning New Respect Today; 2) How You Can Make the Supermarket Your Gold Mine for Health; 3) Special Foods That Exert Amazing Curative Power over Supposedly Incurable Conditions; 4) Foods That Inject Vitality into Your Vital Organs; 5) Foods That Place Your Body in Healthful Balance and Make You Feel Younger; 6) Little Things That You Can Do That Pay off in Health Dividends; 7) Old-Fashioned Remedies That Work Wonders for Stiff Necks and Tricky Backs; 8) What to Do about Frazzled Nerves, the Shakes, and Jumpiness; 9) How to Turn Restless Nights into Solid Sleep; 10) Common Ailments You Can Get Rid of Uncommonly Fast Nature's Way; 11) Digestive and Elimination Problems That Respond to These Safe Home Remedies; 12) How to Harness Nature to Life Your Energy Levels; 13) Simple Ways to Help Yourself to a Longer Life; 14) Nature's Marvelous Health Boosters.

Many remedies suggested are of unproven value and probably worthless. Recent research has even found a few to be harmful. One statement made, though, stands out as fact. The author says the label "superstition" is being changed today to "natural remedy."

706.   **Schuessler's Twelve Biochemic Tissue Remedies.** St. Louis, MO: Formur Inc. (4200 Laclede Ave., St. Louis, MO 63108), 1977. 31p. $0.75pa.

In 1873 Dr. William H. Schuessler of Oldenburg, Germany, published his theory about functional disturbances caused by cell salt deficiency. He believed the body demands a certain amount of each of 12 mineral elements. Consequently, 12 tissue biochemic remedies were made available through homeopathic remedy suppliers.

This booklet lists the remedies and indicates the homeopathic uses and usual dose. Another section lists diseases with the suitable remedy given.

707.   Smith, A. Dwight. **The Home Prescriber.** Chicago, IL: Ehrhart and Karl, Inc. (17 N. Wabash Ave., Chicago, IL 60602), 1964. 42p.

The intent of this booklet is to help the layperson treat minor ailments when a homeopathic physician is not available. It is also hoped that those unfamiliar with the homeopathic system of medicine will become acquainted with it through use of the publication.

The booklet briefly explains homeopathy, provides a list of 22 remedies, and lists some common diseases with suitable remedies. The main section presents, under the names of the remedies, symptoms, conditions, and diseases that suggest the use of the remedy.

708.   Sobel, David S., ed. **Ways of Health: Holistic Approaches to Ancient and Contemporary Medicine.** New York: Harcourt Brace Jovanovich, 1979. 497p. illus. bibliog. $12.95; $7.50pa. LC 78-14081. ISBN 0-15-195308-2; 0-15-694992-Xpa.

This book claims that the modern medicine of Western cultures has, to a large extent, ignored the healing systems of other cultures and other times, overlooking the fact that other cultures could make a contribution. Certain areas have been neglected and undervalued. These areas are discussed in this book, which is a collection of 20 essays by persons advocating a more holistic approach to health and healing.

Many recent books on holistic medicine speak of integrating mind, body, and spirit (some have deeply religious overtones). This one emphasizes another element, environmental factors affecting human health.

Following are the main topics the book covers: 1) Holistic approaches to health; 2) Ancient systems of medicine (includes Navajo Indian and Chinese medicine and selections from Hippocrates); 3) Unconventional medicine (includes religious healing, laying on of hands, and homeopathic medicine); 4) Techniques of self-regulation (such as yoga and biofeedback); and 5) An ecological view of health (includes biological rhythms, air ions, physical activity, and nutritional science).

The book does not launch a serious attack on conventional medicine. The hope is expressed, however, than an integration of our technological achievements with more humanistic and psychological systems can be achieved. It can be argued, of course, that conventional medicine has not undervalued these "systems," that they have been evaluated correctly.

709.   Stanway, Andrew. **Alternative Medicine: A Guide to Natural Therapies.** London: Macdonald and Jane's, 1980. 160p. illus. (some col.). bibliog. index. £6.95. ISBN 0-354-04442-7.

This attractively produced and profusely illustrated book covers 32 alternative medical treatments in an uncritical fashion. Some unusual treatments are included, such as psionic medicine, pyramid healing, and shiatsu.

The author takes the view that there are too few effective conventional medical treatments available, that they are too costly, that they are misused, and that the drugs available have too many side effects. He admits that randomized controlled trials are of some help in evaluating drugs, but he has a bias in favor of uncontrolled trials. He thinks if some treatment seems to work repeatedly, this is sufficient evidence. In addition, he does not think controlled trials are of value in evaluating alternative medical therapies because they are too individualized. In short, Stanway speaks for unevaluated, unproven treatment, although the book contains the usual warning that a physician should be consulted before using a "natural" therapy.

710.   **Therapeutic Index.** St. Louis, MO: Luyties Pharmacal Co., 1976. 12p.

Included in this booklet is a brief history of the Luyties Pharmacal Company, a manufacturer of homeopathic drugs established in 1853, and a list of diseases with appropriate homeopathic remedies.

711.   Thomson, Robert. **Natural Medicine.** New York: McGraw-Hill Book Co., 1978. 329p. illus. bibliog. index. $10.95. LC 78-17598. ISBN 0-07-064513-2.

The author of this book says he is a distant descendant of Samuel Thomson (1769-1845), the first American of European descent to practice "natural" medicine in America. He worked out a "system" of healing based on the same principles of bodily balance the author arrived at himself. Samuel Thomson's system was an unconventional one, called Thomsonianism, which used herbs and steam baths to purify the body. One goal of Thomsonians was "to make every man his own physician."

The first section of the book, "The Theory of Natural Medicine," gives a brief history of natural medicine from the ancient Greeks, enumerates principles of the system, discusses the origin of illness, defines correct nutrition as seen by the author (with recipes), and outlines a detoxification program, the latter to rid the body of "excess waste and toxins." The author evidently derived many ideas from the ancient Persians and the teachings of Avicenna, a physician born in 980 A.D. in present-day Afghanistan.

The second part of the book, "The Formulary," lists 50 basic herbs and gives directions for their preparation. Dosage, fevers, healing, and several types of therapy are discussed. The next section is on "The Well-Being of Children."

The last part of the book contains sections on various parts of the body, e.g., the head, eye, ear, nose, heart, etc., and some miscellaneous matters. There are appendices on "Iridology, the Science of Iris Diagnosis" and "Reflexology (Foot-Zone Therapy)."

Although published by a major publisher, the book cannot be recommended for anything other than as an example of recent publications on "natural" medicine and food.

712.   Thomson, Samuel. **A Narrative of the Life and Medical Discoveries of Samuel Thomson, Containing an Account of His System of Practice and Manner of Curing.** Columbus, OH: Horton Howard, 1822; repr. New York: Arno Press, 1972. 186p. (Medicine and Society in America Series). $11.00. LC 79-180594. ISBN 0-405-03976- ISBN 0-405-03976-X.

This is an autobiographical account of the life, views, and accomplishments of Thomson (1769-1845), who developed a system of medicine called Thomsonianism, an eclectic school of medicine which treated diseases by the application of single remedies ("specifics") to pathological conditions. Special attention was given to the development of indigenous plant remedies. Cases and treatments are discussed. The book also tells of the legal difficulties Thomson encountered as a result of his practice.

713.   Tobe, John H. **The Golden Treasury of Natural Health Knowledge.** St. Catharines, Ontario: Provoker Press, 1973. 619p. index. $20.00. LC 73-83219. ISBN 0-8397-3015-2.

This large volume presents the author's views on health matters and the value of a "natural" life. There are 100 short chapters on a great many subjects. The first chapter expresses the author's philosophy; the other 99 discuss vegetarianism, benefits of a raw food diet, the merits of sprouts, chemical poisoning, herbs and natural healing, heart attacks, a remedy for backache, arthritis, diabetes, cancer, baldness, "the pill" (it will kill millions), baby foods, fasting, sexual virility, and much more.

The author gives opinions on a wide range of health matters, but, in general, his philosophy is that proper food and living will help one achieve a long life free from disease, an idea few would dispute. However, some of his specific beliefs are highly controversial, such as opposition to the use of medicines, vaccines, X-rays, and blood transfusions. In addition, he is against the use of chemicals in food growing and processing. Sometimes he gives medical advice of doubtful validity; other times it seems sensible. Some of his warnings are warranted; others are not.

The last chapter, "Is Back to Nature the Answer," urges the reader to move to a small farm to grow "natural" food. He makes it sound very easy, too easy.

The book is interesting, but it is a curious mixture of good sense and nonsense.

714.   Tubesing, Donald A. **Wholistic Health: A Whole-Person Approach to Primary Health Care.** New York: Human Sciences Press, 1979. 232p. bibliog. index. $14.95. LC 78-3466. ISBN 0-87705-370-7.

"This book is a call for a redefinition of health and illness in the context of a broader view of life, health, and the quality of life to include the whole person—the mental, emotional, and spiritual sides of life as well as the physical." The author's solution is the Wholistic Health Center project. Such centers are church-based, family practice medical care facilities that utilize a team including physicians, pastoral counselors, nurses, and other professionals. The centers emphasize health education, early examination, and prevention.

Following are chapters presented: 1) There's Trouble in Health Care; 2) Everyone Is Dissatisfied with the Quality of Health Care; 3) The System of Health Care Delivery Is Inefficient; 4) Our Concepts of Health and Illness Are Outdated; 5) The Wholistic Health Center: An Alternate Health Care Model; 6) The Wholistic Health Center Philosophy; 7) Introducing the Patient to the Wholistic Health Center Process; 8) The Professions Reexamined in Relation to the Wholistic Health Center; 9) Primary Modalities of Care in the Wholistic Health Center; 10) The Place of the Wholistic Health Center in the American System; 11) Does the Wholistic Health Center Concept Really Work?; and 12) The Future of Health Care.

In meeting the challenge of future health care, the author has defined the basic needs as follows: a need to gather together the professions; a need to develop new models; a need to share knowledge and coordinate efforts; a need to fit into the present health care system; and a need to speak with a united voice.

Perhaps because of the author's background, the book emphasizes pastoral care more than most books on holistic health. The author is articulate and makes a reasonable case for his concept. No extreme views are expressed.

715.   Vithoulkas, George. **Homeopathy: Medicine of the New Man.** New York: Arco Publishing Co., 1979. 154p. bibliog. index. $6.95; $3.95pa. LC 77-29272. ISBN 0-668-04577-9; 0-668-04581-7pa.

A popular work, this book attempts to show that homeopathy is a science which applies laws of nature correctly to stimulate the healing power of the individual. The basic foundations of homeopathy are described. It is based on the Principle of Similars, that is, symptoms are treated with drugs that normally produce the symptoms shown by the patient. (Actually, the drugs are prescribed in such small doses that they do not produce those symptoms, fortunately.) Early founders of the homeopathic system of medicine believed that diluted drugs were more potent than stronger ones, and that the more dilute the more potent. This supposed phenomenon is not explained by chemical mechanisms; some inner "force" is involved, proponents say.

The book also attempts to show that homeopathy is akin to the recently touted holistic school of medicine which is concerned with the whole person.

Chapter titles are: 1) Coming of the New Age; 2) Samuel Hahnemann and the Law of Similars; 3) Preparation of Homeopathic Medicines; 4) The Vital Force; 5) The Dynamic or Subtle Plane; 6) Predisposition to Disease; 7) The homeopathic Interview; 8) A Sample Case: Influenza; 9) The Patient's Responsibility; 10) Does Homeopathy Work?; 11) How Cure Occurs; 12) More Laws of Cure; 13) The State of Homeopathy in the World; 14) Plans for the Future; and 15) Promise of the New Age.

An appendix on materia medica describes such drugs as nux vomica (the poisonous seed of a tree), lycopodium (spores of a club moss), natrum muriaticum (table salt), and phosphorus. Very little is given about their sources or actions. The book describes the symptoms a patient may demonstrate that might call for using such drugs.

The book does not present a convincing case for homeopathic treatment.

716.   Wade, Carlson. **All Natural Pain Relievers.** Foreword by William S. Keezer. West Nyack, NY: Parker Publishing Co., 1975. 227p. index. $8.95. LC 75-19221. ISBN 0-13-022376-X.

The author of this book claims that natural home remedies revealed in his presentation can relieve almost any pain. Many remedies suggested involve exercise, but some require the use of herbs, vitamins, certain foods, meditation, and the like.

Chapter titles are: 1) How Natural Analgesics Can Help You Enjoy Freedom from Aches and Pains; 2) How 5-10-15 Minute Natural Analgesic Home Therapies Help Create Freedom from Headaches; 3) How Back Manipulation Helps Relieve Backaches in a Jiffy; 4) How Simple Flex-Ercises Limber Up and "Untie" Knotted Leg Muscles; 5) How to Revitalize and Reshape Your Feet for Youthful Health; 6) How Natural Analgesics Can Help Free You from Arthritis Pain; 7) Simple Natural Analgesic Healers to Relax-Refresh-Rejuvenate Your Eyes; 8) How to Use Natural Analgesics to Protect Your Ears Against "Noise Pollution"; 9) A Compendium of Natural Pain Relievers for Easing Sore Throat; 10) How Natural Analgesics Can Help "Untie" That Knot in Your Chest; 11) Home Health Tonics, Natural Analgesic Healers to Promote Digestive Health; 12) How Europeans Relieve-Rejuvenate-Relax Aching Muscles; 13) How Natural Isometrics Soothe Aches of the Shoulders-Arms-Wrists-Hands; 14) How Hydro-Helio and Natural Analgesic Remedies Heal Sciatica-Bursitis-Neuralgia; 15) How Natural Postustrengtheners Help Banish Nagging Aches; 16) Heliotherapy—The Soothing Heat; 17) Hydrotherapy—The Natural Healer for Stubborn Aches; 18) How to Use Ice as an All-Natural Pain Reliever; 19) Pain Relieving Secrets from the Mystics; and 20) A Treasury of Herbal and Other Natural Pain Relievers.

Some therapies may prove beneficial, but the claims made for them seem exaggerated, and the author has no qualifications for giving medical advice other than that he is a medical writer. No documentation is included.

717.   Wade, Carlson. **Health Tonics, Elixirs and Potions for the Look and Feel of Youth.** Foreword by Amil J. Johnson. West Nyack, NY: Parker Publishing Co., 1971. 236p. index. $6.95. LC 71-151659. ISBN 0-13-384545-1.

The author of this work has gathered together a number of programs for the treatment of "arthritis pains, sagging skin, faulty digestion, chronic fatigue, sleeplessness, and sluggish kidney-liver functioning." The programs include use of food juices, elixirs made from fresh fruits and vegetables, and potions that are comprised of herbs and seeds.

Following is a sampling of the chapter titles: 1) How Life Food Juices Work to Create Your Internal "Fountain of Youth"; 2) Healthful Elixirs to Help Put Youthful Glamour into Your Skin; 3) How Folk Potions May Help Stimulate Hair Growth on the Head; 4) How to Drink Your Vitamins to Cope with Aging Arthritic Distress; 5) The Raw Juice Program to Help Promote "Happy Glands" for a Youthful Personality; 6) Herb Tonics—Nature's Youth Medicines to Replace Drugs and Patent Medicines; 7) Legendary Aphrodisiacs for Those over 40; and 8) How Herbal Teas Help Invigorate Youthful Mind-Body Power.

Little evidence for the efficacy of suggested remedies is given other than personal testimonials.

718.   Walsh, James J. **Cures: The Story of the Cures That Fail.** New York:
D. Appleton and Co., 1923; repr. Detroit, Gale, 1971. 291p. index. $15.00. LC 70-
137343. ISBN 0-8103-3773-8.

The author of this older work says in the preface that human nature causes
individuals, when ailing, to grasp at straws like the drowning man. The amusing thing
is, he remarks, that the man's mind "often turns the straw into a solid beam of hope
on which he floats into the harbor of good health when he thought he was seriously
ill." That is why so many ridiculous "cures" seem to work at least for a while. This
book is about various "cures" that failed after an initial period of apparent success.

Chapter headings give an indication of the various treatments discussed in the
book: 1) The Cures That Fail; 2) Personal Healers; 3) Drug Cures; 4) "Cures with a
Punch" (cures that possess an extraneous element apart from their real or supposed
physical action, such as drug plants taken from a graveyard); 5) Magnets and Some
Wonderful Cures; 6) Mesmer and His Cures (the process of "mesmerizing" or magne-
tizing patients, later called hypnotism); 7) Dr. Elisha Perkins and His Tractors (the
tractors were two short metallic rods which, when placed in contact with each other
and drawn over the skin of a patient suffering from almost any ailment, brought about
a cure); 8) Absent Treatment: Distance Cures; 9) Andrew Jackson Davis, the Seer of
Poughkeepsie, and a Few Others; 10) Hypnotism; 11) Appliance Cures (such as plaster
and rubber, magnets, electric rings, horse chestnuts, blue light, and liver pads); 12)
Manipulation Cures (such as chiropractic); 13) Mystical Cures; 14) Psychoanalysis and
Coué; 15) Conscious Evolution and Conscious Control; and 16) Conclusion. An appen-
dix, "Galen and the Healer Who Was a Weaver," is included. It is an anecdote about
Galen's experience with a "healer" during the second century in Rome.

Walsh finds the "cures" amusing, but doesn't think their likes can be kept
from developing. He just asks that they not be taken seriously today. So far, fake
cures have seemed funny to succeeding generations only.

719.   Wensel, Louise Oftedal. **Acupuncture in Medical Practice.** Reston, VA: Reston
Publishing Co., 1980. 335p. illus. bibliog. index. $15.95. LC 80-12507. ISBN 0-
8359-0128-9.

This is a difficult book to review because acupuncture is puzzling, and it has
not yet been evaluated by Western scientists. It deserves careful attention, but can be
badly served by authors such as this one who get carried away by their enthusiasm.

The book is in two sections. The first, "A Comprehensive Introduction to
Acupuncture," provides a theoretical, historical, and neurophysiologic basis for acupuncture. One chapter gives precise locations for all points where needles are to be inserted.
There is also a chapter on "Teaching Acupuncture to Americans." Other chapters
deal with conditions in which acupuncture should not be used, its combination with
nutritional therapy, and the need for ingestion of huge amounts of vitamins. There is
also a section on acupuncture as a new health profession. Some scientific material is
presented, some of it well-established fact, and some considered wild conjecture by
scientists.

Part 2, "Acupuncture Treatment of Specific Conditions," covers conditions
that can be treated by acupuncture, a long list including most known ills. Specific
points where needles must be inserted are indicated.

An appendix contains a long list of acupuncture points in Chinese, points for
specific diseases, and an acupuncture quiz. Most sections are followed by brief bibliographies, but a good many references do not seem relevant or are too little-known, non-
scientific publications.

It is of note that acupuncture is known for its analgesic applications. The author of this book has gone far beyond that, recommending it, at least in combination, for treatment of almost everything.

21
MISCELLANEOUS

Listed below are books on miscellaneous aspects of plants. Several works deal with plants used for dyeing cloth, a matter about which some hobby interest prevails. Also included are several books on Biblical plants, a subject that has interested scholars for many years. Remaining works cover a variety of topics, some quite unusual, such as the book by Bengtsson on herbal designs used in embroidery and McDonald's work on growing plants as therapy.

* * * * *

720.   Abbe, Elfriede. **The Plants of Virgil's Georgics: Commentary and Woodcuts.** Ithaca, NY: Cornell University Press, 1965. 217p. illus. bibliog. index. LC 64-8258.

While reading English translations of Virgil's poem *Georgics*, the author of this work became aware of discrepancies in the numerous references to vegetation, that terms were not always clear to readers, and that it was difficult to link the living organism described with what was in the mind's eye. To take care of the latter problem, this book has been illustrated with beautiful woodcuts, done by the author.

The identities of plants mentioned in the poem were determined by comparing existing descriptions, integrating the opinions of other commentators, and using historical and scientific information. Identification was difficult, and Abbe does not claim that his work is definitive.

The plants are listed by scientific name and grouped by family. The main part of the text is made up of quotations from early works, usually arranged in chronological order. There is an illustration for most species. Appended are a list of plants with Virgilian and scientific names, a list of plants by English common names, and a glossary of geographical names. The bibliography lists classical works consulted in preparation of the book, many fifteenth- and sixteenth-century editions.

The book is nicely done. The quotations will interest the gardener, the seeker of herb lore, the student of botanical and horticultural literature, the science historian, and the scholar of the classics.

721.   Bengtsson, Gerda. **Herbs and Medicinal Plants in Cross-Stitch from the Danish Handcraft Guild.** New York: Van Nostrand Reinhold Co., 1978. 64p. illus. (part col.). $6.95pa. LC 78-8618. ISBN 0-442-20677-1.

This booklet presents 26 highly attractive patterns for cross-stitch embroidery. The designs were originally on 1975 and 1977 calendars designed by Gerda Bengtsson, an internationally known textile designer of the Danish Handcraft Guild. Each design has been reproduced in color and again in diagram form so the user can recreate them. In addition, there are section on material and instructions, methods of working, and examples of finished work. Designs are suitable for framing as pictures, pillows, table-cloths, place mats, and napkins.

Only brief information is given on the uses of each herb; the book is primarily a work on decorative designs.

722. Bliss, Anne. **North American Dye Plants.** Illustrated by Robert Bliss. New York: Charles Scribner's Sons, 1980. 288p. illus. index. $5.95pa. LC 79-66891. ISBN 0-684-16393-4.

This is a revised and enlarged edition of a 1976 book called *Rocky Mountain Dye Plants.* It was written for people interested in brewing a pot of dye.

An introductory section gives information on foraging for dye plants; predicting dye colors and variations; yarns and fibers; the mordanting process and common mordants; dyeing procedures; testing for lightfastness; and special techniques.

The main part of the book lists more than 100 plants alphabetically by common name with line drawings for each. Scientific name, a brief description, habitat, uses, and colors produced are given. Also included is a statement about lightfastness of the dye made from the plant.

The book is of convenient size to take on field trips.

723. Bliss, Anne. **Weeds: A Guide for Dyers and Herbalists.** Drawings by Jean Hurley. Boulder, CO: Juniper House (P. O. Box 2094, Boulder, CO 80306), 1978. 113p. illus. bibliog. index. $5.00pa. LC 78-59236. ISBN 0-931870-01-1.

Described here are 50 plants, usually considered weeds, that are able to produce color on wool, the most readily available and easily dyeable fiber. The testing for this book was done with commercially spun 2 ply "unscoured" white worsted rug yarn.

The first part of the book discusses dyeing in general and includes sections on scouring (washing the fiber), mordants (metal salts which assist the bonding of dye to fiber), testing fastness, and instructions for dyeing. The longest part of the work is a listing of the herbal dye plants. Each entry covers about a page and includes scientific and common names, a description of the plant, habitat, flowering season, miscellaneous and historical uses, and instructions for using the plant as a dye. The colors produced are indicated. A nice line drawing is provided for each plant on the pages facing the descriptions.

724. Ford, Richard I., ed. **The Nature and Status of Ethnobotany.** Ann Arbor, MI: University of Michigan Museum of Anthropology, 1978. 428p. illus. bibliog. (Museum of Anthropology, University of Michigan. Anthropological papers. No. 67). $10.00pa. ISBN 0-932206-79-4.

This work is a commemorative work dedicated to Volney H. Jones, an ethnobotanist associated with the Museum of Anthropology at the University of Michigan. As an ethnobotanist, Jones was concerned with the relationship between man and plants as the latter have been used in different societies for food, clothing, shelter, implements, utensils, and medicines. The subject matter of this publication reflects these concerns.

The book contains biographical information about Jones, a list of his publications, and 16 papers by various authors, arranged in the following sections: 1) Theoretical issues in ethnobotany; 2) Native epistemology and ethnobotany; 3) Principles of resource utilization; 4) Anthropogenic plants and communities; 5) Prehistoric economics and paleoethnobotany.

Papers of interest include: "Thinking and Drinking: A Rarámuri Interpretation," "From the Hero's Bones: Three Aguaruna Hallucinogens and Their Uses," "Present and Future Prospects of Herbal Medicine in a Mexican Community," and "Domestication of Sunflower and Sumpweed in Eastern North America."

725.   Grae, Ida. **Nature's Colors: Dyes from Plants.** Photography by Daniel Grae. New York: Collier Books, a Division of Macmillan Publishing Co., 1974. 229p. illus. (part col.). bibliog. index. $14.95; $6.95pa. LC 73-11836. ISBN 0-02-544950-8; 0-02-012390-6pa.

Grae is considered an authority on dyeing with plants, and she teaches dyeing, spinning and weaving. In this book she brings the ancient art of dyeing up to date, providing more than 200 recipes and, in addition, instructions for working out one's own recipes.

Chapter headings are: 1) Let Us Discover Dyeing as the Ancients Did; 2) Types of Natural Dyestuff; Background of Selected Exotic Dyes; 3) Prospecting for Dye Plant Material; 4) Basic Information; 5) Dyeing Procedures; 6) The City Dweller and Natural Dyeing; Foods as Dye Sources; Dyeing Macrame, Crochet, and Embroidery Yarns; 7) Primitive Dyeing Methods: Steeping, Natural Mordants, and Vat Dyeing; 8) How to Work out New Recipes: A Working Method That Leads to Discovery; 9) Natural Dyeing as Design Experience; 10) About the Dye Recipes; 11) Lichen Recipes; 12) Wild Flower and Weed Recipes; 13) Garden Flower Recipes; 14) Wild Shrub Recipes; 15) Garden Shrub Recipes; 16) Tree Recipes; and 17) Food and Food-Related Plant Recipes. In addition, the following appendices are provided: 1) Decreasing and increasing ingredient amounts in a recipe; 2) Percentage method of calculating recipe amounts; 3) Rule-of-thumb estimate of dye plant amounts; 4) Iron buff as a mordant for cotton; 5) Neutralizing machine-spun yarn before mordanting; 6) Over-dyeing; 7) Country-style black ink; 8) Cosmetic recipes; and 9) Sources of chemicals, dyes, fleece, plants, seeds, yarn, and books. The book contains several indexes.

There are eight pages of color plates showing some results of the author's dyeing and art work. This is a practical, inspirational work.

726.   Greenblatt, Robert B. **Search the Scriptures: Modern Medicine and Biblical Personages.** Foreword by Henry King Stanford. 3rd and enl. ed. Philadelphia, PA: J. B. Lippincott, 1977. 173p. index. $8.95. LC 76-50054. ISBN 0-397-59060-1.

The physician who is the author of this well-received work provides insights into illnesses that afflicted various Biblical characters. He sees many instances of forerunners of modern medical practices. A wide range of medical topics are involved, including herbal medicine, forerunners of antibiotics, endocrinology, genetic disorders, uses of wine, fasting, medicinals and religious experience, and much more. Since the author is an obstetrician and gynecologist, the work is somewhat slanted in that direction.

The Biblical characters and some customs and traditions mentioned in the scriptures are given a different interpretation in the light of medical sciences.

727.   Harrison, R. H. **Healing Herbs of the Bible.** Leiden, The Netherlands: E. J. Brill, 1966. 58p.

This small book, which was reprinted from another source, is a study of the materials from which the pharmacopoeia of the Hebrews was drawn. The author points to the difficulty in identifying drugs mentioned in early records. It is virtually impossible, he says, to determine the name of a plant unless it has survived in some way in either Coptic, Arabic, or some other cognate Semitic language. The Hebrews, for the most part, seem to have employed herbs of reputed medicinal value independently of supposed magical properties; their pharmacopoeia was drawn in terms of culinary/hygienic usage or religious/ritual associations.

Following are section headings: 1) Introduction; 2) Glossary of medical terms; 3) Herbs of a general medicinal nature; 4) Culinary and dietary herbs; 5) Narcotics and poisons; 6) Stomachics; 7) Herbs used in religious rites; 8) Ointments and Perfumes; 9) Names of Bible places; 10) Hebrew designation of herbs; and 11) List of quotations from the Old Testament.

The book helps clarify the scope of Hebrew pharmacy.

728.   Jacobs, Betty E. M. **Growing Herbs and Plants for Dyeing.** Illustrations by Kathleen Gough. Tarzana, CA: Select Books (5969 Wilbur Ave., Tarzana, CA 91356), 1977. 126p. illus. bibliog. $6.00pa. LC 77-77943. ISBN 0-910458-12-X.

Presented in two parts, this manual first tells how to grow 23 herbs and seven plants for dyeing. The second part gives instructions on how to use herbs and plants for dyeing, with emphasis on wool dyeing.

In part 1, plants are listed alphabetically by common name, each illustrated with a nice line drawing. Information provided includes botanical name and family, other names, life span, appearance, cultural requirements, propagation, and information about dyeing, such as plant harvesting, part to use, color fastness, and mordant use. Plants listed are: agrimony, barberry, bedstraw, bloodroot, broom, calliopsis/coreopsis, dahlia, dyer's broom, dyer's chamomile, elder, golden rod, heather, hollyhock, lily of the valley, madder, marigold, meadowsweet, mullein, onion, pokeweed, privet, ragwort, safflower, saffron, tansy, tomato, weld, woad, yellow flag, and zinnia.

In part 2, information is given on the following: equipment needed to mordant and dye wool, chemicals needed, dos and dont's when handling wool, quantities, how to wash and mordant wool, and how to dye wool (including a basic dyeing recipe). There is an appendix listing places where seeds and plants can be purchased.

729.   King, Lawrence J. **Weeds of the World: Biology and Control.** London: Leonard Hill; New York: Interscience Publishers, Inc., 1966. 526p. illus. bibliog. index. (Plant Science Monographs).

This comprehensive and scholarly work covers many aspects of weeds. Approximately 5,000 literature references are included throughout the book. Some material presented is not directly related to the subject of this bibliography, but much information is relevant.

There is a chapter on the use of weeds. Included is information on utilization of the plants as food for humans and animals, medical uses of wild plants, examples of plant usage by Indian tribes, and contributions of ethnobotanical studies. A chapter on harmful aspects of weeds includes material on poisonous plants, food-tainting weeds, poisonous and fetish plants used by primitive peoples, and miscellaneous harmful plants.

730.   Krochmal, Arnold, and Connie Krochmal. **The Complete Illustrated Book of Dyes From Natural Sources.** Garden City, NY: Doubleday, 1974. 272p. illus. bibliog. index. $4.95pa. LC 73-9167. ISBN 0-385-05656-7pa.

According to the dust cover, this work is written for craftsmen who "are going back to nature for the vibrant, distinctive colors that no chemical dye can equal." Many plants used as sources, such as goldenrod, coffee, and oak root, are common and readily available. Simple home equipment and supplies are sufficient to use for dyeing, and many recipes provided can be completed in a day or less.

The work begins with chapters on the history of natural dyes and their uses, equipment, supplies, and techniques of preparation. The main text consists of over 220 recipes for dyes grouped by color (yellow, green, blue, purple, red, brown, black, and gray). The recipes are arranged within each group alphabetically by common name of the plant involved. The scientific name is also given, sometimes with either a photograph or simple line drawing. The text is followed by a bibliography and an index.

731.   Lehane, Brendan. **The Power of Plants.** Designed by Amil Bührer and Robert Tobler. New York: McGraw-Hill Book Co., 1977. 288p. illus. (part col.). bibliog. index. $39.95. LC 77-7551. ISBN 0-07-037055-9.

This fine book, with more than 800 beautiful illustrations, is based on the view that plants are the foundation of all existence. "They are the source of our nourishment and health, pleasures and ecstasies; they sustain religions, cultures, civilizations." Among the illustrations are fine old drawings from herbals, electron microscope photographs, cross-sections of vegetables, portraits, scenic views, photographs of flowers and plants, and reproductions of paintings.

There are five chapters: 1) Power to Survive; 2) Power to Sustain; 3) Power to Heal and Kill; 4) Power to Alter Consciousness; and 5) Power over the Spirit.

Each chapter contains historical background material on the subject concerned, and there is emphasis on art, legend, and lore.

732.   Levin, Simon S. **Adam's Rib: Essays on Biblical Medicine.** Los Altos, CA: Geron-X, 1970. 180p. bibliog. index. $6.95. LC 78-111609. ISBN 0-87672-006-8.

This book contains seven essays on Biblical medicine, particularly emphasizing the connection between medicine and religion in those times. An attempt is made to interpret many Biblical passages concerning health, medicine, and the like.

Following are the titles of the papers: 1) The anatomy of Genesis; 2) The physician and disease; 3) Bacteriology; 4) Metabolism and miscellanea; 5) Mothers and babies; 6) Death; and 7) The anatomy of the soul: Dilemmas and difficulties in the soular system.

733.   McDonald, Elvin. **Plants as Therapy.** New York: Popular Library, 1977. 174p. $1.50pa. LC 74-33026. ISBN 0-445-04007-6.

The title of this book may be somewhat misleading because it is not about using herbs and plants as medicine. It is about using the activity of gardening and growing plants as therapy for lessening stress and strain in one's life. It is included here as an example of the increasing interest in this subject.

Most of the book is a narrative of the author's personal experiences and applications in using gardening as therapy. The remainder of the book is a kind of directory including lists of plant societies and garden clubs, university programs in this area, and mail order sources of plants and seeds. Addresses are included. An additional section includes a listing of easy to grow plants and flowers, with complete instructions for each.

734.   Moldenke, Harold N., and Alma L. Moldenke. **Plants of the Bible.** Waltham, MA: Chronica Botanica Co., and New York, Wiley, 1952. 328p. + plates. illus. bibliog. index. (New Series of Plant Science Books, v.28). $15.50. ISBN 0-8260-6170-2.

This well-known work is a comprehensive survey of present-day knowledge of Biblical botany. The authors review past literature on the subject, correct errors, and present evidence about plants and plant products of the Old and New Testaments. Various translations of the Bible were carefully studied in preparation of the work.

The first section is a historical sketch from the earliest writings onward; next there is a description of the Holy Land. The main section of the volume is made up of descriptions of 242 species of plants. Appropriate scripture is quoted, common and Latin names of the plants given, notes on folklore and mythology provided, and evaluations made. The writing has a great deal of popular appeal. The book is quite delightful as well as authoritative and informative. In addition, the many illustrations are beautiful and appropriate. They have been taken from botanical works, Bibles, paintings, woodcuts, and prints.

Information can be found about such plants as cedar-of-Lebanon, crown-of-thorns, date palm, hyssop, manna, myrtle, olive trees, paper reed, pomegranate, Judas tree, passion flower, fig, ebony, bulrush (or papyrus), balsam, and tares.

There is an index of Bible verses and a general index listing Latin and vernacular names. The bibliography contains over 600 references.

735.   Mors, Walter B., and Carlos T. Rizzini. **Useful Plants of Brazil.** San Francisco, CA: Holden-Day, Inc., 1966. 166p. illus. bibliog. index. $10.00. LC 66-17891.

This short book is a concise, but rather comprehensive, review of the useful plants of Brazil. It summarizes knowledge, recent research, and problems concerning the plants. The authors, who are scientists, believe that plants have been "underdeveloped" and hope that their book will be valuable to botanists, chemists, industrial and commercial enterprises, medical students, and laypersons who are interested in the subject.

There is a preliminary section on "Bioclimatic Classification of Brazil," which includes maps of the country. Then 16 chapters are presented, each discussing plants according to their uses: 1) Latex Yielding Plants; 2) Coffee; 3) Oil and Fat Yielding Plants; 4) Wax Producing Plants; 5) Trees with Trunk Exudates; 6) Tannin Supplying Plants; 7) Dye Plants; 8) Aromatic Plants; 9) Spices; 10) Medicinal Plants; 11) Poisonous Plants; 12) Fiber Supplying Plants; 13) Timber; 14) Cork Supplying Plants; 15) Raw Material for the Manufacture of Cellulose and Paper; and 16) Miscellaneous Useful Plants.

There are bibliographies with each chapter, along with a general "supplementary" bibliography. The authors have successfully condensed a large amount of information from scientific literature.

736.   O'Hara-May, Jane. **Foods or Medicines?** London: British Society for the History of Pharmacy, 1971. 61-97p. bibliog. (Transactions of the British Society for the History of Pharmacy. Vol.1, no.2, 1971). 75 pence.

This short monograph is subtitled, "A study in the relationship between foodstuffs and materia medica from the sixteenth to the nineteenth century," and the paper illustrates some changes of viewpoint regarding the relationship. To make the study, the author examines classic works of the period, some of them materia medica works, and a treatise on food.

In conclusion, the author points out that modern research into metabolism has shown that the action of food and most drugs takes place within the same general biochemical framework. She believes the two subjects are complementary to each other in a proper regimen for preserving good health.

737.   Oyle, Irving. **The New American Medicine Show: Discovering the Healing Connection.** Santa Cruz, CA: Unity Press, 1979. 170p. illus. bibliog. $5.95pa. LC 78-31345. ISBN 0-913300-18-7.

The author of this work, a physician, takes the viewpoint that we are entering a new era in medicine. What he describes is, in many respects, a return to the fundamental principles of psychosomatic medicine on a do-it-yourself basis. Oyle believes most illnesses are the result of poor lifestyle or poor habits, and that one has control over his/her own health. He places emphasis on mental attitude, although nutrition and physical exercise are also said to be determinants of health.

The book suggests achieving better health through improvement of outlook and viewing the world in a new light. Frequent references are made to current research and theoretical findings in such areas as consciousness and reality.

738. Preuss, Julius. **Julius Preuss' Biblical and Talmudic Medicine.** Translated and edited by Fred Rosner. New York and London: Sanhedrin Press, 1978. 652p. bibliog. index. $35.00. LC 78-7430. ISBN 0-88482-861-1. (Translation of Biblisch-talmudische Medizin).

This classic work has for almost 70 years served as a guide to the highly developed concepts of medical knowledge and practice found in Biblical and Talmudic literature. Since German is no longer widely spoken among Jews or in most Western countries, this English translation of the 1911 work is welcome. Preuss, a physician, was a great Jewish historian of medicine, and this work is highly authoritative. It contains elaborate documentation with many literature citations and an index of passages cited in the Hebrew Bible and Talmud. (A subject index has also been provided.)

As can be seen by the chapter headings following, more than herbal medicine is covered. However, plant remedies were a major source of medicine in this period of Jewish civilization.

Chapter headings are: 1) The Physician and Other Medical Personnel; 2) The Parts of the Body and Their Functions; 3) Illness and Its Healing; 4) Sicknesses and Their Treatment; 5) Injuries and Malformations; 6) Diseases of the Eyes; 7) Dentistry; 8) Diseases of the Ears; 9) Disorders of the Nose; 10) Neurological Disorders; 11) Mental Disorders; 12) Skin Diseases; 13) Gynecology; 14) Obstetrics; 15) Materia Medica; 16) Legal Medicine; 17) Regimen of Health; 18) Dietetics; and 19) Writing on Medicine in the Bible and Talmud (bibliography).

739. Quinn, Vernon. **Shrubs in the Garden and Their Legends.** Illustrated by Marie A. Lawson. New York: Frederick A. Stokes Co., 1940. 308p. illus. index.

Thirty shrubs arranged alphabetically by common name are described in this work. Emphasis is on the history, legends, and myths surrounding the plants, but scientific names, habitat, and uses are also included.

Among the shrubs discussed are: azalea, barberry, boxwood, burning-bush, dogwood, forsythia, hawthorn, holly, hydrangea, japonica, laurel, mock-orange, spirea, winterberry, snowberry, and many others.

The book is well written. No bibliography has been provided, but references to authorities and classics are made throughout the text.

740. Rice, Miriam C. **How to Use Mushrooms for Color.** Illustrations by Dorothy Beebee. Eureka, CA: Mad River Press (Route 2, Box 151-B, Eureka, CA 95501), 1980. 145p. illus. $7.95pa. ISBN 0-916422-19.4. (Revised and enlarged edition of **Let's Try Mushrooms for Color**).

This is a manual on how to use mushrooms for dyeing cloth. The material is presented in three sections. Part 1 introduces the reader to the techniques of dyeing; part 2 provides information on identifying the fungi used as a source for the dye, and part 3 describes the mushrooms in lay terms for those with no experience in identifying the fungi. About 115 species are listed with line drawings. Also included are eight pages of color plates and five pages of charts showing the full range of colors obtainable from mushrooms.

741. Rolfe, R. T., and F. W. Rolfe. **The Romance of the Fungus World: An Account of Fungus Life in Its Numerous Guises, Both Real and Legendary.** With a Foreword by J. Ramsbottom. London: Chapman and Hall, 1925; repr. New York: Dover Publications, 1974. 308p. illus. index. $3.50pa. LC 74-81401. ISBN 0-486-23105-4.

This book was written to demonstrate all the ways fungi have concerned mankind, such as economically and in literature and fantasy. References to literature, scientific and literary, are given in footnotes.

A glance at the contents of the book shows the variety of areas covered: 1) Introduction; 2) The fungi in mythology and folklore; 3) The fungi in fiction; 4) The fungi in reality: their structure and characteristics; 5) The fungi in reality: their modes of existence; 6) The damage caused by fungi and its effect on mankind; 7) The uses of fungi: in medicine; 8) The uses of fungi: in industry; 9) The uses of fungi: as foods; 10) The cultivated fungi and other fungus foods of commerce; 11) The poisonous fungi; 12) The curious phenomena exhibited by fungi; 13) The study of the fungi as a hobby; 14) Some further historical aspects of the fungi; and 15) The derivation of fungus names.

This is a very interesting as well as informative book.

742. Sapeika, N. **Food Pharmacology.** Springfield, IL: Charles C. Thomas, 1969. 183p. illus. bibliog. index. (American Lecture Series, Publication No. 732). LC 68-25978.

This book is somewhat outside the subject area considered in this bibliography, but it helps place chemical and biological hazards of foods in proper perspective. The foreword points out that every meal contains deliberate or accidental additions of dozens of possibly injurious non-nutritive materials. These include chemical additions, spices, condiments, toxicants, natural bioactive and pharmaco-active compounds, and synthetic substances. In addition, there are the ever-present micro-organisms not yet possible to eliminate, and radioactive fallout from the environment. Many foods containing these materials are used regularly with little or no obvious effects. Some only occasionally produce disturbances in health. A few are always harmful and are generally avoided, but cause discomfort, disease, and death when eaten by persons ignorant of the danger. This book takes a comprehensive view of the subject and provides an account of a wide variety of substances.

Following are chapter headings: 1) General Considerations; 2) Foods of Plant Origin; 3) Foods of Animal Origin; 4) Food of Marine Animal Origin; 5) Food Additives; 6) Food Contaminants; and 7) Water, Soft Drinks, and Alcoholic Beverages.

Among foods of plant origin considered are ackee fruit, almonds, apricot, asparagus, bamboo shoots, bananas, beans, betel nut, buckwheat, cabbage, carrots, cashew nuts, clover, cress, cycad seeds, figs, garlic, gums, pectin, hemlock, honey, horseradish, jenghol seed, licorice, maize, manchineel, mango, manioc, manna, marmite, marrows, squashes, melons, mushrooms, mustard, nutmeg, oak, onions, peanuts, peas, pepper, pineapples, potatoes, prunes, rhubarb, rice, seaweed, strawberries, tamarind, tomatoes, tung nuts, yams, and wheat. In each case the potentially harmful compounds found in the foods are discussed.

743.   Schery, Robert W. **Plants for Man.** 2d ed. Englewood Cliffs, NJ: Prentic-
Hall, Inc., 1972. 657p. illus. bibliog. index. $22.50. LC 72-140.
ISBN 0-13-681254-6.

This book is an encyclopedic treatment of plants that serve and sustain man.
The aim of the work is to bring together scattered information, provide a vew of plant-
man interdependency, and make the reader aware of how fundamental plants are for
society.

The presentation is in four parts: 1) Introduction; 2) Products from the plant
cell wall; 3) Cell exudates and extractions; and 4) Plants and plant parts used primarily
for food and beverages. Chapter headings are: 1) Man's Relationship with Plants; 2)
Man's Economic Interest in Plants; 3) Forests Available to Man; 4) The Forest Belts of
North America; 5) Wood and Its Uses; 6) Forests, Man, and the Future; 7) Fibers;
8) Latex Products; 9) Pectins, Gums, Resins, Oleoresins, and Similar Exudates; 10) Vegetable Tannins and Dyes; 11) Essential Oils for Perfumes, Flavors, and Industrial Uses;
12) Biodynamic Plants: Medicinals, Insecticides, Growth Regulants, Tobacco, etc.;
13) Vegetable Oils, Fats, and Waxes; 14) Carbohydrate Extractives: Sugars and Starches;
15) Food Plants; 16) The Cereals; 17) Other Food Seeds and Forages; 18) "Vegetables":
From Root, Stem, and Leaf; 19) Fruits; 20) Beverage Plants; and 21) From Micro-
organisms to Miscellanea.

Each chapter elaborates on relatively few plants of major economic importance
in the category indicated by the title. Condensed listings of less widely used sources follow the major discussions. Some of the discussions present new discoveries and developments such as hallucinatory drugs, the population explosion, and the modern importance of gardening and landscaping cultivators. Historical importance and future prospects of the plants and their products are covered.

The book is illustrated with good photographs of plants, scenes, and people,
and includes maps, tables, and graphs. It is a fine source for a variety of information.
Of particular value is material on less-familiar tropical plants.

744.   Sherwood, Martha. **Collecting Roots and Herbs for Fun and Profit.** Chicago,
IL: Contemporary Books Inc. (180 North Michigan Ave., Chicago, IL 60601), 1978.
282p. illus. bibliog. index. $5.95pa. LC 77-91190. ISBN 0-8092-7674-7.

Presented here are nine chapters on a wide variety of topics related to the cultivation, harvest, preservation, and marketing of approximately 80 fairly well known
herbs and plants. Some specific topics covered are: how to get started in the herb business; how to preserve various kinds of herbs; and herbal treatment of diseases. There
is a listing of dealers who buy and sell herbs and a short listing of periodicals on the
subject.

Most of the discussions about the herbs include comments on habitat, description of the plant, culinary and medicinal uses, and an unusual bit of information—the
market value. Even though market prices obviously fluctuate widely, this figure will
give some idea of relative value.

Exact preparations, recipes, and dosages are given for many of the herbs.

745.   Tippo, Oswald, and William Louis Stern. **Humanistic Botany.** With illustrations by Alice R. Tangerini. New York: W. W. Norton and Co., 1977. 605p. illus.
(part col.). bibliog. index. $13.95. ISBN 0-393-09126-0.

This work was written primarily as a textbook for undergraduate courses in
botany for students not majoring in science. Technical language has been kept to a
minimum, and the book has a good deal of popular appeal. Emphasis is on the relationship between plants and people. Stress is given to such areas as poisonous plants,

marijuana, narcotic plants, hallucinogenic plants, medicinal plants, and food plants. Also included are biographical sketches of significant figures in the botanical field, and the historical development of botany is outlined. In addition, the book includes a solid core of scientific material.

Chapter headings are: 1) The Nature of Botany; 2) Form and Function; 3) On Names and Naming; 4) Linnaeus; 5) The Cell; 6) Wood; 7) Poisonous Plants; 8) Marijuana; 9) Medicinal Plants; 10) Plant Hallucinogens; 11) Food Plants; 12) Spices; 13) Algae; 14) Fungi; 15) Mosses and Ferns; 16) Seed Plants; 17) Genetics; 18) Mendel; 19) Evolution; 20) Darwin; 21) Ecology; 22) Man's Influence over His Environment; and 23) Exploring for Plants. A 20-page glossary has been provided.

The book is interesting and nicely done. It includes about 100 line drawings and 275 photographs, some in color.

746.   U.S. Department of Agriculture. **Drying Crude Drugs.** By G. A. Russell. Washington, DC: GPO, 1921. 16p. illus. (U.S. Department of Agriculture. Farmers' Bulletin No. 1231).

Although quite old, this pamphlet is still used by people involved in the revival of collecting and drying crude drugs.

The bulletin discusses principles and methods of drying, drying equipment, drying with artificial heat, and the care of dried crude drugs. The methods of construction of two driers which use artificial heat are described, a large-type drier and a small stove drier.

747.   Verrill, A. Hyatt. **Wonder Plants and Plant Wonders.** New York: D. Appleton-Century Co., 1939. 296p. illus. index.

The author of this work says he has tried to tell the stories of some of the strangest plants known as well as stories of others that are remarkable for various other reasons. Plants from all over the world are included, and the accounts are interesting. Illustrations, many of them photographs, add a great deal to the novelty of the book.

Contents is as follows: 1) What is a plant?; 2) The plant department store (includes plants that furnish cloth, paper, rope, and gum); 3) The most useful trees (palms); 4) Trees that grow while you wait (banana, willow, and resurrection plants); 5) Plants that cure and kill (herbs, medicinal plants, and toxic plants); 6) Plant giants (includes sequoia, cypress, giant cacti, apa-apa, etc.); 7) Intelligent plants (eucalyptus trees, ivy, sensitive plants); 8) Plants that build rafts (such as reed balsa); 9) Strange partners (discusses pollination, the pitcher-plant, Venus's fly-trap, etc.); 10) Plants that sail seas (cecropia tree, reeds, etc.); 11) Plants that we eat (potatoes, sweet potatoes, yams, tomatoes, sweet peppers, pimentoes, sugar cane, corn, and grains); 12) Wonder plants that we drink (fruit beverages, cocoa, tea, and fermented beverages); 13) Magic plants (plants believed to possess magical power such as mandrake); 14) Plants with strange uses (catnip, lavender, castor bean plant, sandalwood tree, tobacco, white poppy, Indian hemp, and others); 15) Plant travelers (burs, cotton, Milkwort, touch-me-nots, and mangrove tree); 16) Plant public enemies (weeds); 17) Wonder plants of commerce and industry (flax, hemp, sisal, dyes, and waxy plants); 18) The first of all calendars (day lilies, morning-glories, and four-o'-clocks); and 19) The most wonderful plants (microscopic plants).

748.   Walker, Winifred. **All the Plants of the Bible.** Garden City, NY: Doubleday and Co., 1979. 240p. illus. (col.). $14.95. LC 78-22802. ISBN 0-385-14964-6.

This is a new edition of a work originally published in 1957. The late author, a trained artist, served as official artist to the Royal Horticultural Society of Westminster and as artist-in-residence at the University of California. She painted all 113 fine water-color illustrations in the book. In producing the work, she used a descriptive list of the plants issued by the New York Botanical Garden and compiled by Dr. Harold Moldenke, a noted authority on Biblical plants.

The plants are arranged alphabetically by common (Biblical) name with the illustration on the facing page. The appropriate scripture is given, followed by a description of the plant with history, growing habits, and present-day uses.

There is a short supplement that contains plants mentioned in the Apocrypha, listed separately because many Christian churches do not consider the apocryphal books part of the Scriptures. A second supplement lists and describes briefly a few Biblical plants that are not pictured.

This is a most attractive as well as interesting book.

749. Wigginton, Eliot, ed. **Foxfire 1-.** Garden City, NY: Anchor Press/Doubleday, 1973-. Most vols. 400-500 pages. (no.1). $5.95, ISBN 0-385-07353-4; (No.2). $5.95, ISBN 0-385-02267-0; (No.3). $6.95, ISBN 0-385-02272-7; (No.4). $6.95, ISBN 0-385-12087-7; (No.5). $6.95, ISBN 0-385-14308-7; (No.6). $7.95, ISBN 0-385-15272-8. All vols. paperback.

These are fascinating books about how to live a simple, uncomplicated life away from the modern, technical, fast-paced lifestyle. They are books about the "affairs of plain living." Each discussion is on a different topic and is based on interviews with people who lived the simple life as a youngster, or who are still living such a life, and have had first-hand experience in the particular subject. Most individuals interviewed are living or have lived in the Appalachian Region of the United States.

Topics covered are varied, e.g., knife making, gardening, cheese making, and horse trading. Specific instructions included in many of the articles and interviews provide both interesting and nostalgic reading and practical advice. Although these books are not exclusively concerned with herbs, there is considerable herb lore and discussion of the uses of the plants throughout the volumes. Herbs are very much a part of the simple life where one has to depend on his own resources for survival.

The first volume was published in 1972, and five others are available at this writing—all with entirely new articles and interviews on new subjects. These books are highly recommended for a unique reading experience and for the valuable practical instructions included. The reviewer is personally acquainted with a case where the technique of hog butchering was learned solely from these *Foxfire* volumes.

APPENDIX

DIRECTORY
OF ORGANIZATIONS,
ASSOCIATIONS, AND GROUPS

Following is a list of organizations, associations, and groups concerned with the subjects treated in this bibliography. Some are old, well-established organizations whose members are in scientific pursuits. Most, however, are recently established groups of laypersons who have merely an interest in the subject considered. An attempt has been made to supply current addresses, but many of the groups are small and may have no permanent address.

Acupuncture Association
34 Alderney St.
London, SW1V 4EU
England

Acupuncture International Association
2330 S. Brentwood Blvd.
St. Louis, MO 63144

Acupuncture Research Institute
P.O. Box 7534
Long Beach, CA 90807

American Academy of Medical Preventics
11311 Camarillo St.
North Hollywood, CA 91602

American Association of Constitutional
   Medicine
c/o Kenneth L. Sanders
405 Appleway Ave.
Coeur D'Alene, ID 83814

American Association of Homoeopathic
   Pharmacists
6231 Leesburg Pike, Suite 506
Falls Church, VA 22044

American Board of Homoeotherapeutics
6231 Leesburg Pike, Suite 506
Falls Church, VA 22044

American Center for Herb Study
P.O. Box 454
Mountain View, AK 72560

American Chiropractic Association
2200 Grand
Des Moines, IA 50312

American Council of Women Chiropractors
c/o Elizabeth C. Gerlt
3169 S. Grand Blvd.
St. Louis, MO 63118

American Foundation for Homeopathy
7297-H Lee Hwy.
Falls Church, VA 22042

American Healing Association
Box 6311
Yucca St.
Los Angeles, CA 90028

American Holistic Medical Association
Rt. 2
Welsh Coulee
La Crosse, WI 54601

American Institute for Research and Education
   in Naturopathy
c/o Kenneth M. Rofrano
N.Y.C. Community College
300 Jay St.
Brooklyn, NY 11201

311

American Institute of Homeopathy
6231 Leesburg Pike, Suite 506
Falls Church, VA 22044

American Medical-Psychic Research
    Association
135 Madison Ave. NE
Albuquerque, NM 87123

American Naprapathic Association
330 N. Milwaukee Ave.
Chicago, IL 60641

American Natural Hygiene Society, Inc.
National Headquarters
1920 Irving Park Road
Chicago, IL 60613

American Society of Pharmacognosy
President: Jack K. Wier
School of Pharmacy
University of North Carolina
Chapel Hill, NC 27514

American Spice and Trade Association
Box 1267
Englewood Cliffs, NJ 07632

American Vegan Society
Box H
Malaga, NJ 08328

American Vegetarian Union
P.O. Box 68
Duncannon, PA 17020

Association for Holistic Health
P.O. Box 9532
San Diego, CA 92109

Australian Chiropractors, Osteopaths and
    Natural Physicians Association
c/o Mrs. A. Downer, Secretary
6/102, Kirribilli Ave.
Kirribilli, New South Wales
Australia

Australian Institute of Homeopathy
c/o Mrs. G. Reynolds, Secretary
7 Hampton Road
Artarmon 2064, Australia

Bay Area Homoeopathic Study Group
c/o Randall Neustaedter
645 62nd St.
Oakland, CA 94609

Bio-Dynamic Farming and Gardening
    Association
17240 Los Alamos St.
Granada Hills, CA 91344

Biogenic Institute of America
Rt. 2
Welsh Coulee
La Crosse, WI 54601

British Acupuncture Association and Register
34 Alderney St.
London SW 1V 4EU
England

British Herbal Medicine Association
Walter House
418/422 Strand
London W.C. 1

British Homoeopathic Association
43 Russell Square
London WC1, England

British Naturopathic and Osteopathic
    Association
Frazer House, 6 Netherhall Gardens
London NW3 5RR
England

California Certified Organic Farmers
1920 Maciel Ave.
Santa Cruz, CA 95860

California Orthomolecular Medical Society
2340 Parker St.
Berkeley, CA 94704

Canadian Association for the Preventive and
    Orthomolecular Medicine
2177 Park Crescent
Coquitlam, British Columbia
Canada V3J 6T1

Canadian Health Food Association
c/o Mrs. Florence Hogg
20440 Douglas Crescent
Langley, British Columbia
Canada V3A 4B4

Canadian Organic Certification Association
Box 269
St. Jacobs
Ontario, Canada NOB 2NO

Cancer Control Society (and other
    nutritionally related diseases)
2043 No. Berendo St.
Los Angeles, CA 90027

Carolina Farm Stewardship Association
c/o Frank Porter Graham Center
Rt. 3, Box 95
Wadesboro, NC 28170

Colorado Organic Growers and Marketing
    Association
2555 West 37th Ave.
Denver, CO 80211

The Committee for Freedom of Choice in
    Cancer Therapy
146 Main St., Suite 408
Los Altos, CA 94022

Consumers for Nutrition Action
3404 St. Paul, Ste 1-B
Baltimore, MD 21218

Denver Homoeopathic Laymen's League
c/o Orville Hudley
229 S. Franklin St.
Denver, CO 80209

East/West Center for Holistic Health
275 Madison Ave., Suite 500
New York, NY 10016

Ecologos
80 Martin Road
Milton, MA 02186

Economic and Medicinal Plants Research
    Association
8 Grange Gardens
Cambridge CB3 9AT
Great Britain

Foundation for Alternative Cancer
    Therapy, Ltd.
P.O. Box HH, Old Chelsea Station
New York, NY 10011

Foundation for Chiropractic Education and
    Research
3209 Ingersoll Ave.
Des Moines, IA 50312

Foundation for Natural Living
P.O. Box 189
Monte Rio, CA 95462

Fruitarian Network
c/o Nellie Shriver
Box 4333
Washington, DC 20012

Hawaii Health Net
2535 S. King St.
Honolulu, HI 96814

The Healing Research Trust
Field House, Peaslake, Guildfort
Surrey GU5 9SS
England

Health Corps
P.O. Box 333
Venice, CA 90291

Herb Society of America
Horticulture Hall
300 Massachusetts Ave.
Boston, MA 02115

Herb Trade Association
4302 Airport Blvd.
Austin, TX 78722

Herbal Medicine Research Foundation
P.O. Box 29187
San Antonio, TX 78229

Holistic Education Network
P.O. Box 1233
Del Mar, CA 92014

Holistic Health Organizing Committee
Village Design
1545 Dwight Way
Berkeley, CA 94703

Holistic Life Foundation
1627 Tenth Ave.
San Francisco, CA 94122

Homeopathic Council for Research and
Education
66 E. 83rd St.
New York, NY 10028

Homeopathic Foundation
Three E. 85th St.
New York, NY 10028

Homoeopathic Laymen's League,
Manheim, PA
c/o David Fidlers
R. D. No. 5
Manheim, PA 17545

Homoeopathic Laymen's League of
New York
c/o Mrs. L. C. Becker
90 La Salle St., Apt. 18-D
New York, NY 10027

Homoeopathic Laymen's League of the
Northeast
c/o Lorina Cooper
Hawley Road
North Salem, NY 10560

Homoeopathic Laymen's League,
Pittsburgh, PA
c/o Steffne Witney
120 Genessee Road
Pittsburgh, PA 15241

Homoeopathic Study Group of
Rochester, NY
c/o Jeffrey Van Riper
60 East Ave.
Brockport, NY 14420

Homoeopathic Study Group of Westchester
and Fairfield Counties
c/o Phyllis Freeman
27 Spicer Road
Westport, CT 06880

Howey Foundation
2a Lebanon Road
Croydon, Surrey CRO 6UR
England

Incorporated Society of Registered
Naturopaths
1 Albemarle Road
The Mount
York YO2 1EN, England

Independent Cancer Research Foundation, Inc.
468 Ashford Ave.
Ardsley, NY 10502

International Academy of Biological
Medicine, Inc.
P.O. Box 31313
Phoenix, AZ 85046

International Academy of Preventive Medicine
10409 Town & Country Way, Suite 200
Houston, TX 77024

International Association of Cancer Victims
and Friends, Inc.
7740 W. Manchester Ave., No. 110
Playa Del Rey, CA 90291

International Chiropractors Association
1901 L St. N. W., Suite 800
Washington, DC 20036

International Federation for Practitioners of
Natural Therapeutics
21, Bingham Place
London, WIM 3FH
England

International Federation of Organic
Agriculture Movements
c/o Coolidge Center, Riverhill Farm
17 Bradstreet Ln.
Topsfield, MA 01983

International Homeopathic League and the
San Francisco Homeopathic
Medical Society
6200 Greary Blvd.
Medical Building at 26th Ave.
San Francisco, CA 94121

International Institute for Biological and
Botanical Research Ltd.
P.O. Box 912
Brooklyn, NY 11202

International Institute of Integral Human
Sciences
P.O. Box 1387
Station H
Montreal, Quebec
Canada H3G 2N3

International Naturopathic Association
3519 Thom Blvd.
Las Vegas, NV 89106

International Vegetarian Union
10 Kings Dr.
Marple
Stockport, Cheshire SK6 6NQ, England

Jewish Vegetarian Society
855 Finchley Road
London NW11 8LX
England

Lehigh Valley Natural Healing
c/o Bill Brodhead
R. D. No. 1
Box 298A
Northampton, PA 18067

Los Angeles County Homeopathic Medical
Society
c/o G. Brunler
435 South Curson, Apt. MJ
Los Angeles, CA 90036

Maine Organic Farmers and Gardeners
Association
Certification Committee Director
Johnny's Selected Seeds
Albion, ME 04010

Michigan Homeopathic Laymen's Society
c/o Leonard Lystad
29546 Norma
Warren, MI 48093

Mid American Health Organization
13620 W. Capitol Dr.
Brookfield, WI 53005

National Acupuncture Association
P.O. Box 24509
Los Angeles, CA 90024

National Acupuncture Research Society
1841 Broadway
New York, NY 10023

National Association of Naturopathic
Physicians
2613 N. Stevens
Tacoma, WA 98407

National Center for Homeopathy
7297-H Lee Hwy.
Falls Church, VA 22042

National Council on Wholistic Therapeutics
and Medicine
P.O. Box 15859
Philadelphia, PA 19103

National Health Federation
212 W. Foothill Blvd.
Monrovia, CA 91016

National Herbalist Association
271 Fifth Ave., Suite 3
New York, NY 10016

National Institute of Medical Herbalists
148 Forest Rd.
Turnbridge Wells
Kent TN2 5EY, England

National Nutritional Foods Association
15041 Moran St.
Westminster, CA 92683

Natural Organic Farmers Association
70 Highland Ave.
Newport, VT 05855

Nebraska Organic Agriculture Association
Route 1, Box 61
Marquette, NE 68854

New Mexico Organic Growers Association
1312 Lobo Place NE
Albuquerque, NM 87106

New York Natural Food Associates
363 Hamilton St.
Albany, NY 12210

North American Vegetarian Society
P.O. Box 72
Dolgeville, NY 13329

Northwest Provender Alliance
1505 10th Ave.
Seattle, WA 98122

Nutritional Research Association
610 Third Ave.
Bradley Beach, NJ 07720

Ohio Ecological Food and Farm Association
567 Montgomery Court
Columbus, OH 43210

Organic Gardening Clubs of America
33 East Minor St.
Emmaus, PA 18049

Organic Growers and Buyers Association
P.O. Box 9747
Minneapolis, MN 55401

Organic Growers of Michigan
Route 1, Box 56
Lawrence, MI 49067

Oriental Healing Arts Institute
8820 Sepulveda Blvd., Suite 210
Los Angeles, CA 90045

Phytochemistry Society of North American
Biology Dept.
University of South Florida
Tampa, FL 33620

Quest of Carmel
P.O. Box 6301
Carmel, CA 93921

Research Society for Natural Therapeutics
8 Stokewood Road
Bournemouth, Dorset
England

Rocky Mountain Nutritional Foods
  Association
8800 W. 14th Ave.
Lakewood, CO 80215

Sacro Occipital Research Society
  International
Box 358
Sedan, KS 67361

Salt Lake City Homoeopathic League
c/o Edith S. Willes
2603 S. Eighth St. East
Salt Lake City, UT 84106

San Francisco Vegetarian Society
1450 Broadway, No. 4
San Francisco, CA 94109

Santa Cruz Homoeopathic Lay League
c/o Lucinda Concannon
131 Sunnyside Ave.
Santa Cruz, CA 95062

Shiatsu Education Center of America
52 W. 55th St.
New York, NY 10019

Society for Economic Botany
c/o Edward S. Mika
College of Pharmacy, University of Illinois
833 S. Wood St.
Chicago, IL 60612

South Pacific Federation of Natural
  Therapeutics, Ltd.
c/o Mrs. Clare Gulson, Secretary
1, Sage St.
St. Ives, New South Wales 2075, Australia

Tilth Producers Cooperative
Washington Small Farm Resources Network
Blue Mountain Action Council
19 East Poplar
Walla Walla, WA 99362

Touch for Health Foundation
1174 N. Lake Ave.
Pasadena, CA 91104

United Acupuncturists of California
125 Quincy
St. Mary's Square
San Francisco, CA 94108

Vegetarian Information Service
P.O. Box 5888
Washington, DC 20014

Vegetarian Society of New York
277 Broadway
New York, NY 10007

Willamette Valley Tilth Association
Rt. 1, Box 308
Sheridan, OR 97378

Women's National Homeopathic League, Inc.
1911 Walnut St.
Dover, OH 44622

AUTHOR AND TITLE INDEX

SUBJECT INDEX